THE CASE OF SIGMUND FREUD

SANDER L. GILMAN

THE CASE OF SIGMUND FREUD

MEDICINE AND IDENTITY AT THE FIN DE SIÈCLE

THE JOHNS HOPKINS UNIVERSITY PRESS
BALTIMORE AND LONDON

Printed in the United States of America on acid-free paper

The Johns Hopkins University Press
2715 North Charles Street
Baltimore, Maryland 21218-4319
The Johns Hopkins Press Ltd., London

Library of Congress Cataloguing-in-Publication Data

Gilman, Sander L.
The case of Sigmund Freud : medicine and identity at the fin de siècle / Sander L. Gilman
p. cm.
Includes bibliographical references and index.
ISBN 0-8018-4535-1 (hc : alk. paper)
1. Freud, Sigmund, 1856–1939—Religion. 2. Judaism and psychoanalysis. 3. Antisemitism—Austria—Vienna—History. 4. Medicine—Austria—Vienna—History. 5. Freud, Sigmund, 1856–1939. I. Title.
[DNLM: 1. Cultural Characteristics. 2. History of Medicine, 19th cent. 3. Identification (Psychology) 4. Jews—psychology. 5. Psychoanalytic Interpretation. WM 460.5.I4 G487c]
BF109.F74G55 1993
305.8′924—dc20
DNLM/DLC
for Library of Congress 92-39662

A catalog record for this book is available from the British Library.

FOR

J. Edward Chamberlin

IN FRIENDSHIP

In estimating the position of Israel in the human values we must remember that the quest for righteousness is oriental, the quest for knowledge occidental. With the great prophets of the East—Moses, Isaiah, Mahomet—the word was "Thus saith the Lord"; with the great seers of the West, from Thales and Aristotle to Archimedes and Lucretius, it was "What says Nature?" They illustrate two opposite views of man and his destiny—in the one he is an "angelus sepultus" in a muddy vesture of decay; in the other, he is the "young light-hearted master" of the world, in it to know it, and by knowing to conquer.

William Osler, "Israel and Medicine" (1914)

▪

"Tell me," he says. "I've often wondered how you know . . . how you recognize one another. I mean, how did you know that [he] was a Jew? Did you give each other signals, or are there secret signs, or what? I mean, what do you do when you are introduced?" . . . I raise my trouser leg. "That's what we do," I say, "we show each other our cloven hooves."

Clive Sinclair, "Bulgarian Notes" (1990)

CONTENTS

PREFACE

This book originated as a lecture series in the fall of 1988 during my stay as the visiting senior fellow of the Council of the Humanities and Old Dominion Foundation Fellow in English at Princeton University. I am indebted to Elaine Showalter of Princeton, whose scholarly work, friendship, and intellectual rigor helped shape this book.

These lectures became a graduate seminar during my tenure in the spring of 1989 as the Northrop Frye Visiting Professor of Literary Theory at the University of Toronto. My presence there was made possible by J. Edward Chamberlin, with whom I have written on topics closely related to this book and for whose intensive criticism and intelligent comments I am always grateful.

The material was then presented during the academic year 1989–90 as an undergraduate lecture course held under the auspices of the Departments of German Studies, Psychology, and Comparative Literature and the Program in Biology and Society at Cornell University and as a graduate seminar in the Departments of Psychology, History, English, and Religious Studies during my tenure as the B. G. Rudolph Visiting Professor of Jewish Studies at Syracuse University in fall 1991. I was substantially aided in my research by the students in all of these classes at all of these institutions. I am grateful for their attentive questions and their contributions.

The final draft of the book was written while I was the visiting historical scholar at the National Library of Medicine, National Institutes of Health, Bethesda, Maryland, during 1990–91 and the director of a National Endowment for the Humanities seminar on Freud and the culture of his time at the Freud Museum in London in summer 1991. Funding for the overall project was provided by the Lucius Littauer Foundation and the National Endowment for the Humanities. I am grateful to the director of the Museum, Erica Davies, and its former director, Richard Wells, for their help.

I am also grateful to William Griffiths at Toronto and Marjorie Howes at Princeton, and to Heather Munro, Chandak Seengoopta, John Davidson, and Catharine Gelbin at Cornell for the work they put into the preparation of the book. Alice M. Bennett undertook to turn my prose into understandable English, and Jane Dieckmann prepared the index that helps make the volume useful.

At the National Library of Medicine, the Library of Congress, and the Library of the University of Maryland (College Park), I was able to examine all the materials Freud cites in all of his references. At the rare book room of the College of Physicians and Surgeons, Columbia University, and the Library of Congress I had access to those books purchased from Freud's library (as well as the other books included in that sale). At the Freud Museum I was able to consult the bulk of Freud's library.

The question of what volumes actually belonged to Freud remains a complicated one. Nolan D. C. Lewis and Carney Landis ("Freud's Library," *Psychoanalytic Review* 44 [1957]: 327–28 and catalog) provided a reprint of the bookseller's catalog for the volumes purchased in 1938 for the Psychiatric Institute (which are now at Columbia). David Bakan ("The Authenticity of the Freud Memorial Collection," *Journal of the History of the Behavioral Sciences* 11 [1975]: 365–67) called the attribution of some of these titles into question, showing that several of them had simply been added by the bookseller to those books he had purchased from Freud. K. R. Eissler ("Bericht über die sich in den Vereinigten Staaten befindenen Bücher aus Sigmund Freuds Bibliothek," *Jahrbuch der Psychoanalyse* 9 [1977]: 10–50) provided further information about the origin of some of the volumes now at the Columbia Medical College and reproduced the bookseller's catalog. Eissler also listed those titles now at the Library of Congress. Further comments on Freud's books in New York are to be found in the work of Ernest Harms, "A Fragment of Freud's Library," *Psychoanalytic Quarterly* 40(1971): 491–95, and, concerning the small number of books in Freud Museum in Vienna, the essay by Hans Lobner ("Some Additional Remarks on Freud's Library," *Sigmund Freud House Bulletin* 1 [1975]: 18–29). The library that Freud retained and that is now housed at the Freud Museum, 20 Maresfield Gardens, London, was first cataloged by Harry Trosman and Roger Dennis Simmons ("The Freud Library," *Journal of the American Psychoanalytic Association* 21 [1973]: 646–87). A more complete catalog is now available at the museum, compiled by Keith Davies. My notes to the volumes in these collections are reflected in the documentation to each chapter; I have ignored only those titles in the New York collection that were clearly not part of the Freud library. It is clear that Freud did not read all the books in his possession (some of them are uncut dedication copies).

In addition, I want to thank the staff at Olin Library, Cornell University; the Wellcome Institute for the History of Medicine; the Library of the Royal Society of Medicine; and the British Library for their help in locating materials. The visual sources are from several collections, as noted in the legends. I thank the owners for giving me the permission to reproduce them.

All the quotations from Freud's works in this book, unless otherwise noted, are taken from the *Standard Edition of the Complete Psychological Works of Sigmund Freud,* ed. and trans. J. Strachey, A. Freud, A. Strachey, and A. Tyson, 24 vols. (London: Hogarth, 1955–74, referred to in the notes as *SE.* I have compared each quotation with the original as it appears in Sigmund Freud, *Gesammelte Werke: Chronologisch Geordnet,* 19 vols. (Frankfurt am Main: S. Fischer, 1952–87), referred to in the notes as *GW.* Changes in the translations are noted. Although I have criticized the existing English translation (and continue to do so), it is the one most widely available and is the format in which Freud is best known in the English-speaking world. Unless I cite translations in my notes, all the other translations in this book are mine. Where possible I have used contemporary English translations.

Versions of some sections of this book have appeared in the *Bulletin of the History of Medicine,* and the *International Journal of Psycho-Analysis* as well as in my *Difference and Pathology* (1985) and *The Jew's Body* (1991). These sections have been thoroughly reworked for inclusion in this larger work.

THE CASE OF SIGMUND FREUD

INTRODUCTION: ON MEDICINE AND RACE

The Covert Meaning of Race

During spring 1990 an article in the *New York Times* called attention to the radical difference in life expectancy between white Americans (75.5 years) and African Americans (69.5 years).[1] Similar reports appeared in scholarly publications stressing "race" as *the* precipitating factor accounting for the difference in the mortality rates.[2] In these contexts, "race" was meant to signify the economic consequences of belonging to a marginalized group. It was nurture rather than nature. But at the close of the twentieth century race not only is a social category reflecting the medical consequences of belonging to a specific group but retains its older, biological implications.[3] In fall 1990, the *New York Times* led its "Science Times" section with a banner headline: "Uneasy Doctors Add Race-Consciousness to Diagnostic Tools."[4] The theme of this essay was that doctors were "showing a cautious resurgence of interest in giving more consideration to their patients' racial or ethnic backgrounds when diagnosing and treating illnesses." Here it is evident that race is employed (ever so cautiously) in the biological sense.

Race, as a leading biological anthropologist remarked, "has always been a troublesome issue for human biologists [and physicians, we might add], aside from the social and political problems that have been involved."[5] The author goes on, however, to cite "the convenience which the social scientist finds in the term race." And this reflects the social scientist's emphasis on "the problems engendered by race relations." C. Loring Brace's praise of the use of race within sociology stressed its social component rather than its biological one. This was clearly nurture rather than nature. But there is a confusion in medical use between "biological" and "sociological" definitions of race that leads to the complicated overlapping of both definitions. In addition, in the 1990s there is the added dimension of whether such constructions are to be understood as positive or negative ones. Is it good or bad to belong to or believe you belong to a race?

All aspects of the discussion of race within medical science had been suppressed for decades. Given its abuse in the Shoah as well as in neocolonial policies throughout the world, it is clear that the concept of race is a poisoned one.[6] By the 1960s race came to be understood as a constructed category; it had no validity. As Theodosius Dobzhansky noted in 1967, "Every person has a genotype and a life history different from any other person, be that person a member of his family, clan, race, or mankind. Beyond the universal rights of all human beings (which may be a typological notion!), a person ought to be evaluated on his own merits."[7] This view resuscitated the earlier views of nineteenth-century thinkers such as John Stuart Mill, who wrote that "of all vulgar modes of escaping from the consideration of the effect of social and moral influences on the human mind, the most vulgar is that of attributing the diversities of conduct and character to inherent natural differences."[8] Mill was responding to the rationales for black slavery. Race has been dismissed as a category of scientific evaluation, especially in areas such as the practice of medicine, where its inclusion historically led to horrible abuses.[9]

We at the end of the twentieth century have not suddenly become callous to the medicalization of the concept of race. It is also evident that the meanings associated with race affect those included within these constructed categories. The concept forms them and shapes them. It is clear that there are "real," that is, shared, genetic distinctions within and between groups. But the rhetoric of how the "group" is defined becomes central. The discovery of the "depression" gene in the "Amish" (actually a single extended family in Pennsylvania) or the presence of sickle-cell disease among "blacks" (actually only those individuals who inhabit or whose ancestors inhabited malarial water areas, primarily in tropical Africa and the Middle East) have been evoked as models for the creation of the idea of race as an important feature of the perception of disease. Likewise, the social context of urban African Americans has been evoked as the explanation for the appearance of specific pathologies. The range of the pathologies "explained" by either biological predisposition or social location has ranged from the genetic to the epidemic to the sociopathic. The attempt to provide a single cause for specific types of perceived or real illnesses understood as appearing in a single race ignores the complexity of both diagnosing and defining what illness is. For the "cause" of illness is multidimensional and reflects the self-understanding of the individual with the disease as well as the overt signs and symptoms of a disease. Indeed, the form and structure of these signs and symptoms may be shaped by the very comprehension of the meaning of the disease.

Once the rhetoric of race is evoked, its ideological context is also present. The long-held association between race and disease and its internalization within an individual belonging to such a race is the basis for this book. It traces the idea of the special risk led by members of a specific race, the Jews, as defined in the biological and medical science of post-Enlightenment Europe. It is evident to me that the nineteenth-century concept of race, with its stress on the perfected prototype, is different from the contemporary biological view of race as a probabilistic aggregate.[10] The debates about medical probability in the late nineteenth century are tainted with the image of perfectibility or degeneration. But the discussion of race today, within and outside medicine, has inherited many of the hidden assumptions about the meaning of such difference. The use of the concept of race as a primary cause of illness is fraught with the consequences of its own history.

The complexity of reintroducing the concept of race into medicine does not mean dismissing the biological underpinnings of some diseases. One can speak of genetic cohorts of varying sizes without evoking race. Thus Henry Rothschild can note that though "there are no 'Jewish' diseases as such, unquestionably some disease alleles have a higher frequency in the various Jewish subgroups or subpopulations of these subgroups."[11] And, one might add, in seemingly unrelated populations (as in the case of Kaposi's sarcoma as found among various "peoples" of the Mediterranean basin). The interaction between the biological and the social sources of illnesses is perceived through the complex psychological structures that enable us to explain and deal with the anxiety of being at risk for disease and, ultimately and inevitably, death.

There is little sense in denying that there are diseases that haunt any given cohort. "The Jews" as an ideological construct may not have any given diseases, but Jews may and indeed do.[12] The problem is not the debate about the "kernel of truth," as some sociologists seem to want it to be. Admittedly there are diseases that seem to be predominantly if not exclusively "Jewish," and there are moments in time when Jews evince certain specific patterns of disease. Thus today the "reality" of the higher incidence of Bloom's syndrome among certain cohorts of Jews in Europe and their descendants can be shown to be a reflex of patterns of genetic transmission. Whether hysteria was indeed a dominant illness among European Jews of the nineteenth century can only be extrapolated from the discussions of the period. Is one more real than the other? Can we ignore the one and take the other more seriously because it is "real"?[13] Or must we take each of them seriously in the case of the individuals as well as the groups afflicted? But most important, is not the understanding of both types of illness by those who manifest them colored by the meaning ascribed to the illness within the culture in which they function?[14] Likewise, there is the question of social practice. European Jews, especially in the course of the nineteenth century, were multilingual. They were forced to move from country to country and they (in most cases) brought with them their "Jewish" languages—Yiddish and Hebrew. They practiced infant male circumcision and had specific eating and sexual practices. What is of interest is what these practices came to mean within the medical discourse of the nineteenth and early twentieth centuries.

The initial project of this book is to sketch the contemporary understanding of how race determines the risk of a group—here the Jews—for specific diseases. The anti-Semite, it has been noted, responds viscerally to the Jew: "Through a process of unconscious empathy, the sight of a Jew gives him a sense of being mutilated."[15] This anxiety generated by the circumcised body of the male Jew colors the very meaning of the diseases associated with the Jew. As the German Jewish neurologist Bernhard Berliner, who trained in Berlin under Hermann Oppenheim from 1910 to 1914, noted in the mid-1940s: "The total appearance of the Jew, physical and spiritual, inspires the Gentile with a secret fear which is in tune with his own fear of the father of his childhood."[16] Berliner's statement evoked the body of the uncircumcised adult male as the source for the German's anxiety about masculine identity. This is precisely the reversal of the claim that the Jewish male, circumcised (in reality or in fantasy), was the real source of danger for the Aryan. The male Jew understood *himself* as the object that inspired the anxiety of his Other. This sense of discomfort with one's own body, visible in a way that only such a stress on one's own real or imagined difference can provide, is the manifestation of the internalization of the charge of the diseased nature of the Jew's body.

The diseases thus take on specific meaning because they are associated with aspects of the "racial" definition of the Jew's body and mind. The "diseases" are Jewish, and the Jews are "diseased." In this context it is unimportant whether the diseases are indeed transmitted genetically, are acquired because of the social or family milieu of the individual, or are invented out of whole (or partial) cloth. The central question to ask is how the category of "Jewish diseases" was employed to create the image of the Jew as an infected and therefore potentially infecting member of the body politic. The diseases examined, from hysteria to cancer, in no way exhaust the list of "Jewish" diseases, but they serve as exemplary markers to outline the meaning associated with specific disease entities at the fin de siècle.

That the medical establishment of the fin de siècle needed hysteria, with all its implications, to be a "Jewish" disease is clear. But the claim for the physical and mental incapacity of the Jews is in no way tied to the problem of reality testing. Jewish diseases seem to exist across time and space regardless of the actual status of the Jews. When a group of Jews can be found that matches the image of the pathological nature of the Jews, this is evoked as evidence; when statistics are generated, they are used; when neither case material nor statistics can be evoked, the argument is still present, still evoked, and evidently still powerful enough to shape the self-image of the Jew. It is not the reality of the Jews as a group afflicted with certain illnesses, but rather the meaning attributed to these illnesses that is central.

My thesis is rather simple: given that the biology of race stands at the center of the nineteenth-century "science of man" (which would include biology, medicine, and anthropology), it is extraordinary to imagine that anyone who thought of himself as a "scientist" during this period could have avoided confronting this aspect of science. And those male scientists (such as Jews) who were labeled as different within this science had to come to terms with the fact that the arena of endeavor that gave them status as scientists also demanded that they acknowledge (or refute) their inherent inferiority.

My approach is very different from the one first suggested by Robert Merton in 1942.[17] Merton struggled to understand the presence within German science, in terms of both practice and theory, of rampant anti-Semitism. He saw this as a process of infiltration, by which the "caste standards" of the general society are introduced into a "pure" science. This introduction not only sets the standards for the theory but also provides the rationale for the exclusion of "inferiors" as incapable of doing science. My argument presupposes that inherent in the very definition of the biological and medical sciences of the day are the "caste standards" that label Jews as unable to undertake the task of science because of their inherently pathological nature. At the same time the claims for "universalism" made by the science of the day gave these claims a neutral face. It was as if science spoke in one voice and said: "What I speak is true because it is neutral. And what I say is that you are sick. And my neutrality gives me a special (and powerful) status in this new world now defined by the importance of science." The Jewish physician[18] was forced to deal with this claim if he (and physicians were primarily men until the beginning of this century)[19] was to share in the social status of the physicians, a status open to him only during the nineteenth century and the rise of civil emancipation.

The abyss between the "sick" and the "healthy" within the model of race clearly reflects the need for physicians who see themselves as members of the "better" race to also understand themselves as "healthy."[20]

The generation of a purified self-image in the creation of a social space where disease can, indeed, must occur shapes the image of the sick Jew. And the Jew, physician or not, responds. For these constructs are not merely perceptual or cognitive structures. As such they could be dismissed as peripheral to the self-definition of the Jew. Rather, they reflect the social realities of the world in which the Jew functions and that are internalized into the self-representation of the Jew. They form the "scientific laws" that govern the realities of this world. They are reflected in the actions of the people in the world and also help determine those actions.

Freud as a Jewish Physician-Scientist

My test case is the association of the Jews with specific forms of disease and the response of one Jewish scientist, Sigmund Freud, to this special status. Freud is not typical in his response. Indeed, there are a number of Jewish physician-scientists, both within and outside psychoanalysis, who come to play a role in this book. Their response to ideas of disease and risk becomes a litmus test for one means by which a group of scientists can deal with a science that labels them at risk for the very illnesses they are treating. It is analogous (but not identical) to the position of the woman physician in regard to the views about female risk in the medicine of the late nineteenth century. Much of the work by Regina Morantz-Sanchez on women in the history of American medicine already presents many of the conflicts and the means attempted to resolve this double bind.[21] The question of responses to theories of biological or social determinism during this period has been often raised, but as of now there are few detailed studies of the structural response to these images of pathology by those scientists belonging to stigmatized groups.

The answers of other Jewish biological and medical scientists are either slightly or radically different from Freud's. But all resist the authority of biological determinism in complicated and interesting ways. This is therefore a case study that highlights the "science of race" in the latter half of the nineteenth century and the first half of the twentieth. It looks at it with the very specific focus of the implication of the idea of "race" for the model of disease and the response of one caught in the web of this association. But Freud was not merely a "Jew"; he was also a physician.[22] Here a conflict arises that is not at first evident.

Such a study is valuable not only as an important source study for the history of medicine as well as the history of psychoanalysis, but as a detailed presentation of individual responses to the professional claims of the human sciences. The very status of science as a profession in the late nineteenth century gives those designated as different hope of transcending their social inferiority. It is also within the innate claims of that science to validate the difference among specific groups of human beings that places such scientists in an impossible position: if the claims of the science are valid, then members of the race are condemned to a life of often stigmatizing disease even if they share in the status of being one who can "research" and "cure."

To date there has been only a limited examination of the extensive medical literature on the pathologies attributed to the Jews in nineteenth- and early twentieth-century medicine and on their social and ideological significance. (This question has not been examined in any systematic manner even in the most recent studies of German eugenics.)[23] I have documented the argument about the somatic and psychological pathologies of the Jews as found in the medical literature of the time and will relate this to Freud and the language of psychoanalysis. Little or no attention has been given to the strategies through which those scientists, labeled by their science as inherently different, have dealt with this idea of difference. This is especially true within the understanding of theories of biological determinism by those groups (including male Jewish scientists) who are seen as innately pathological. Such a detailed study of the strategic devices that one nineteenth-century scientist, Sigmund Freud, evolved can help set the stage for an understanding of how stigmatized individuals, who wished to function within the professionally defined world of medical science (as a thought-collective) have had to generate explanatory models that helped free them from stigma.

The importance of the tension between the "real" possibility that Jews may be (or become) ill and the charge that Jews are essentially diseased provides the affective dimension for this book. Freud's world was the world of European Jewry. Philip Rieff did not exaggerate when he commented that "despite his irreligion, Freud felt intensely Jewish and lived his life in largely Jewish society. His is the familiar history of the European Jewish intellectual. His friends were all Jews, his patients mostly so; his private culture—jokes and familiar sentiment—exemplify a Jewishness more binding than religious orthodoxy."[24] And, one must add, he was a Jewish physician in a time when the question of the relation between medicine and race had a powerful hold on the science of the day. Freud struggled with the problem of what form of resistance would be open to him. It is true that he was not in general a "tough Jew," in that he was not a political activist, though in his private life he could be aggressive toward those showing anti-Semitic attitudes.[25] He was an individual whose response to the anti-Semitic violence of his world became part of his manner of coping with all aspects of his life. But his response was not that of some of his generation, "an over-intense admiration or indeed worship," to evoke Isaiah Berlin's phrase, for the Aryan majority. He understood himself as a Jew, as different.[26] And this for him (as for Jewish contemporaries such as Theodor Herzl) was in no way negative. But his own "neurotic distortion of the facts" came about in his choice of profession, where, according to the ideology of nineteenth-century science, the distinctions of race should have had no impact. Freud's own distinction between a life devoted to politics and one devoted to science is worth evoking in this context.[27] He explained his desire to study medicine rather than law because he felt himself disqualified for a life of political activism as a Jew, but he felt he could function within the sphere of science. This image of medical science as a safe place for Jews is one that will be called into question. Indeed, Freud's struggle with the rhetoric of race within the world of medical science marked his science and his life.

In examining Freud's response to the special status of the Jewish body and the Jewish mind we can see how a Jewish physician in a specific Diaspora setting, here German-speaking medical culture, responded to the assumed risk of disease and death associated with being Jewish. (This risk, which was given medical definition within the scientific literature of the age, was paralleled by the very intense sense of the risk associated with being Jewish on the very streets of Vienna.) Each of the chapters therefore traces, often back into the "prescientific" literature, the ideas of Jewish physical and psychological difference and shows how this difference was medicalized in the course of the nineteenth century. To understand how this discourse is transformed as part of Freud's resistance to the underlying presuppositions of the medical science of his time, I have applied an interpretive model that is both psychoanalytic (rooted in the concepts of projection and transference) and also sociological (rooted in the question of the meaning and function of groups). I want to understand how the individual variations on the broader themes of resistance are shaped as well as to determine the place of such individual perceptions within a broader framework.

I am especially interested in the link between the problem of identification (especially "identification with the aggressor") and the possibility of resistance (in Foucaultian terms) to the implications of such aggression. What I see being worked out (at least in part) within the rhetoric of psychoanalysis is a complicated answer to the stigmatization of the Jew, especially the Jewish male, in the science of the nineteenth century. The new science of psychoanalysis provided status for the Jew as scientist while re-forming the idea of medical science to exclude the debate about the implication of race. The question of the constitution of the subject within psychoanalysis is linked to the problem of identification.

Mikkel Borch-Jacobsen writes of the primary drive toward "identification, a primordial tendency which then gives rise to desire; and this desire is, from the outset, a (mimetic, rivalrous) desire to oust the incommodious other from the place the pseudo-subject already occupies in fantasy."[28] I read this primacy of identification (and its concomitant use of the tools of projection and transference) as the underlying structure that shapes the generation of the self and the Other. Here I see the link between the constitution of the subject as a means of dealing with the stigmatization of the self and the initial pre-Oedipal and ungendered constitution of the self. To understand this later (post-Oedipal) development (which is bound by the rhetoric of the subject's localization in history, class, and geography), one must turn to the replacement of the bifurcated, introjected image of the caregiver (as the "good" and "bad" Other) in the adult by the peer group (in Freud's case, the world of science). It is the peer group that assumes the bipolar structure of the caregiver.

To understand the constitution and structuring of this moment I have relied on the work of the great Polish Jewish sociologist of science Ludwik Fleck.[29] Fleck pointed out in an essay in 1947 how very much our preception of the world about us is structured by the apparent givens of that group (which he calls a thought-collective) whose language, rhetoric, and idealizations we share (or believe we share). One of the givens in Freud's scientific thought-collective is the factor of race. How then does the racially marked individual, identifying with the power of that thought-collective, deal with it in order to provide a safe emotional space for his own sense of identity?

My attempt to sketch one of the many factors that shaped the questions and rhetoric of a science is in no way to be understood as a means of denigrating the basic model of the psyche that Freud and his contemporaries evolved. Indeed, the psychological mechanisms for coping with the risk assumed to be attendant on being Jewish are those first (or at least best) described in psychoanalytic theory. It is necessary to comprehend the cultural and textual context of the development of a science. This in no way calls the science itself into question. To frame the representation of the Jew in the science in which Freud was trained and the culture in which he lived, it will be necessary to reconstruct, if pointillistically, images from that discourse of science that are reflected in Freud's construction of the rhetoric of psychoanalysis. No comprehensive reconstruction is possible within these limits. Rather, the first chapter looks at the scientific construction of the idea of the Jew as a means of framing the overall path of Freud's incorporation of as well as resistance to the rhetoric of the science of race. The subsequent chapters examine the three contexts of the Jew within the medical literature of the period: the medical construction of the psychopathology of the Jew (in the debates about conversion and circumcision), of the pathophysiology of the Jew (in a reading of the meaning ascribed to the Jewish foot), and the sociopathy of the Jew (in a reading of the charges of criminality lodged against the Jews). All three are shown to be adumbrated within the rhetoric of psychoanalysis, as Freud carefully frames these particular charges into universal attributes of his definition of a human being. Central to his displacement is the dominant medical and anthropological denotation of the Jew in Freud's own time as well as his sense of himself as necessarily included within that highly charged debate.

1

PSYCHOANALYSIS, RACE, AND IDENTITY

The Anthropological Construction of the Jew and the Meaning of Disease

Peter Altenberg (1859–1919, pseudonym for Richard Engländer) was one of those self-consciously marginal figures in the cultural world of turn-of-the-century Vienna. Altenberg was a highly idiosyncratic essayist who sold handmade jewelry in the cafés of Vienna as an excuse to receive patronage from a wide range of admirers. He lived, like many other marginal *Luftmenschen,* who lived by their wits and not much else, in the middle of Vienna, at the Café Central. For all his self-styled marginality, in one respect he strove to be a member of the Viennese majority. In 1900 he converted from Judaism to Catholicism. What conversion meant for Altenberg can be seen in an undated "begging" letter from home to one of his patrons that sketches the central dimensions for the self-understanding of the Jew in late nineteenth-century Vienna:

> Since you have not even acknowledged that you received my gift, I can assume that you have been influenced by the dark, evil soul of that person, an absolute liar, who once called himself my friend and admirer. For you, a Christian, are naïve, full of belief and agreeable. He, however, that incarnation of Jewishness, is full of uncontrollable tricks!!! I must suffer for the fact that nature and fate have made me *Christian* in my *external* and internal organization, in my body, my posture, my pronunciation, my nose, my soul, my spirit, while this person attempts unsuccessfully to disguise the sign of Cain of an inferior race through hairsplitting and pseudoidealism!!![1]

Altenberg's image of the difference between the Christian and the Jew has to do with "external" (his stress) and "internal" differences: differences in the meaning of the body, of stance, of language, of the mind, and of the soul. Altenberg's list moves from the observable to the hidden, from the external to the internal. This is a morphological definition of race rather than a genetic one, yet it also incorporates all those invisible qualities that we later associate with the genetic idea of race. What is created is the genotype of the Jew.[2] Conversion is possible only because Altenberg was created by "nature and fate" as a Christian, that is, as an Aryan. In Altenberg's letter one can see how traditional religious labels ("Jew" and "Christian") take on the properties of categories of race ("Jew" and "Aryan") or, better said, how categories of religious difference are transformed into categories of racial science.[3] It is the confusion at the turn of the century of these two interlocked but conceptually separate categories of religion and race that can introduce our problem.

Peter Altenberg's categories represent his contemporary European views of Jewishness as neither a religion (Judaism) nor a political movement (Zionism) nor an ethnic identity (as an "Austrian or German of the Mosaic persuasion") but a race (the Jews). It is, to quote the Viennese proverb of the time, not religion but race that defines the Jew: "Was der Jude glaubt ist einerlei / in der Rasse liegt der Schweinerei!" (The Jew's belief is nothing / it's race that makes him swinish!)[4] Or as the displaced Austrian painter and politician Adolf Hitler rephrased it in *Mein Kampf* (1925), "The whole existence [of the Jews] is based on one single great lie, to wit, that they are a religious community while actually they are a race—and what a race!"[5] Thus the double bind of fin-de-siècle Jewry is the desire to go "beyond Judaism" paired with the impossibility of this undertaking once "Judaism" is defined racially (fig. 1).[6] And it is in the science of the time that the debate about the racial identity of the Jews was joined.

By the fin de siècle it is no longer religion that in any way defines the Jew in terms of the self-perception of the Jewish scientist. As the German Jewish sexologist Max Marcuse noted in 1912: "What earlier differentiated the Jew from the non-Jew, as well as unified the Jews—was their religion and what evolved from their religious laws. This connection has been destroyed. The Jews no longer claim to be the 'chosen people,' no longer believe in the God of the Jews, and understand the laws of Moses to be only social and hygienic directives."[7] Peter Altenberg's views, and those of many of his "Jewish" contemporaries of the fin de siècle (those designated as Jewish in the cultures in which they lived), reflect the internalization of this basic definition of the Jew as a member of a different and lower race.

The Jew as a member of a different race was as distant from the Aryan = Christian as was the Hottentot, the "lowest" rung on the *scala naturae,* the scale of perfection, of eighteenth-century biological science.[8] The categories of race were understood as mutually exclusive. Although the Jew was placed elsewhere on the ladder of development than the

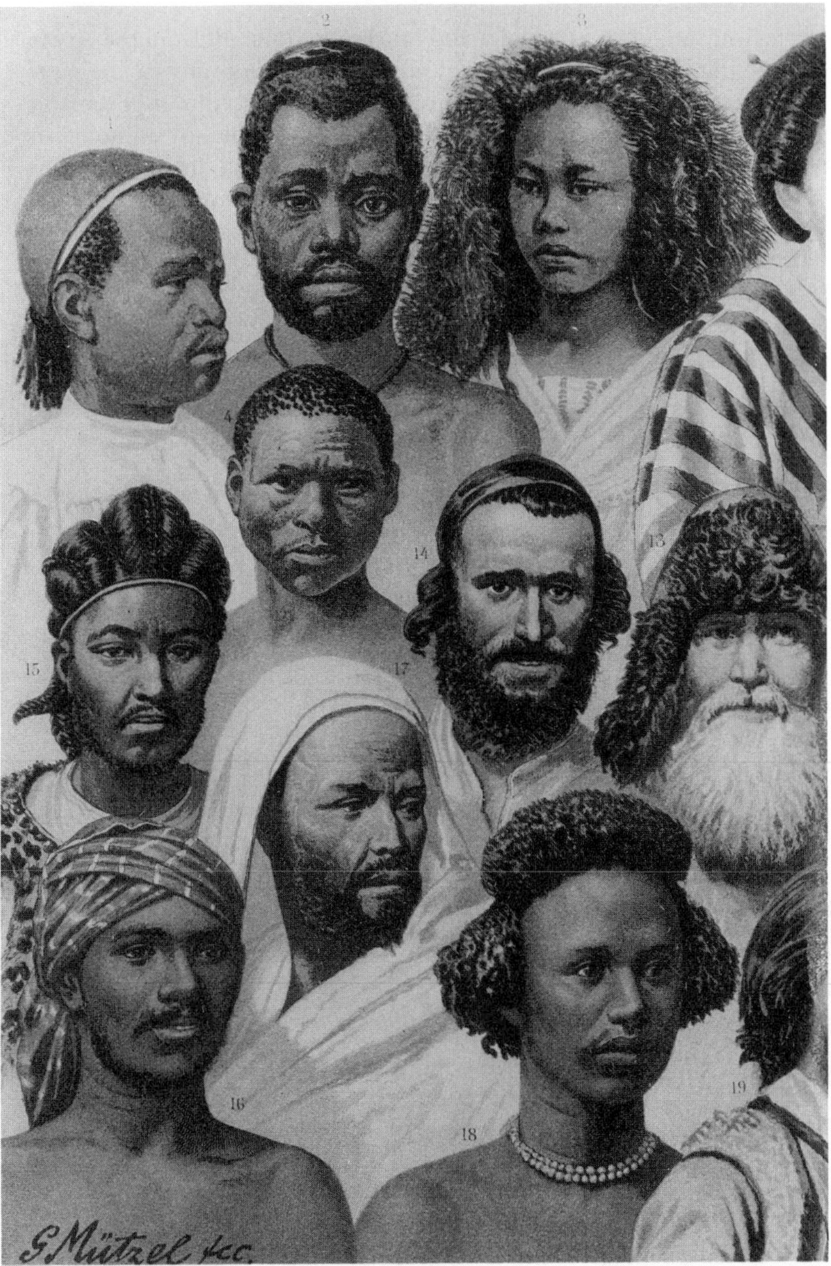

Figure 1. The physiognomy of race in the medical anthropology of the late nineteenth century. The Eastern Jew as the exemplary member of the "dark-skinned" races. Part of the frontispiece of Carl Ernst Bock, *Das Buch vom gesunden und kranken Menschen* (Leipzig: Ernst Keil, 1893). (National Library of Medicine, Bethesda, Md.)

Hottentot, the Jew was equally and inherently different from the Aryan (and by implication less good). Given the basic philosophy of late nineteenth-century science, this difference was defined in terms of observable phenomena (or phenomena suggested to be observable) by ethnologists and those they influenced, such as the physicians of the period. The "human" science of the period claimed that Jewish anthropometric difference was an absolute that could be seen and measured. And it was mirrored as well in the diseases from which the Jew was understood to suffer.

As usual, Heinrich Heine said it best. He introduced his 1842 poem on the endowment of the Jewish hospital in Hamburg with the verses:

> A hospital for poor, sick Jews,
> for people afflicted with threefold misery,
> with three evil maladies
> poverty, physical pain, and Jewishness.
>
> The last-named is the worst of all the three:
> that thousand-year-old family complaint,
> the plague they dragged with them from the Nile valley,
> the unhealthy faith from ancient Egypt.
>
> Incurable, profound suffering. No help can be looked for
> from steam-baths, shower-baths, or all the
> implements of surgery, or all the medicines
> which this house offers its sick inmates.[9]

For Heine, being Jewish was an illness, an illness equal to if not greater than physical illness. In *The Genealogy of Morals* (1887) Friedrich Nietzsche accepted Heine's view, seeing Jews as glorifying their own state of illness. For it is "the Jew who, with frightening consistency, dared to invert the aristocratic value equations . . . and maintain that only the poor, the powerless, are good; only the suffering, sick and ugly, truly blessed."[10] Jewish thinkers needed to universalize this charge that the Jews glorify their own weaknesses. They needed to see the disease of the Jews as a reflex of the human condition. But they were often able to articulate this only when the realities of political anti-Semitism had proved their inability to function within the political system of European science. Sigmund Freud felt himself constrained to respond to this evocation of the difference of the Jew's body in *Moses and Monotheism* (1939 [1934–38]). In discussing the practice of infant male circumcision, he quoted Heine's image of the disease of Judaism:

> Herodotus, who visited Egypt about 450 B.C., enumerates in his account of his journey characteristics of the Egyptian people which exhibit an aston-

> ishing similarity to traits familiar to us in later Jewry: "They are altogether more religious in every respect than any other people, and differ from them too in a number of their customs. Thus they practise circumcision, which they were the first to introduce, and on grounds of cleanliness. . . . They look down in narrow-minded pride on other people, who are unclean and are not so close to the gods as they are." . . . And, incidentally, who suggested to the Jewish poet Heine in the nineteenth century A.D. that he should complain of his religion as "the plague dragged along from the Nile valley, the unhealthy beliefs of Ancient Egypt"?[11]

The act of circumcision sets apart the Jewish male, even the scientist-physician (in that he is no longer fully a male). The Hungarian Jewish psychoanalyst Franz Alexander, in commenting on Heine's verses in 1940, notes that "Judaism, *per se,* is not a disease. The Jewish ailment is nothing but a reflex of the crisis in the world's morale."[12] But even Franz Alexander recognized that projecting the diseases attributed to the Jew to the world would not cure the Jew. For within the medical world of the nineteenth and early twentieth centuries, "Jewishness" is an illness that cannot be cured through the ministrations of medicine, for it is embedded in the very core of the Jew.

For fin-de-siècle medical science Jewish racial difference was statistically measurable; Jewish pathologies were statistically evident. These pathologies could be illnesses of the body or of the mind. Carl Heinrich Stratz, the non-Jewish ethnologist who wrote a slim pamphlet on the anthropology of the Jews in fin-de-siècle Vienna (a pamphlet owned and read by Sigmund Freud), dismissed as "full of half and complete untruths" the typical definition of the Jews as "a hated and despised people of a Semitic race and Mosaic faith, defined by a long nose and numerous physical frailties such as a hunched back, knock knees, flat feet, etc."[13] Yet he also tabulates in great detail the diseases attendant on being a Jew. The idea of a morphology of the Jewish race was contingent upon the image of the unique construction of the Jewish body and the Jewish psyche. Within most of these theories of difference, the concepts of "soma" and "psyche" are presumed to be inherently linked, after the mind-body model that dominated nineteenth-century medicine. The most radical example of this epiphenomenalism viewed the mind simply as a product of the brain, much as bile is a product of the liver. (This parallel is the favorite of mid-nineteenth-century physicians, such as P. J. G. Cabanis.) Diseases of the mind were diseases of the brain. By the close of the nineteenth century, European physicians were convinced that most mental illnesses were of organic origin and that racial (as well as familial) degeneracy played a major role in predisposing any individual to risk.[14] The key phrase was coined by Wilhelm Griesinger in 1868: "The so-called mental illnesses are found in individuals suffering from brain and nerve illness."[15] Even in those cases where no clear somatic illness could be shown, where only a functional deficit was known, one assumed some underlying organic lesion. The explanation for Jewish difference, within the mainstream of European medicine, came to be found within the nature of the Jewish body. Jewish brains, therefore, were seen as being at the source of Jewish intellectual and emotional pathology.[16] The merging of the racial with the medical arguments was, as we will see, general.

Now it made little difference if one agreed, as did "Aryan" as well as "Jewish" scholars, for or against the "racial purity" of the Jews.[17] Either the Jews were a "pure" race, and this gave them certain unmistakable qualities of physiognomy, physiology, and psyche (usually negative) that were associated with certain signs or stigmata, or they were a "mixed" race in which the least positive qualities of both groups dominated, as indicated by observable phenomena. As Charles Darwin's cousin, the eugenicist Francis Galton, stated it: "The difference of origin would betray itself in his descendants; they would revert towards the typical center of their race."[18] The first view meant that the immutability of the Jew across time and space could be stressed, for good or for ill. Robert Knox, in one of the most widely cited and republished studies on race, expressed this view at midcentury: He looked "attentively at the Jewish physiognomy on the streets, as he perambulates our pavements, and with a hoarse, unmusical voice, proclaims to you his willingness to purchase cast-off clothes of others; or assuming the air of a person of a different stamp, he saunters about Cornhill in quest of business; or, losing sight of his origin for a moment, he dresses himself up as the flash man about town; but never to be mistaken for a moment—never to be confounded with any other race."[19] The debate about the immutability of the Jew was again raised in the public press in 1902 when the professor of archaeology at the University of Berlin, Friedrich Delitzsch, gave his lecture "Babel and Bible" before Emperor Wilhelm II.[20] Delitzsch argued for the importance of the Assyrian excavations being undertaken at the time for an understanding of the background to biblical history.

Delitzsch also argued, with telling visual images from Babylonian sources, that it was quite possible to distinguish the image of the Jews depicted on these ancient monuments because of their similarity to the appearance of Wilhelmenian Jews. Central to Delitzsch's argument was the physiognomy of the Jew. But it had been a striking feature of Jewish self-representation during the 1890s that Jews, such as Freud and Herzl, adopted the "Assyrian" (as it was referred to by contemporaries) style of long, spade-shaped, black beard, which marked them visually as "Oriental" rather than "Occidental."[21] This style was the result of the popularization of the German archaeological discoveries in Mesopotamia. But Delitzsch's presentation caused an uproar even in Vienna because of his visual "proof" of the immutability of the Jewish body rather than the culturally determined style of the Jewish beard.

The second view, of the "mixed" nature of the Jewish race, was espoused by such notable figures as the polygeneticist Paul Broca. This should have provided an escape from the charge of the inherent difference of the Jews, since it seemed to argue the mutability of "Jewish" racial characteristics, and it was in the very body of the Jew that this mutability could be seen. The great French historian Anatole Leroy-Beaulieu, in his often-cited attack on anti-Semitism (1893), commented that "there is in every Jew a secret power of metamorphosis which has often amazed me. He is able to undergo any transformation while scarcely ever losing the impress of his race, just as he preserves on his body the mark of his religion. He has the remarkable faculty of taking on a new skin, without at bottom ceasing to be a Jew. There is something Protean in him. The ease with which he transforms himself borders on the miraculous. He is like a metal in constant state of fusion; he may be cast into any mould and is able to assume any shape, without changing his substance."[22] Such a view is echoed as the basic assumption of the nature of the Jews in one of Sigmund Freud's sources, the extensively illustrated ethnology compiled by the anthropologist-physician Georg Buschan in the 1920s. For him the "Jews are a distinct and clearly differentiated people who possess a rigid, immutable religious, typological, and blood consciousness."[23] Carl Heinrich Stratz argued that even though the Jews were a mixed race, there were sufficient "traits in their physical structure to enable them to be labeled as Semitic. These racial characteristics are the remains of their original racial character and remind one of the southern branch of the white race."[24] The assumption in these texts was that even though there were subcategories of the Jewish racial types, these subcategories had limited, fixed, immutable "Jewish" qualities.

Just as "Christian" came to mean "Aryan" over the course of the nineteenth century, so too did those scientists who argued the existence of subcategories of the Jewish race come to employ religious labels for its difference.[25] Ashkenazim and Sephardim were the favorite racial subtypes, since they were already terms in the religious division of the Jews into roughly "northern" and "southern" groups. This reflected the crudest anthropological division of the European into northern types (Jews with "red hair, short beard, short concave nose, small gray, lustrous eyes") and southern types (Jews with "long black hair and beard, large almond eyes, a melancholy cast of countenance, with a long face and a prominent nose—in short, the type we find represented in the paintings of Rembrandt").[26] A variation on this theme saw three rather than two subtypes. This was most forcefully argued by the leading German anthropologist of the late nineteenth century to deal with this question, the Viennese-trained physician Felix von Luschan, who held the chair of anthropology in Berlin.[27] Physiognomy becomes the core for such racial differentiations among Jews, and it will be of little surprise that even these seemingly benign classifications come to be associated with the categories of the healthy and the ill. The "Jewish type" was seen to "consist of a hooked nose, curling nasal folds (ali nasi), thick prominent lips, receding forehead and chin, large ears, curly black hair, dark skin, stooped shoulders, and piercing, cunning eyes. This is the typical Jew featured in cartoons, and these characteristics, when present in an individual, mark him as a 'Jew.'"[28]

The separateness of the Jews continued to dominate the debates about the morphology of race in Europe throughout the later nineteenth century, even in those theories where "race" was viewed as mutable.[29] The qualities of race, even as seen by those who argued for the greatest range of mutability, were understood as determined by or associated with models of disease. Such was the case even in the relatively late work of Jewish anthropologists such as Maurice Fishberg, who highly problematized the existence of a single, uniform Jewish race.[30] (This later becomes a central problem for another German Jewish anthropologist, Franz Boas.)[31] For Fishberg, to quote a review of his book, "The Jew has, so to speak been pressed into shape by his religion on the one hand and the Gentile on the other, and it is only when the pressure is maintained that the type remains constant, and any relaxation of either constraining force is sufficient to denationalize the Jew."[32] But this very view of the mutability of Jewish types becomes one of the qualities seen as immutable—Jews can shift their external form, they can come to look like everyone else in a national culture, yet they still preserve their essence as Jews. And that essence is tied to their diseased nature and their role as the cause of disease. No matter what the strategy used, the Jews remain identifiable and different.

One can find this discussion even in the work of the founder of political geography, Friedrich Ratzel, who in the 1880s espoused the view that the Jews are a mixed race whose negative qualities were exacerbated by their having been displaced from their original home in the Near East.[33] (Ratzel saw geographic location as the prime determiner of racial attributes. His view suggested the inheritance of acquired characteristics dependent on the local climate and geography.) The result of Jews' being out of their proper spaces, like the parallel arguments about the nature of the Jewish body, was that the Jews represented a pathology—in terms of either their social maladaption (qualities that evolved in response to the environment in the Near East were not appropriate for life in Europe) or a physical maladaption (skin color, body structure). Especially, the Jewish mind is seen as a reflection of this pathology. Richard Wagner's notorious son-in-law Houston Stewart Chamberlain adapted Ratzel's views when he commented that "race is not an original phenomenon, it is produced; physiologically by characteristic mixture of blood, followed by inbreeding; physically by the influence which long-lasting historical and geographical conditions exercise upon that special, specific, physiological foundation."[34] And this meant that the Jew had a special status as one at risk for specific diseases present in Europe. It also meant that Jews were supposed to be immune to those tropical diseases that dominated their original home.[35] The debate about the immunity of Jews to certain diseases, such as tuberculosis, is reflected in the fascination of European science with the special status of the Jewish body.[36]

One Jewish response is to begin to doubt the very meaning of one's own mind and body. Jacob Wassermann chronicled in the 1920s the ambivalence of the German Jews toward their own bodies, toward their own differences. And this difference is articulated within the terms of the biology of race. He writes: "I have known many Jews who have languished with longing for the fair-haired and blue-eyed individual. They knelt before him, burned incense before him, believed his every word; every blink of his eye was heroic; and when he spoke of his native soil, when he beat his Aryan breast, they broke into a hysterical shriek of triumph."[37] Their response is to feel disgust with their own body, which even when it is identical in *all* respects to the body of the Aryan remains different: "I was once greatly diverted by a young Viennese Jew, elegant, full of suppressed ambition, rather melancholy, something of an artist, and something of a charlatan. Providence itself had given him fair hair and blue eyes; but lo, he had no confidence in his fair hair and blue eyes: in his heart of hearts he felt that they were spurious" (156). The Viennese Jewish poet Fritz Löhner, famous for his poetry and his opera libretti (such as Franz Lehár's *Land of Smiles*), summarized this response in his extraordinary poem of 1909 entitled "Jewish." In it the speaking voice addresses the "doctor," asking what he meant when he said there was very much Jewish about her. The doctor lists the speaker's best attributes: her satin eyes, her lustrous hair, her bright mouth, such as Solomon sings about in the Song of Songs. But, the doctor says, what is truly Jewish about you, what "burns the deepest wounds in me,' is that "you deny what is Jewish in you, and that is too, too Jewish" ("Missachten, was man 'jüdisch' nennt, / Ist leider, leider jüdisch!").[38] The Jews' experience of their own bodies was so deeply affected by the anti-Semitic rhetoric that even when they met the expectations for perfection of their community Jews experienced their bodies as flawed, as diseased.[39]

The Jews' Diseases

The signs of disease (or immunity to disease) had long marked the Jews as different. Johannes Buxtorf, writing for a fearful Christian audience about the inner nature of the Jews in an account of their nature and practices, cataloged their diseases (such as epilepsy, the plague, leprosy) in 1643.[40] Johann Jakob Schudt, the late seventeenth-century Orientalist who was *the* authority on the nature of the difference of the Jews for his time, cited their physical form as diseased and repellent: "Among several hundred of their kind he had not encountered a single person without a blemish or other repulsive feature: for they are either pale and yellow or swarthy; they have in general big heads, big mouths, everted lips, protruding eyes and bristle-like eyelashes, large ears, crooked feet, hands that hang below their knees, and big shapeless warts, or are otherwise asymmetrical and malproportional in their limbs."[41] Schudt's view saw the diseases of the Jews as a reflex of their "Jewishness," of their stubborn refusal to acknowledge the truth of Christianity.

The view that the Jewish body was different, but not necessarily predetermined to be different, also existed in the medical literature of the eighteenth century. Bernadino Ramazzini, professor of medicine in Padua, published a study of occupational diseases in 1700. The one group represented that was both a religious and an occupational group was the Jews. The Jews of Padua were traditionally cleaners of mattresses and collectors of rags, and they developed specific diseases associated with that task. But even Ramazzini, who notes that "these people are pursued by various diseases which result from the trades that they pursue, and not, as is commonly believed, from some infirmity of the race or from their unwholesome diet," begins his account with the racial image of the Jews as "people whose like is not to be found on the face of the earth; nowhere have they a fixed abode, but they are in every country; they are a lazy race, but active in business; they do not plough, harrow, or sow, but they always reap."[42] Even within an environmental discussion of the nature of the Jews, there is the argument that there is always some component that sets the Jews inherently apart.

Ramazzini's environmental view was accepted and repeated by the Jewish physician Elcan Isaac Wolf in 1777. Wolf had graduated from the medical faculty at Giessen in 1763 and was to move to Metz in 1781.

In Wolf's work there is a further revision of the traditional argument, for Buxtorf and Schudt saw Jews' difference as the mark of Jewish guilt in their original denial of Christ as well as their consistent refusal to acknowledge the truth of Christianity. For Wolf, following the environmental views of Ramazzini, Jews in Germany are more diseased, especially in terms of their mental illness, than their fellow country people—not because of any inherent biological difference, but because of the "horrible persecution of heathen tyrants" and the religious practices of the Jews.[43] Not their biological nature but Christian society and the religion of the Jews make the Jews different. Wolf translated the Enlightenment social and antireligious program into a means of reforming the physical and mental disabilities of the Jews. But different the Jew is. This is quite a bit further than Ramazzini was willing to go. For him the status of the Jews, like the status of all the occupations he examined in Italian society, was determined by divine order. Wolf's view is the position Jewish savants must take to free themselves from the taint of inherited disability. But the limitation on Wolf and other Jewish physicians was that they had to admit the inherent physical difference of the Jew. True or not, the acknowledgment from Jewish physicians of a primary sign of Jewish difference, the diseased nature of the Jewish body (and mind), provided further proof for the special category in which the Jew was placed. For the non-Jewish scientist the Jew was different, and this difference presented itself as a disease, a disease that affected the Jew directly but could also affect the culture in which the diseased Jew dwelt. Wolf's view was that the poor food and limited activity of the Jews led to their illnesses. The diseases of the Jews were thus caused by the environment in which they were forced to dwell. Given the status of German Jewry before emancipation and the opening of the ghettos, Wolf's reading was most probably accurate. However, it was stated within a scientific tradition, that of Western medicine, that was highly influenced by Christian theological models of Jewish difference.

In a medical survey of Poland (1792) written by F. L. de La Fontaine, a German who was the personal physician of King August of Poland at the close of the eighteenth century, the Polish Jew, the reification of anti-Semitic caricatures of the Jew, especially Western Jews, was the subject of a separate essay.[44] The filthy environment of the Jews, their food, and their sexual practices caused a catalog of illnesses ranging from syphilis to conjunctivitis. La Fontaine's criticism labeled the Jews as ill, more diseased than their contemporaries even though they had greater public freedom and security" (147). The sense of the special disposition of the Jews toward specific illnesses was stressed as a means of articulating their differences from their Christian neighbors. Central for La Fontaine was that their "all-too-early marriage in their thirteenth, fourteenth, or fifteenth year, with their weak bodies, takes from them the necessary fluid of life [*Lebenssaft*] of lasting health; therefore a Jew at forty looks much older than a healthy peasant or citizen at sixty or seventy" (151–52). The importance of the conservation of semen as one of the Brownian fluids paralleled much of the late eighteenth-century discussion of the evils of masturbation and other sexual excesses.[45] Here it was early marriage that sapped the individual's stamina, and the result was similar to that catalog of diseases ascribed to "the heinous sin of self-pollution." But for the Enlightenment physician La Fontaine, it was not the inherent nature of the Jews but their social environment and religious practices that predisposed them to specific forms of illness.

How intensively this image of the Jew as the diseased member of society became the central means of representing the Jew can be seen in a description by the "liberal" Bavarian writer Johann Pezzl, who traveled to Vienna in the 1780s and described the typical Viennese Jew of his time:

> There are about five hundred Jews in Vienna. Their sole and eternal occupation is to counterfeit [*Mauscheln*], salvage, trade in coins, and cheat Christians, Turks, heathens, indeed themselves. . . . This is only the beggarly filth from Canaan, which can be exceeded in filth, uncleanliness, stench, disgust, poverty, dishonesty, pushiness, and other things only by the trash of the twelve tribes from Galicia. Excluding the Indian fakirs, there is no category of supposed human beings that comes closer to the orangutan than does a Polish Jew. . . . Covered from foot to head in filth, dirt, rags, covered in a type of black sack . . . their necks exposed, the color of a black, their faces covered up to the eyes with a beard, which would have given the high priest in the temple chills, the hair turned and knotted as if they all suffered from the *plica polonica*.[46]

The image of the Viennese Jew is of the Eastern Jew, suffering from the diseases of the East, such as the *Judenkratze,* the fabled skin and hair disease also attributed to the Poles under the designation *plica polonica*.[47] The Jews' disease is written on the skin. It is appearance, skin color, and external manifestations that mark the Jews as different. There is no question upon first seeing Jews that they suffer from Jewishness. Pezzl's contemporary Josef Rohrer stresses the "disgusting skin diseases" of the Jews as a sign of the group's general infirmity.[48] And the essential Jew for Pezzl, even worse than the Polish Jew, is the Galician Jew, the Jew from the eastern reaches of the Habsburg empire.[49] This theme reappears in Arthur Schopenhauer's mid-nineteenth-century evocation of the Jews as "a sneaking dirty race afflicted with filthy diseases (scabies) that threaten to prove infectious."[50]

What is of interest in La Fontaine's and Pezzl's presentation of the Eastern Jew is that, even though it seems to be phrased entirely within the medical discourse of its time, it has specific political overtones. Both writers reflect the debates about the social status of the Jew and its reflection in the Jews' physical state. In 1788, in a widely circulated paper presented to the Royal Society in Metz concerning the status of the Jews, the Abbé Grégoire discussed the "physical" as well as the "moral and political regeneration of the Jews." He echoed much of Wolf's earlier "liberal" argument about Jewish difference, but like many of his contemporaries he placed the physical collapse of the Jew primarily at the door of Jews' social practices, specifically the early marriages they arranged for their offspring.[51] Here we have a charge that sees not the external prejudice against the Jew, the centuries of confinement in the ghetto, as the cause of Jewish difference and disease, but the group practices Jews engaged in. And it is the sexuality of the Jew that is labeled as different, as "perverse." This document became the focus for all the later (both revolutionary and antirevolutionary) images of the Jews as "diseased." It lists five causes of the physical decay of the Jews, including the early marriages practiced within the Jewish community. All the etiologies proposed by Grégoire are based on the social inequality imposed upon the Jews or on their religious practices. La Fontaine's views echo Grégoire's observations and their underlying ideology, that if the Jews were given social equality and if they altered their particularly Jewish practices, they would be freed from illness. In the eyes of many Germans, such as the philosopher Johann Gottlieb Fichte, no such alteration could take place. Jews remained Jews no matter what changes were made in their status, their religion, or their physical well-being.

During the late eighteenth century these views were paralleled by other calls for the "physiological transformation" of the Jews, to use Jakob Katz's felicitous phrase.[52] Jews had to become new human beings by shedding their Jewishness and, therefore, their risk for disease. In contrast to Grégoire's views, a number of European writers assumed that the nature of the Jew was immutable. Karl Wilhelm Friedrich Grattenauer, in a pamphlet titled *Concerning the Physical and Moral Characteristics of Contemporary Jews* (1791), argued that the mentality of the Jew was unalterable, even through the act of baptism.[53] Grattenauer and many other contemporary anti-Jewish pamphleteers saw in the movement toward Jewish emancipation a threat to their means of distancing themselves from the powerless Jews. Grattenauer was reacting to the claims by proponents of emancipation, such as the Abbé Grégoire, that the diseased aspects of Jewish life, language, and mentality were merely artifacts of the repression of the Jews or of their religious practice. Grattenauer reversed this. He labels the advocates of Jewish emancipation as ill, consumed by the disease of equality (131)! Both, however, relate the Jews' special nature to their sexuality. Grégoire sees the sexual selectivity of Jewish religious practices as one of the sources of their illness; Grattenauer sees their "whoredom and shamelessness" as a sign of their moral corruption (3). Both relate sexuality to disease and disease to the special nature of the Jews.

By the early nineteenth century the theme of the diseased nature of the Jews becomes part of the discussion within the medical establishment of Jews' dissimilarity to other inhabitants of Europe. This demanded some type of state action, for one of the roles of nineteenth-century medical science in the newly powerful nation-state was as the medical policing authority. At least one local official in Württemberg in the middle of the nineteenth century saw the diseased nature of the Jews as a major problem for the public health authorities of his time.[54] Jewish physicians agreed, accepting the charge of Jewish physical inferiority but seeing the setting of the Jews, the political repression under which they had been forced to live, as the sole cause. The Viennese physican Martin Engländer concludes his study of the "diseases of the Jewish race" with the cry: "The Jews need land, air, and light for their physical regeneration!"[55] The call for regeneration means that the Jews are indeed a "degenerate" people, no matter what the proximate cause, and this is inscribed on their bodies and minds across generations.

But more so, it was sensed that the Jews not only were diseased, but were corrupting. Remember that Nietzsche argued, in *The Genealogy of Morals* (1887), that "it was the Jew who, with frightening consistency, dared to invert the aristocratic value equations good/noble/powerful/beautiful/happy/favored-of-the-gods and maintain that only the poor, the powerless, are good; only the suffering, sick, and ugly, truly blessed."[56] The Jew glorifies all the qualities of his own body and makes out of them the norms for the new world. Just as the image of the Jew's body is that of the carrier of disease, so too does the Jew become the corrupting disease within the body politic.[57] This view was espoused by Adolf Hitler as early as 1919 when he wrote that "Judaism is first and foremost a racial and not a religious community. . . . Its effect is that of a racial tuberculosis among the peoples of the world."[58] Hitler, in looking back at the Vienna of the turn of the century, could characterize the Jews as the infection hidden within the body: "If you cut even cautiously into such an abscess, you found, like a maggot in a rotting body, often dazzled by the sudden light—a kike! . . . This was pestilence, spiritual pestilence, worse than the Black Death of olden times, and the people were being infected by it."[59] Ludwig Wittgenstein, the fin-de-siècle Austrian philosopher with his own roots in Viennese Jewish culture, echoed this image when he commented that within European history the Jews "are experienced as a sort of disease, an anomaly, and no one wants to put a disease on the same level as normal life [and no one wants to speak of a disease as if it had the same rights as healthy bodily processes (even painful ones)]."[60] The Jews are not merely diseased themselves but present a palpable danger to the entire society in which they dwell: "There is a contradiction in expecting someone *both* to retain his former aesthetic feeling for the body and *also* to make the tumor welcome" (20).

The sense that one simultaneously was diseased and was the source of the disease in the body politic is echoed in Sigmund Freud's comment to Roman Rolland that "I, of course, belong to a race which in the Middle Ages was held responsible for all epidemics (*Volksseuchen*) and which today is blamed for the disintegration of the Austrian Empire and the German defeat."[61] The reversal and extension of this view, that the diseases of the Jew are transmuted into the diseases of all human beings, is one of the underlying mechanisms in the establishment of the discourse of psychoanalysis. It is not solely that as a neurologist Freud employed an essentially pathological model to define the normal (for Freud the normal is what is not sick). The very association between the idea of the potential illness ascribed to his own cohort becomes the pathology that is potentially evident in all human beings.

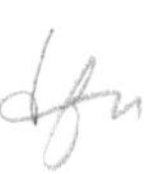

One must remember the age-old tradition within medicine that the physican must appear healthy. Hippocrates opens his description of *The Physician* with the observation that "the dignity of a physician requires that he should look healthy, and as plump as nature intended him to be; for the common crowd consider those who are not of excellent bodily condition to be unable to take care of others."[62] This tradition dominates even the modern view of the physician, in which the doctor must have "a sound constitution and a healthy look, which indeed seem as necessary qualifications for a physician as a good life and virtuous behaviour for a divine."[63] Members of a race such as the Jews, whose physical ugliness was a sign of their inherent pathology, were thus disqualified by their very bodies from assuming the role of physician.

Other Jewish psychoanalysts dealt with the charge of the diseased nature of the Jews in different ways. The image of the Jew as the source of disease is reversed in Otto Rank's essay "The Essence of Judaism" (1905), where he describes the Jews as having a "parasitic existence among the people with whom they were living." He provides a footnote to this phrase, observing: "The psychic-parasitic existence of the Jews has its biological analogy in the parasites, of which the sexual component makes up the most considerable part of the body."[64] The "primitive" sexuality of the Jew, for Rank a sign that the Jew is not as repressed as the Christian, becomes the marker of the Jew as parasite, as the source of disease.

The Cultural Construction of Jewish Difference and the Discourse on Disease

The difference of the Jew from the Aryan was thus the subject of interest not only to the anthropologists but also to the physician and to the physician as an agent of state authority. Echoes of the polygenetic arguments about the origin of the races remained substantially anchored in the popular representation of the Jew, as well as the Jew's representation in "high" science (including medicine) at the fin de siècle. It is in the interaction of late nineteenth-century ethnologists and medical scientists (so very many worked in both fields, such as Georg Buschan, Felix von Luschan, Adolf Bastian, Cesare Lombroso, and Emil Kraepelin) that this becomes of vital importance.

One can take two exemplary works, one from anthropology and the other from medical science of the period, as examples of their interaction in the science of the fin de siècle. In Richard Andree's 1881 study of Jewish folklore and in the 1882 medical dissertation on the anthropology of the Jews by Bernard Blechmann (see below), the central question is the relation between ideas of who the Jews are and of what their bodies mean. Andree's discussion centers on the permanence of the Jewish racial type, but more important, on its implications. Andree is the most widely cited German expert who argued for the immutability of the Jew. He was a strong advocate of the view that the Jews were a pure (but defective) race. He observed concerning the conservative nature of the Jewish body and soul: "No other race but the Jews can be traced with such certainty backward for thousands of years, and no other race displays such a constancy of form, none resisted to such an extent the effects of time, as the Jews. Even when he adopts the language, dress, habits, and customs of the people among whom he lives, he still remains everywhere the same. All he adopts is but a cloak, under which the eternal Hebrew survives; he is the same in his facial features, in the structure of his body, his temperament, his character."[65] And it is the body of the Jew that is the sign of this immutability.

It is important to acknowledge that "scientists" of the late nineteenth century, like Andree, drew on earlier, quasi-theological works for their proof. Andree cites the passage quoted earlier from Johann Jakob Schudt on the significance of the Jew's body as proof of the immutability but also the diseased nature of the Jew (27). This is remarkable, for even Andree comments that Schudt is hardly a "scientific source." But Schudt and other older studies of the physical anthropology of the Jews permit Andree to stress the physical anomalies of the Jews, such as their small stature (only the Hottentots, the Malays, and the Japanese are smaller) (32). And these physical stigmata are signs of the particular diseases such as hemorrhoids, scrofula, tuberculosis, and poor vision that afflict them, illnesses that are as much the result of their social practices (such as early marriage) as of their constitution (33).

But it is not just the pathophysiology of the Jews that is a reflection of their nature. Even the hatred they occasion is a direct result of their innate difference. Andree cites the "natural hatred of the Jews" as the result of the Jews' inherent inability to integrate themselves into the peoples they dwell among, even when they are culturally integrated into their world (60–67). The overt sign of this is the sexual separateness of the Jews. Jewish sexuality, as represented by the practices of endogenous marriage and of infant male circumcision, becomes the touchstone for the debates about Jewish social practice as the cause of the biological differences of the Jew (68). It is the act of circumcision that most sets off the Jewish male's body from that of his neighbors (as seen from a European perspective) (152–60). It is a sign of the special relationship that the Jews claim with the deity. But in the Diaspora it became a sign of the inferiority of the Jews, the source of the derision of the Romans and the desire of the Jews to reconstruct the prepuce or wear artificial prepuces so as to look like everyone else in the society. But in spite of the barbaric nature of this custom, they have maintained this tradition in Germany. He cites one side of the raging debate concerning the abolition of circumcision in the 1840s, Leopold Zunz's opposition to the abolition of the act, as if it were the only position his Jewish contemporaries took on this issue. The image of the Jew becomes more and more the image of the male Jew, though Andree does provide long descriptions of the physiology and physiognomy of the Jewish woman.

For Andree, the Jew must remain separate even when he illogically wishes to become part of the society he dwells in. The social sign of this difference, itself a result of the Jew's physiology, is inscribed on his tongue just as his sexual difference is inscribed on his genitalia. This is the *Mauscheln* (speaking with a Jewish accent) or *Jüdeln* (speaking with Jewish words) of the Jew.[66] (These terms are clearly pejorative. *Mauscheln* in its original usage in German means to counterfeit, as we saw in the quotation from Pezzl cited above.) His language retains the "unique lisp or disgusting language, which, even if one should shut one's eyes and without seeing the physiognomy, would enable one to recognize the Jew."[67] This special sign is embedded in the nature of the Jew's language—no matter what language he speaks. "The average German," a German-Jewish commentator noted, "regards Jewish language and dress not only as 'strange,' but as a caricature, a ridiculing of his own language and dress. The Jewish language is, to him, 'German in an ugly disguise.'"[68] Andree's views mirror those of Arthur de Gobineau, the most important theoretician of race in nineteenth-century Europe, who claimed that one of the salient features of the Jews was their lack of an "ancestral language." Jews have never had a real language; even Hebrew was simply borrowed from the "black Hamites." "Jews used the tongue of the country where they settled; and, further, these exiles were known everywhere by their special accent. They never succeeded in fitting their vocal organs to their adopted language, even when they had learnt it from childhood."[69] And Gobineau, in turn, reflected the views of the eighteenth-century physiognomists, such as Johann Caspar Lavater (quoting his friend, the poet J. M. R. Lenz): "It is evident to me that the Jews bear the sign of their fatherland, the Orient, throughout the world. I mean their short, black, curly hair, their brown skin color. Their rapid speech, their brusque and precipitous actions also come from this source. I believe that the Jews have more gall than other people"[70] Or as Georg Buschan notes in the 1920s, the Jews in Europe speak a "grotesque mix of Old Franconian dialect mixed with Jewish linguistic elements."[71] It is this link between language and physiology that marks the meaning of *Mauscheln* as a pathological sign. By the mid-nineteenth century this attribute, while part of the overall caricature of the Jew in Western Europe, is powerfully associated by Western Jews with the Eastern Jews, who had maintained Yiddish as their primary language.

Jews were themselves very concerned about being identified as different by the very quality of their language and their voice. The renowned Jewish conductor Hermann Levi, best known for his advocacy of Wagner, was reported by Hans von Bülow in 1884 as rushing out of the theater, having just conducted an opera by the Jewish composer Meyerbeer, exclaiming: "If I have to conduct this damned *Mauschel*-opera again, I'll join an anti-Semitic society!"[72] Bülow sees Levi's sensitivity to the inherent difference of the "Jewish tone" of Meyerbeer as a sign of the struggle between *Gemauschel* and *Nichtmauschel* that characterized contemporary culture. Arthur Schnitzler, the playwright, was struck the first time he heard his recorded voice played back by its "nasal, Jewish character."[73] For it was language, more than any other factor associated with race, that was traditionally understood in Germany as determining race or nationhood.[74] For the Germans of the nineteenth century language was the mirror of the origin of civilization. It is no surprise that the linguistic label "Semite," rather than any other racial designation, is applied to the Jews during the course of the nineteenth century.[75] When Theodor Lessing, then teaching philosophy and pedagogy at the Technical College in Hannover, visited Galicia in 1909, the eastern reaches of the Austro-Hungarian empire, he was struck that the character (or rather the lack of character) of the Eastern Jews was so directly expressed in their language.[76] Their language revealed their nastiness, superstitiousness, fanaticism, selfishness, and the absence of noble virtues such as naturalness, naïveté, and honesty. Lessing's Galician critic Binjamin Segel quite rightly notes that this image of the language of the Jews "is taken from the newspapers of the Viennese anti-Semites."[77]

It is the acquisition of language, the leading nineteenth-century anthropologist Ludwig Woltmann states, that provides the human ability for "invention, imitation, and transmittal," all of which define human society.[78] Moreover, language, according to Woltmann, is necessary for "logical thought" (113). This is all part of Woltmann's argument about the basis for the difference of the races. Thus he notes that it is true that "a black child can learn a foreign language as easily and as quickly as his mother tongue. But it is questionable whether a black could absorb the rich vocabulary of a highly developed race, for example, the style and the fullness of the language of Shakespeare." This is seen as the result of the "physical (i.e., construction of the larynx, the gums, the tongue, the teeth) and the spiritual-psychological inheritance" (113–14). Jews are in an identical situation. For it is in the claimed inability of the Jew to speak the language of culture that the weakness of the Jew is to be found. Adolf Bastian, the great explorer of Siberia, commented that languages "carry the local character of the race."[79] And one of Freud's anthropological sources, John Lubbock, pointed out the close relation between evolved gestural patterns and the primitive nature of the races that use them.[80] No matter how the race changes, these inherited linguistic features are preserved.

Even those Jewish physicians such as Moses Julius Gutmann, citing the anthropologist Felix von Luschan as his authority, who argue that "language is not a sign of race," provide a caveat. For Gutmann "it is the better language, the better grammar, the better religion, perhaps also the better alphabet that survives."[81] In terms of the language of the Jews, the "better" German drives out the corrupt Yiddish, especially in terms of its intermediate (or bastard) form, *Mauscheln*. It is in the work of Heymann Steinthal, the Jewish cofounder of ethnopsychology, that this debate about the nature of the Jew's language is focused. In 1893 Steinthal published an essay in the *General Newspaper of the Jews* arguing that *Mauscheln* was a more or less indelible sign of Jewish identity.[82] *Mauscheln* is the "means of speech by which a listener knows a speaker is a Jew without looking at him." The origin of the language lies in the "organ of speech, the intonation as well as in the articulation" of language. (Indeed, Jews even *mauscheln* when they speak "our holy Hebrew"!) Although Steinthal advocates the linguistic assimilation of the Jews into the German-speaking world, and as far possible, the abandonment of *Mauscheln,* he also wishes to preserve the use of Hebrew words in the language of German Jewry. Hebrew is to be preserved, Yiddish and other languages and dialects, such as *Mauscheln,* are to be abandoned. The reason is that Hebrew is a "real" language, representing a newly reborn national identity. It was seen as belonging to the nature of the "race" or, in Steinthal's terms (as I shall discuss below), the *Volk.* It was no accident that the major battle among the Zionists was whether Hebrew or Yiddish would become the language of the future Jewish state. Hebrew won, since it was seen as a "real" language.[83] In a survey of the languages Jews spoke in Austria, published in 1905, the overwhelming majority of Jews in all the lands spoke German! This was accomplished by having "Jewish-German" count as a German dialect.[84]

Andree's image of the Jew is an anthropological one: it stresses the relation between the biological core of the Jew—race—and the resultant social acts. He seems to offer sociological explanations for some phenomena. Thus he seems to reject as unprovable the view of at least one distinguished German biologist of the time, Gustav Jaeger, that the Jewish soul was marked by a specific smell, a version of the stench, the *foetor judaicus,* associated with the Jew as early as the Roman poet Martial, but of central importance in defining the image of the Jew in the Middle Ages (68–69).[85] Rather, he associated the smell of the Jew with the Jew's consumption of garlic. But even this he saw as a reflex of the Jews' "southern" nature, acquired from the long exposure to their original Mediterranean homeland, for only "southern" peoples indulge in this disgusting habit. (This confusion between the "acquired" smell of the Jew and the Jew's inherent "stench" is paralleled by Johann Jakob Schudt, who described the "stench" of the Frankfurt Jews as inherent, for even their infants smelled, but also as a result of their dietary habits.)[86]

The smell of the Jew acquires importance as a marker of sexual difference for the racial biology of the period. Jaeger's evocation of the different smell of the Jew's soul and Andree's attempt to see this smell as a reflex of the Jew's culture do not negate one another. Acquired characteristics become part of the essence of the Jews; thus their smell is a sign of the measurable, observable difference attributed to them. Given the centrality of olfactory impressions in the debates about the nature of human sexual attraction (from Darwin on), it is not surprising that the question of the Jew's smell comes to have clinical significance. One striking document, a letter of 1912 from a young man to a professor of medicine in Bohemia, reflects the assumptions among non-Jews about the smell of the Jew's body: "My brother, a Christian, wishes to marry a Jewess. I would like to draw your attention to one thing that could make this difficult, to wit, that the Jews have a specific racial smell, which in our terms can be outspokenly unpleasant. I would like to ask whether through this a certain aversion might arise that in the course of time could have a negative impact on their psychological harmony. One cannot, of course, give this a trial run; our doctors seem to have no knowledge or experience of this, as mixed marriages rarely occur here."[87] This statement is taken quite seriously by the physician who cites it. He refers to the biology of sexual attraction, ignoring the discourse of racial difference inherent in this view.

The assumptions of racial science become part of the underpinings of the medical science of the fin de siècle. Bernard Blechmann's medical dissertation, written under Carl Schmidt in the medical faculty of the University of Dorpat in 1882, draws heavily on Andree's work.[88] But it is a medical dissertation, written to document the knowledge the physician must have about the Jews. Blechmann, like Andree, begins by stating how little is really known about their nature (8). He documents the existing literature on the physical anthropology of the Jews, stressing the physical anomalies—such as the narrow chest measurement of the Russian Jews, which is less than the prescribed width for recruitment into the army (9). Such a view would have been very much in keeping with the general tendency of "modern" medical knowledge, with its roots in pathological anatomy. As Erna Lesky noted about the "second Viennese" school of medicine, which dominated the teaching of medicine in Vienna during the late nineteenth century: "First [they sorted] the facts scientifically on a purely anatomical basis . . . [and] second, [they demonstrated] the applicability of the facts and their utilization for diagnosis in live patients."[89] First one describes the "reality" of the Jew's body—then one proceeds to therapy.

Central to Blechmann's concern is the question of the relation of the Jew's body to the common good of the state. He reports on every possible study that documents the physical inability of Jews to serve in the army (15–17, 50–51). Healthy means being able to fulfill the role of the good citizen, and that role is defined by the ability to serve in the army. And he comments on the sources of his insufficiency in the biology as well as the social practices and conditions under which the Jews live. These are linked for Blechmann, as they are for Andree, not in the model Wolf uses, which attributes the illnesses of the Jews to inferior social status, but rather by assuming that the nature of the Jews determines their social practices and therefore their physiological results.

Blechmann also provides physiological explanations for some of the manifestations of Jewish difference Andree notes as givens. Thus Andree's discussion of the *Mauscheln* of the Jews, their inability to speak with other than a Jewish intonation, is understood by Blechmann (and others) as having a specifically anatomical origin. Jews speak differently because the "muscles, which are used for speaking and laughing are used inherently differently from those of Christians, and that this use can be traced . . . to the great difference in their nose and chin" (11). It is important to note that by the 1880s at least western European Jews were well enough integrated into the linguistic communities where they lived that they spoke the regional dialects. Blechmann's view underlies the ongoing assumption that Jews can be recognized by their manner of speech as much as by the nature of their bodies. The Viennese Jewish literary critic Theodor Reik, one of the first generation of psychoanalysts, commented on the attitude toward the Jew's language. He described the "natural" ability of the Jew to command the language of the Jews (here, Yiddish) but only that language: "A Gentile Viennese journalist spoke such excellent Yiddish that he was often considered a Jew. When one of his colleagues once teased him about his facility in speaking Yiddish, he said: "I can, you must."[90] This is a standard topos for the anti-Semitic attitude toward the Jewish presence in German-language culture: "The Jews Jew in their speech even when they do not *Mauscheln,* and this Jewing is virtually impossible for an Aryan to copy in either its intonation or its logic. Julius Korngold, the father of the composer Erich Wolfgang Korngold, once praised the Aryan journalist Hans Liebstöckl, who could Jew extraordinarily well, by saying that one could hardly note any difference between him and a Jew. Thereupon Hans Liebstöckl replied, using his Jew accent: 'There is a difference: I can Jew; you've got to.'"[91] This is echoed in Theodor Adorno's interview with a telephone operator in the 1940s who claims that "you get so you always know a Jewish voice."[92] The immutability of the Jewish voice was a reflex of the biology of the Jew but was also a mirror of the Jew's inherently different psychology.

Blechmann's dissertation is a typical medical dissertation of the time. It is in no way original; indeed, it relies on the published literature of the period. He undertakes to examine the anthropological literature of the nature of the Jews and excerpt the materials that are relevant for the medicine of his time. It is important to note that most studies in anthropology on the late nineteenth-century Jews (and the medicalization of this information) are based, like Blechmann's dissertation, on studies of Jews in eastern Europe and the Russian empire. In Freud's own library, the sole illustrated monograph about the Jews as a race, that by Carl Heinrich Stratz, presents visual images of "exotic" Jews, Jews from the East or the Middle East. Indeed, a commentator in 1912 remarked on the bias this indicates but also on the paucity of studies of Jews in western Europe.[93] It also stresses where the unchanging, diseased Jew was supposed to lie—in the East.[94] This image, so strongly present in the literature on Jewish difference in a period of Jewish acculturation and assimilation in western Europe, used the Eastern Jew as the example of inherent Jewish difference.[95] With millions of Eastern Jews streaming across central and western Europe beginning in the 1880s, the claim of Jewish difference could be substantiated by daily experience. Here were Jews who looked different, who acted differently, and who suffered from a wide range of diseases.[96] The last was of special importance given the fear of contamination (real or imagined) that haunted Germans and Austrians at the close of the nineteenth century. Special train stations were created in Berlin and Hamburg through which these Jews were processed—herded into huge barracks, ordered to strip, moved into communal showers, their clothing disinfected, and then moved onto ships as quickly as possible and sent out into the world. All of this was because of the fear of contagious diseases spreading to the general population, and the Jew was understood as the source of disease.

The debates about the special relationship of the Jews to disease at the close of the nineteenth century can be placed in a broader, more theoretical framework. Beginning in the work undertaken in 1848 by Rudolf Virchow, examining the typhus epidemic in Upper Silesia, the distinction between "natural" and "artificial" epidemics had been gradually accepted into the overall structure of medical thought about the transmission of disease.[97] Virchow, building on earlier work, distinguished between those diseases that were "natural" in that they were spread evenly across a population and were due to "natural" conditions (such as dysentery, malaria, pneumonia) and "artificial" diseases that were located in a specific, definable subgroup of society and were "attributes of society, products of a false culture, that is not distributed to all classes (such as typhus, scurvy, tuberculosis, and mental illness). They point toward deficiencies produced by the structure of state or society, and strike therefore primarily those classes which do not enjoy the advantages of the culture."[98] Clearly, Jewish and liberal physicians needed to see the diseases ascribed to the Jews as "artificial," for then they could be altered, if only over time. Other scientists saw these diseases as "natural," reflecting a predisposition of the Jew for such illnesses. In one of the first systematic studies of "the nature of anti-Semitism" during the fin de siècle, the Catholic Heinrich Coundenhove-Kalergi presented in 1901 such an image of the "artificial" origin of the Jews' disability:

> What would we think of a person who incarcerated refugees who had come to him for help in moldy cellar rooms, cut them off from all human contact, and forced them to undertake the filthiest and basest occupations in order to preserve their lives! After years these unhappy prisoners would be physically and morally ruined. They had acquired a foolish jargon, comic gestures, their clothing was in tatters, their eyes dripped, their spines were deformed, their aspirations had become low and common. Such a crime would be horrible but could be comprehended as a result of the base nature of mankind. If the torturer also trampled on these artificially degenerated individuals, amused himself about their physical and moral fragility, and mocked them, this would be no longer human but diabolical.[99]

The assumption of such liberal discourse is that the state of the Jews can be described as diseased and that the disease can be clearly attributed to specific historical cause. It reversed the assumption of a Jewish predisposition to disease without calling into question the basically diseased nature of the Jews.

We can turn for some elaboration of this problem to Talcott Parsons's model of the patient role, a model that reflects the medical practices and assumptions of late nineteenth- and early twentieth-century medicine.[100] Parsons divides the medical model of disease into four stages: the "patient's" failure to function; the acknowledgment by all that the patient is not responsible for the failure; excusing the patient from the obligations attendant on the assumptions of the social role; and the requirement that the patient attempt to achieve health. The debates about the diseases of the Jews are usually reflected in two quite different readings of this paradigm. First, the Jews show their inability to function in society through the presence of the overt signs of disease; the disease is, however, the Jews' responsibility in that it is part of their inherent "nature" (a "natural" disease); this disqualifies Jews from the social roles of the "healthy" society and places them in the permanent liminal role of the chronically ill and permanently infectious; there can be no cure, no attempt to get well. The opposing argument is complicated and in no way the simple antithesis. The Jew is sick, does show a failure to function, which reveals a weakness in the Jew; but this is an "artificial" disease that is the reflection of the society in which the Jew lives. Jews as a group may not be excused from social roles because of these disabilities. Any excuse of an individual would be taken as an admission of the permanent nature of the disease in the collective. The Jew must try to regain a state of health as defined by the world of science. But that state of health is defined as not being Jewish. It is important to stress that the sick roles in the late nineteenth century were much more rigid than they became in the course of the twentieth century.[101] The line between the patient and the doctor, as well as the sense of the patient as passive object of manipulation and the physician as agent of change, was much more defined.

Jewish scientists of the late nineteenth and early twentieth centuries found themselves trapped by such views. Like Wolf, who was forced to accept the charges of Jewish difference but attributed it to social rather than biological difference, they were constrained by the "realities" of their professional definitions as scientists to accept as valid the charges of Jewish biological inferiority. The eugenicist and Zionist Elias Auerbach, who by World War I had already emigrated to Palestine, could write in 1914 that "the Jews are without a doubt one of the most interesting objects of the biology of race. In the midst of the limitless racial mixing in Europe they still represent a relatively clear racial unity (for the offspring of mixed marriages usually leave the Jewish community). . . . The multitudinous signs of disease, which long have been attributed to the Jews because of their racial identity or their inbreeding, have been proved to be an artifact of their occupation."[102] They are sick, but this is a reflex of their social role. But it is vital to realize that for savants such as Auerbach, who accepted versions of the traditional so-called Lamarckian view of the inheritance of acquired characteristics, this mark upon the Jew was neither superficial nor trivial. As Philip Rieff has noted, "The connection between psychoanalysis and Lamarckianism cannot be overestimated. Freud, Freudians, and schismatics—including [C. G.] Jung, [Alfred] Adler, [Wilhelm] Reich—are thoroughly and consciously Lamarckian, and assert their science would be impossible if shorn of that strain."[103] It was not a quality that could be overcome in the generation that was itself afflicted; nor, perhaps, could it be overcome by the biblical sevenfold generations into the future. The refutation of this model, beginning with August Weismann in the 1880s, did not provide a sufficiently powerful explanatory model to displace it completely.

Even beyond the bounds of traditional racial science at the turn of the century, the assumption of the link between Jews and disease is made, as in the work of the German Marxist Karl Kautsky. It is true that Kautsky, much like Elias Auerbach, attributes this to the "citification" of the Jew and the resultant urban ills: "Jewish nature . . . is the exaggerated nature of the city dweller."[104] (This view was part of the debate triggered at the beginning of the century by the work of the German economist Werner Sombart on the role of Jews in shaping capitalism and on the special status of the city in this process.) Even the special language attributed to the Jew, the Jew's *Mauscheln,* is but an acquired characteristic, an urban accent, no different from the Swabian spoken by the Swabians or the Saxon spoken by the Saxons (52). It is the result of Jews' having been cut off from contact with their fellow citizens. Kautsky tells the story of the Jewish child who is sent to a village by his father so that he will stop speaking *Mauscheln* and learn the local dialect. After a year he goes back to the village to retrieve the child and is horrified to find that not only does the child still *mauscheln,* but so does the entire village (52). The assumption, which Kautsky wishes to dismiss but finds difficult, is that there is a biological model of inheritance that passes such attributes from generation to generation and that these attributes can infect the world in which the Jews are to be found. This argument is taken quite seriously in "scientific" studies such as the anthropologist Hans F. K. Günther's ethnology of the Jews. Günther claimed that *Mauscheln* is infectious and can be contracted from prolonged contact with the Jews. This can be seen in the fact that the non-Jewish inhabitants of cities such as Frankfurt and Breslau "show the influence of a phonetics of *Mauscheln.*"[105] Given the cryptobiological arguments of late nineteenth-century Marxism (as exemplified by Friedrich Engels's late studies of "historical materialism," that amalgam of Marx and Darwin), it is not surprising that there is as much nature as nurture in these arguments of adaption. For the story Kautsky tells is a tale of the impossibility of Jewish adaptability and the inherent nature of Jewish difference.

Mauscheln is one of the central signs of the difference of the Jews. It can be a sign of biological immutability or of the social impact that formed them. Sigmund Freud's use of *Mauscheln* in many of the jokes in his study of humor (1905) reflects the complexity of such a sign of difference.[106] The power of linguistic dissonance can be seen in Freud's using one of the punch lines from his study of humor in a text written almost two decades after the publication of that study, illustrating how entrenched the sense of language is as a marker for Jewish difference.[107] The Eastern Jew's language is written on the Jew's tongue, is identifiable through the Jew's speech, and represents the hidden disease of the Jew. Freud "dispenses with the comic element of dialect" ("das komische Element des Jargons," the pejorative term for Yiddish) (*SE* 8:108; *GW* 6:119). Yet such jokes are told in *Mauscheln* as the "comic Jewish dialect" ("im scherzhaft gebrauchten jüdischen Jargon") (*SE* 4:297; *GW* 2/

3:302), but even more so, for Freud (like Albert Einstein) was a compulsive teller of such dialect jokes.[108] All of his contemporaries comment on this fact. Theodor Reik recounts returning with Freud from the memorial service for Karl Abraham. Freud commends Reik for balancing his praise of Abraham with an acknowledgment of his weakness: "And to illustrate his remarks, he told me one of those Jewish jokes which so unmercifully expose the psychic motives of our exaggerated eulogies of the dead."[109] Freud told Jewish dialect jokes to signify that he could choose to use this narrative mode but that it was not intrinsic to his nature. Wilhelm Reich, who like Reik and Freud, was a central European Jew who suffered under the charge of his own inability to command the language and substance of science, noted that "he used to quote Jewish jokes. . . . He made these jokes, but he was not anti-Semitic. Surely not. Much of his Judaism was protest, not genuine. . . . His German was perfect. His thinking was German. It was not Jewish, even though [Pierre] Janet had proclaimed that psychoanalysis was a Jewish science."[110] Reich's claim that Freud's "Jewishness" was only a facade since he really did have command of the language of high culture, echoes the insecurity of the Jew in his own language. For Reich, Freud was not "characterologically, religiously or nationally" a Jew (62). For a Jew, according to Reich, is "somebody who behaves in a Jewish way, either nationally or religiously, who is bound up with his customs, who speaks the Jewish language, who lives in it, thrives in it, and so on" (61). Reich, like Freud, was quite simply, in many people's eyes, a member of the Jewish race. A. A. Brill noted that after the publication of his translations of Freud's works "[he] received letters from so-called Jewish scientists accusing Freud of crypto-anti-Semitism. One of them was angry because Freud used many Jewish jokes to illustrate some of his theories on wit and humor."[111] In writing his scholarly work Freud could also choose not to use *Mauscheln*. He framed the telling of such stories in the purest of German academic prose, as he does in his study of wit. But Jews of his age found even such an evocation troubling. But what is most striking is that the new discourse of psychoanalysis, that scientific language that Freud evolves (among other reasons) to exorcise the demon of anti-Semitism from the world of the human sciences, becomes stereotyped (even in Freud's mind) as the language of Jews. This tension between the universalizing desire of psychoanalysis and the particularistic charge that this discourse is but the masked language of the Jews exemplifies the burden under which the Jewish scientist of the fin de siècle struggled. The terms of that struggle were inscribed on the Jew's body, not only in the world of science but also in the general culture in which Jews lived.

Representing the Jewish Body in the Literary Culture

The fantasy of Jewish difference and disease permeates all aspects of central European culture in the late nineteenth and early twentieth centuries. We can call upon a turn-of-the-century literary work that represents the reconstruction of the Jewish body and psyche. Written by the German physician-author Oskar Panizza (1853–1921) in 1893, it depicts the careful reconstruction of the Jew Itzig Feitel Stern (one of the classic anti-Semitic literary characters of the mid-nineteenth century) into an "Aryan." The story begins with a detailed description of Stern's physiognomy—his Jewish "antelope's eye," his nose, his eyebrows, his "fleshy and overly creased" lips, his "violet fatty tongue," his "bow-legs," his "curly, thick black locks of hair."[112] But it is not just his body that marks him as a Jew. His language, whether French or High German, is "warped" by his "Palatinate-Yiddish." He "meeowed, rattled, bleated and also liked to produce sneezing sounds." His speech was a "mixture of Palatinate Semitic babble, French nasal noises and some High German vocal sounds which he had fortuitously overheard and articulated with an open position of the mouth." His body language was equally marked. His gait marked him as a Jew, and it bore a striking resemblance to the way "people with spinal diseases" walked (64, 65, 68). His gesticulation was equally "Jewish." All of Stern's physiognomy points toward the perverted nature of the Jew.

Stern goes to Professor Klotz, the famous Heidelberg anatomist, and has his body reshaped. He is forced into orthopedic appliances and has his movements retrained in order, in his own words, to "become such a fine gentilman just like a goymenera and to geeve up all fizonomie of Jewishness" (68). His "Palatinate-Yiddish" is rehabilitated and formed into a pure High German. But his Jewish soul remains. Stern desires a "chaste, undefiled Germanic soul which shrouded the possessor like an aroma." To accomplish this he undertakes his own medicalized version of the ancient libel concerning the Jews' need for Christian blood. He buys the blood of Christians and has it exchanged for his own. Having been transformed into an Aryan, Stern decides to marry a "blond Germanic lass" (77). Indeed, all the physical changes that are necessary to make him into the ideal image of the Aryan have taken place—all but one. Feitel Stern remains circumcised. At least Panizza never mentions this phenomenon, even though there are procedures, many of them ancient, for the reversal of circumcision and though, as I mentioned in my discussion of Andree's work, these procedures were again in circulation at the close of the century.[113] The circumcision of the genitals is the outward sign of the immutability of the Jew within.

On his wedding night Stern becomes intoxicated, and in his drunkenness all his newly acquired qualities of body, tongue, and mind disintegrate. The *foetor judaicus* that had been masked by the Christian blood he bought reappears and marks his final collapse as he lies "crumpled and quivering, a convoluted Asiatic image in a wedding dress, a counterfeit of human flesh."[114] All the changes the Jew acquires are useless. He unravels under the influence of drink. As Immanuel Kant had observed in his *Anthropology,* "Women, clergymen, and Jews ordinarily do not become drunk, at least they carefully avoid all appearance of it, because they are weak in civic life and must restrain themselves (for which sobriety is required)."[115] Jews become their true selves when the constraints of civilization are removed.

How intensely the view that the Jew can see (and represent) the world just as well as the Aryan dominates the Jewish response can be seen in an answer to Oskar Panizza's tale, called "The Operated Goy," a story published in 1922 by the writer-philosopher Mynona (Salomo Friedlaender [1871–1946]).[116] Mynona's tale represents an assimilated Jew's response to Panizza's message about the immutability of the Jew. But Mynona's fable still relies on images of the Jewish body and the meanings associated with it within fin-de-siècle society. In Mynona's story the protagonist is the Aryan Count Reschock, whose noble family of anti-Semites can trace its roots back to the destruction of Jerusalem by the emperor Titus. His body is that of the essential Aryan: "Thin lips, Prussian chin, proud nape of the neck, extraordinarily stiff posture; legs that in their innocence were neither knock-kneed nor bowed; . . . that stood on aristocratic and simultaneously pan-Germanic feet and walked about as if descending from Mount Olympus." Through his anti-Semitic demeanor, he captures the interest of the beautiful but very Jewish heiress Rebecka Gold-Isak, with her "almond eyes, ebony hair, ivory skin, etc." (280, 282). She presents her father with the ultimatum: she must marry Count Reschock. (She is the prototype of the seemingly unique American stereotype of the 1950s, the Jewish American princess.) Her father insists that if such a wedding is to be, the bridegroom must totally become a Jew.

Central to his physical transformation is his ritual circumcision (185–86). But this is not sufficient. Rebecka must "convert" the anti-Semite into a philo-Semite. Her means are psychological rather than physiological. Mynona's satiric reversal of the blood libel is seen in the means by which the count's soul is to become Jewish. He undergoes the application of what was understood in the 1920s as an essentially Jewish science:

> Wasn't his radical hatred of the Jews precisely the most uncanny means of generating the opposite: the most radical shift from one extreme to another? Anti-Semitism is possibly even more Jewish than Judaism. In general, those who hate and discriminate predispose themselves in all secretiveness slowly but surely to the most intimate blood relationship, even to an identification with the object of negation. If she could bring the young count to self-realization, then she could be sure of him. One had to force him to undertake psychoanalysis. She bribed his servant Bör, more with her charm than with money, and sought aid among feudal nobles, who again following her lead, quietly but irresistibly influenced young Reschock until he himself appeared with mysterious psychic inhibitions in the examination room of the famous Freud. This veritable destroyer of fig leaves so anatomically robbed the noble Reschockish soul of its protective covering that the count fell into the arms of his servant, who hurried to him with a horrendous cry. He pulled himself together and stared into the dark eyes of his fate in the form of the beautiful Jewess, with inherited bravery, yes audacity. At first in his fantasy, then in reality. (286–87)

Mynona, along with Karl Kraus, one of the most articulate early critics of psychoanalysis, parodies the use of psychoanalysis as a means of altering the soul.[117] Here it becomes the means of effecting the alteration of the body. The question of who can be cured and who is diseased lies at the heart of the matter. Kraus confronted the question of the meaning of psychoanalysis in a 1924 essay in which he used the epistemological conflict between the physician and the patient as his model for the impossibility of psychoanalysis: "There are real psychoanalysts where one cannot know whether they are the doctors or the patients. It is of the nature of this disease and its therapy that an illness is a therapy and the therapy an illness, that those who are healthy leave the office as patients and the patients as physicians."[118] This is, of course, the conflict the Jewish physician, such as Freud, finds when he is confronted with his own Jewishness as a pathological factor, a factor that the Jewish writer Kraus cannot, or indeed will not, evoke when he speaks of the "plague" of psychoanalysis but that is present in the origin of his own rhetoric. But it is made crystal clear in the work of Kraus's non-Jewish contemporary, the Czech novelist Ladislaw Klima, in 1928, when he has the protagonist of his novel disguise himself as an old Jew, "because he already has knock-knees," in order to visit the most famous psychopathologist in all of Germany—who turns out to speak in *Mauscheln*.[119] The Jewish psychotherapist is the disease he wishes to cure.

In order finally to win her hand, Reschock is physically transformed by the famed orthopedist Professor Friedländer into the physical form of "a Jewish Talmudic scholar." He studies Hebrew. He is finally circumcised, and he changes his name to Count Moshe. By the close of the story, he and his beloved have moved to Jerusalem, where they raise a family of Orthodox children. Professor Friedländer's practice has blossomed. He has become the scourge of all anti-Semites, for he has shown how easily a member of one race can be transformed into another.

The problem with Mynona's retelling of Panizza's story is that the basic ethnographic assumptions, the biological basis of defining the Jew, persist even in his rebuttal. It is in the necessary physical transformation of the count, in his change from an Aryan body type to that of the Jew, that the realities should be undermined. Unlike Feitel Stern, whose image unravels at the conclusion of Panizza's tale, Count Reschock becomes a "real" Jew. It is the shaping of the psyche of the Aryan through the Jewish means of psychoanalysis that creates "Count Moshe." It is necessary for him to be given a Jewish "soul." There is a powerful belief, even among assimilated Jewish thinkers such as Mynona, in the biological basis of reality, a biology that is mutable but real and that affects an individual's understanding and response to the world. This is revealed in many of the satiric underpinnings of the tale. When the count first sees his future bride, disguised an an Aryan, his dog immediately "smells" her as a Jew. The reason for her disguise: she had heard about this new arrival in her community, about his anti-Semitic attitude, and had decided to capture him "even if she had to marry him out of vengeance."[120] The hidden, malevolent nature of the Jew is manifest here in the representation of the Jewish woman even in a tale whose point should be the malleability of the physical. Hidden beneath a "red-blond" wig Rebecka wears is the "ebony hair" that marks her true difference. And it is the difference of race as well as the difference of gender.

These texts transform the scientific debate about the racial nature of the Jew into the stuff of literature and thereby give it a safe locus in which to be played out. Mynona and Panizza relate to the idea of their racial difference in quite different ways. Panizza saw the diseased Jewish body as even more repellent than his own. Trained as a physician at the University of Munich, Panizza's own personal life reflected the central problem we will examine in the course of this study: the identity of the physician as separate, or at least separable, from the patient. For Panizza not only was a physician but also morbidly believed himself to be syphilitic. His fantasy about his own diseased body becomes the reality of the body of the Jew. In 1895 the publication of his play *The Council of Love* led him to be sentenced to a year in prison in Munich. In that work he represented the introduction of syphilis into the Renaissance world through the Jewish princess Salome, who was the vehicle by which the devil corrupted the flesh. The devil, like Salome, is visible as a Jew: "His features wear an expression that is decadent, worn and embittered. He has a yellowish complexion. His manners recall those of a Jew of high breeding."[121] Thus syphilis is introduced into the debauched world of Renaissance Rome and the history of Europe by the Jews.

Panizza's text and Sigmund Freud's reading of it can serve as an example of the blindness necessary for fin-de-siècle Jews to function within a world of high culture that presents them as the source of disease and contagion. Freud selectively read this play, citing it in the notes to *The Intepretation of Dreams* (1900) as a "strongly revolutionary literary play" and remarking only that "God the father is ignominiously treated as a paralytic old man."[122] Freud reads Panizza's image as a universal one and incorporates it in his own personal critique of religion (not Judaism). However, this image is evoked within the context of a dream image of Freud's father, the dying Jew, who soiled his bed during the last days of his life. On November 13, 1907, Freud again comments on Panizza and his drama, repressing Panizza's clearly anti-Semitic images.[123] Panizza's image of God the Father as the limping, syphilitic Jew whose tubercular son, Jesus Christ, has inherited his disease and shows symptoms of locomotor ataxia and mental deficiency employs much of the vocabulary that comes to categorize the hidden nature of the Jew in the medical science of the fin de siècle. Freud ignored these aspects of the representation of the Jew, focusing on Panizza's critique of religion. Freud does not see the representation of the Jew—of himself—in this text, because to acknowledge it would be to question the very nature of his role as the neutral physician. How can he simultaneously be the diseased patient, the source of the disease, and the healer? To see the devil and Salome as Jews (which his contemporaries clearly did) would be to admit that his own gaze was poisoned by the inherent nature of the Jew. The very act of "seeing" Jews in these contexts meant being aware of the difference ascribed to his perceptual framework.

The Gaze of the Jew

Other transformations in the theme of the special nature of the Jew's body take place at the fin de siècle in other cultural spaces, including that of science. The impact of such fantasies of the biological nature of the Jew—the Jew's body, psyche, and soul—on the development of psychoanalysis is at the core of this book. The special nature of the Jew, the diseases and sociopathic acts ascribed to it, are a universal in the general culture of the nineteenth century. It is no surprise that the Jew is seen in terms of this dominant paradigm of the late nineteenth century, since this age saw the biologizing of all arenas of culture. We find Jewish biological and medical scientists of the late nineteenth century forced to deal with what is for them the unstated central epistemological problem of late nineteenth-century biological science: how one could be the potential subject of a scientific study at the same time that one had the role of the observer; how one could be the potential patient at the same moment one was supposed to be the physician.[124] This was especially a problem in Vienna, where the domination of the "second Viennese" school stressed the central role of the physician as scientist and the independent, neutral role of its physician-scientist as diagnostician.[125]

Being a Jew is indelible. To again quote the seventeenth-century scholar Johann Jakob Schudt: "The Jewish people remain so identifiable that among a thousand people one can immediately know the Jew."[126] Or Johann Friedrich Blumenbach's variation on this: "Even a layman could identify the Jew's skull among the many skulls in my collection."[127] The Dutch anatomist Peter Camper, the great advocate of the equality of the races, even in his establishment of the relative nature of their physiognomies, saw that the Dutch Jews looked "different" from his other contemporaries, but he could not quite localize this difference. Where it was to be found Camper was not sure, but it was not in the "nose" of the Jew:

> There is no nation that is as clearly identifiable as the Jews: men, women, children, even when they are first born, bear the sign of their origin. I have often spoken about this with the famed painter of historical subjects [Benjamin] West, to whom I mentioned my difficulty in capturing the national essence of the Jews. He was of the opinion that this must be sought in the curvature of the nose. I cannot deny that the nose has much to do with this, and that it bears a resemblance to the form of the Mongol (whom I had often observed in London and of which I possess a facial cast), but this is not sufficient for me. For this reason, I feel that the famed painter J[acob] de Wit has painted many men with beards in the meeting room of the Inner Council [in Amsterdam], but no Jews.[128]

This view continues, in various forms, to Charles Darwin, who sees a "uniform appearance" of the Jews, which is independent of their geographic location.[129] Try to suppress the Jew without, the Jewish body, and all that will happen is that the Jew within will be preserved and will appear or be seen by the sharp eye of the scientist trained to spy out the difference between the Jew and all others.

The Jew was immediately visible. Francis Galton tried to capture this

"Jewish physiognomy" in his composite photographs of "boys in the Jews' Free School, Bell Lane (figs. 2 and 3).[130] Galton photographed a number of pupils in this school and used a form of multiple exposure to create an image of the "essence" of the Jew—not just physiognomy but the Jew's very nature. Called forth by two papers to be given before the Anthropological Institute "on the race characteristics of the Jews," Galton believed the experiment had captured the "typical features of the modern Jewish face." Galton's trip to the Bell Lane school confronted him with the "children of poor parents, dirty little fellows individually, but wonderfully beautiful, as I think, in these composites." There, and in the adjacent "Jewish Quarter," he saw the "cold, scanning gaze of man, woman, and child" of the Jew as the sign of their difference, of their potential pathology, of their inherent nature. "There was no sign of diffidence in any of their looks, nor of surprise at the unwonted intrusion. I felt, rightly or wrongly, that every one of them was coolly appraising me at market value, without the slightest interest of any other kind."[131] It is in the Jews' gaze that the pathology of their souls can be found.[132] At the turn of the century, Sigmund Freud read this view of the "vivacity of the eye" as a sign of the "remarkable persistence" of the Jew's physiognomy.[133] Using Galton's photographs, Hans F. K. Günther later attempted to describe the "sensual," "threatening," and "crafty" gaze of the Jew as the direct result of the physiology of the Jewish face and reflecting the essence of the Jewish soul.[134] This view is at least as old as the seventeenth century. Robert Burton writes in *The Anatomy of Melancholy* of the "goggle eyes" of the Jews, as well as "their voice, pace, gesture, [and] looks" as a sign of "their conditions and infirmities."[135] (Burton's authority is our old friend, the German theologian Buxtorf.) It is not merely that Jews "look Jewish," but that this look marks them as inferior: "Who has not heard people characterize such and such a man or woman they see in the streets as Jewish without in the least knowing anything about them? The street arab who calls out 'Jew' as some child hurries on to school is unconsciously giving the best and most disinterested proof that there is a reality in the Jewish expression."[136] The gaze of the non-Jew seeing the Jew is immediately translated into action; the gaze of the Jew becomes the functional equivalent of the damaged language, the *Mauscheln,* of the Jew.

And this gaze is dangerous. The Germans believed that the Jews possessed the evil eye, as S. Seligmann observed.[137] Freud commented on Seligmann's work in his essay "The Uncanny" (1919). He cited the fantasy about the evil eye, that "whoever possesses something that is at once valuable and fragile is afraid of other people's envy, in so far as he projects on to them the envy he would have felt in their place. A feeling like this betrays itself by a look even though it is not put into words; and when a man is prominent owing to noticeable, and particularly owing to unattractive, attributes, other people are ready to believe that his envy is rising to a more than usual degree of intensity and that this intensity will convert it into effective action" (*SE* 17:240). This is the "look" of the Jew, but placed by Freud into the broadest, most universal category of the gaze.

As the Jewish social scientist Joseph Jacobs notes in his discussion of Galton's finding of the absolute Jewishness of the gaze:

> Cover up every part of composite A but the eyes, and yet I fancy anyone familiar with Jews would say: "Those are Jewish eyes." I am less able to analyze this effect than the case of the nose. . . . I fail to see any of the cold calculation which Mr. Galton noticed in the boys at the school, at any rate in the composites A, B, and C. There is something more like the dreamer and thinker than the merchant in A. In fact, on my showing this to an eminent painter of my acquaintance, he exclaimed, "I imagine that is how Spinoza looked when a lad," a piece of artistic insight which is remarkably confirmed by the portraits of the philosopher, though the artist had never seen one. The cold, somewhat hard look in composite D, however, is more confirmatory of Mr. Galton's impression. It is noteworthy that this is seen in a composite of young fellows between seventeen and twenty, who have had to fight a hard battle of life even by that early age."[138]

For the Jewish social scientist such as Jacobs, the inexplicable nature of the Jewish gaze exists (even more than the "nostrility" that characterizes the Jewish nose) to mark the Jew. His rationale is quite different from that of Galton—he seeks a social reason for the "hard and calculating" glance seen by Galton, but he claims to see it nevertheless. The Jewish "race," as was the commonplace in the anthropological literature of the age, could never be truly beautiful.[139] And it is the Jewish gaze that most of the writers fix on. Arthur de Gobineau noted that the "French, German and Polish Jews—they all look alike. I have had the opportunity of examining closely one of the last kind. His features and profile clearly betrayed his origin. His eyes especially were unforgettable."[140] This gaze is documented in the physiognomies of the fin de siècle, such as that of the German physiognomist Carl Huter (fig. 4).[141] Huter, an artist who evolved his "psychophysiognomy" under the influence of spiritualism, presents a chart of the gaze, reaching from the eye in the moment of aesthetic perception (1) to the aggressive and destructive gaze (12). It is this gaze that is attributed to the Jew.

It is the meaning of these eyes that haunts the Jewish scientist. Jacobs noted in the essay "Anthropological Types" in the *Jewish Encyclopedia* that these "eyes themselves are generally brilliant, both eyelids are heavy

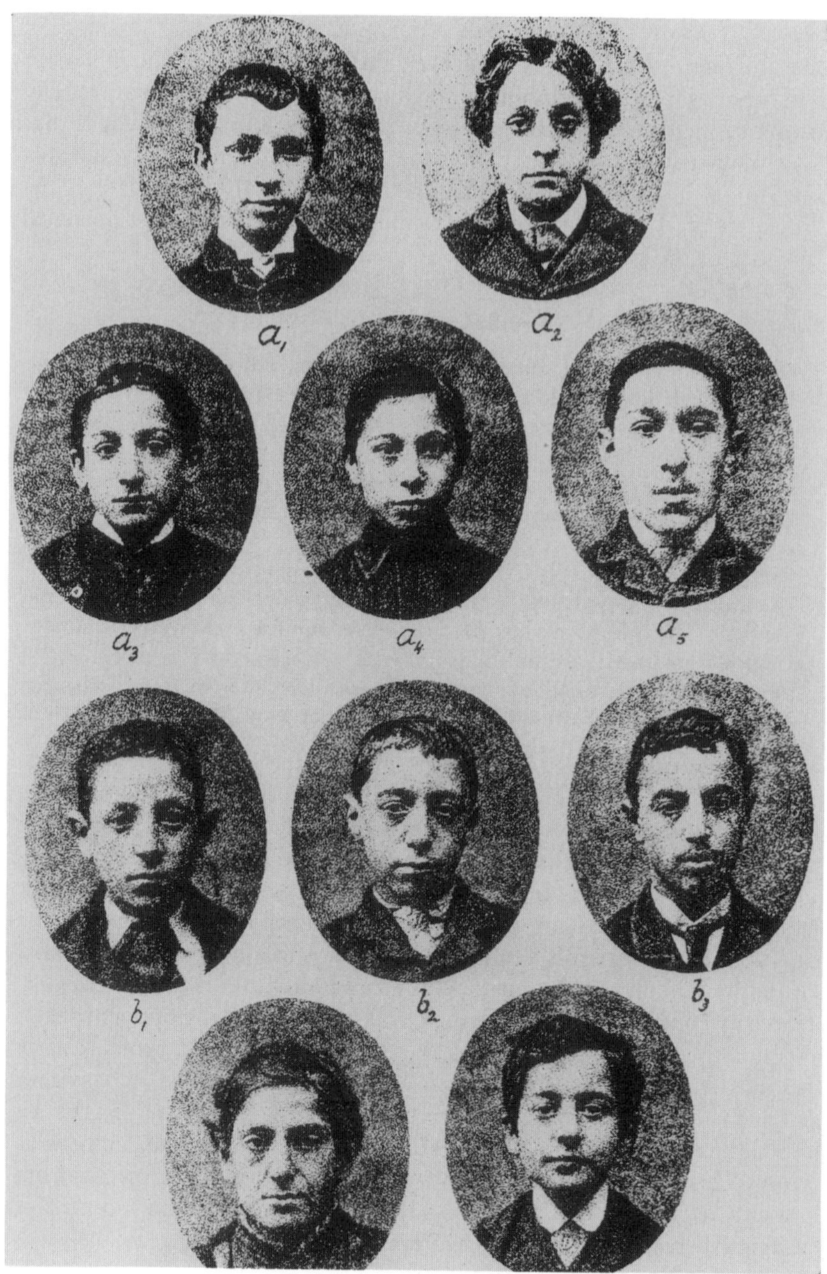

Figure 2. Francis Galton's original photographs of Jewish students at a London school. From Joseph Jacobs, *Studies in Jewish Statistics* (London: D. Nutt, 1891). (Private collection, Ithaca, N.Y.)

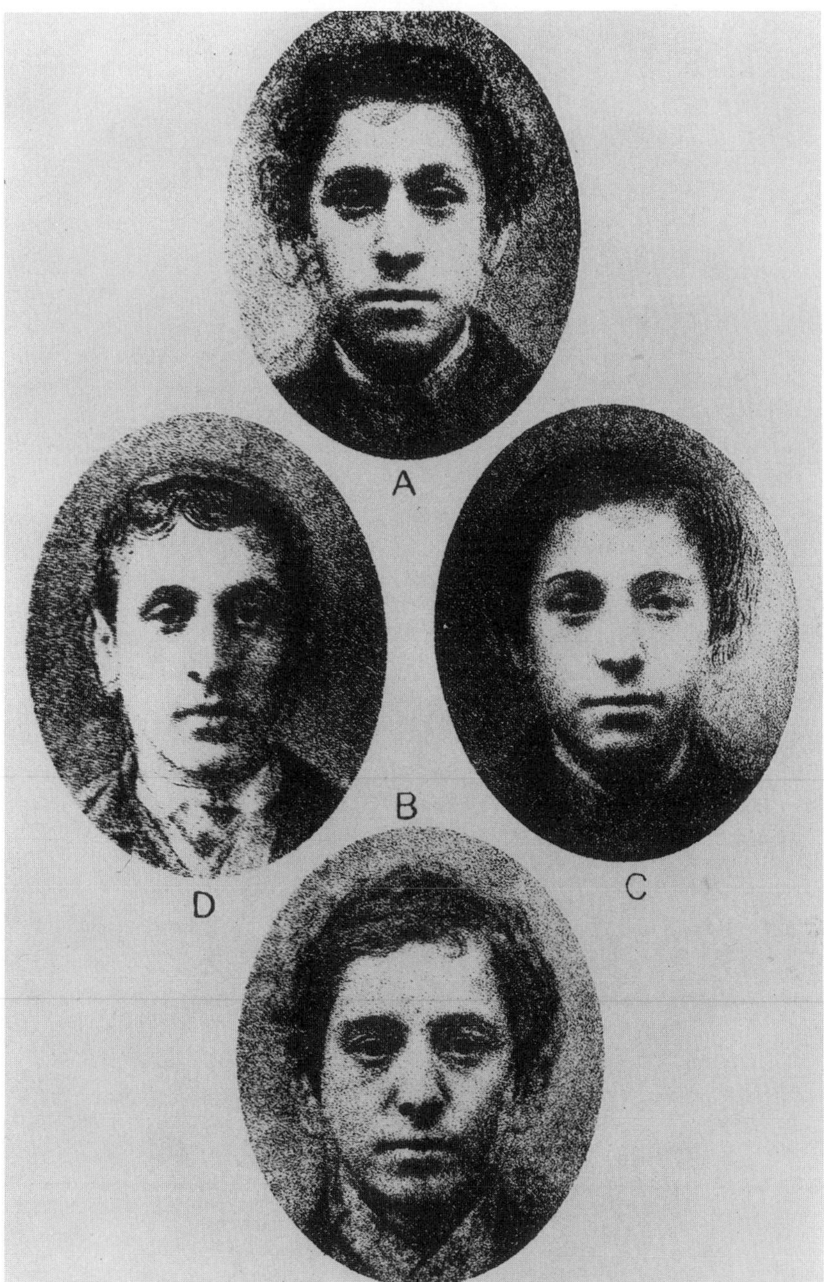

Figure 3. Galton superimposed the original photographs to produce a form of multiple exposure and created an image of the "essence" of the Jew. From Joseph Jacobs, *Studies in Jewish Statistics* (London: D. Nutt, 1891). (Private collection, Ithaca, N.Y.)

Tafel 100. Die Augensprache als Grundlage eines wissenschaftlichen Charakter- und Gedankenlesens.

Die 12 hauptsächlichsten Blickrichtungen.

1. **Beobachtender Blick.** Der Augapfel steht wenig unter der Achse. Beide Lider treten etwas zusammen, so daß fast nur die Pupille sichtbar ist.

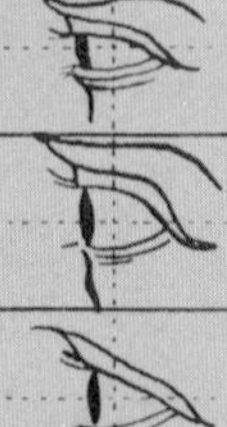

2. **Vorstellender Blick.** Der Augapfel liegt auf der Achse. Die Lider sind mehr geöffnet, so daß die halbe Iris sichtbar ist.

3. **Denkender Blick.** Der Augapfel liegt auf der Achse, die Lider sind offen.

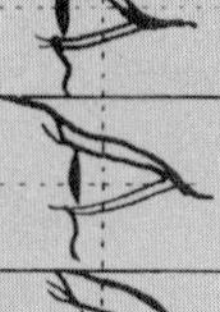

4. **Juristischer Blick.** Der Augapfel ist herausgedrängt, so daß die Iris ganz sichtbar wird. Die Lider sind energisch offen.

5. **Philosophischer Blick.** Der Augapfel liegt etwas über der Achse nach oben gerichtet. Die Lider gehen etwas nach oben.

6. **Weiser Blick.** Der Augapfel liegt noch höher über der Achse. Das Oberlid ist groß, auch die Wimpern gehen nach oben.

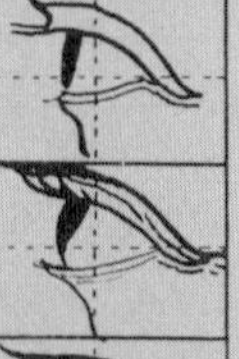

7. **Ethischer Blick.** Der Augapfel ist sehr stark hochgestellt, das Oberlid legt sich weit über denselben.

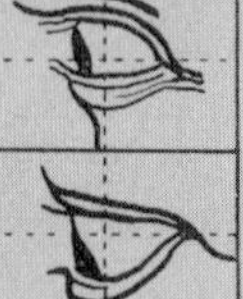

8. **Religiöser Blick.** Es ist der verstärkte ethische Blick. Die Lider sind noch mehr aufwärts gerichtet.

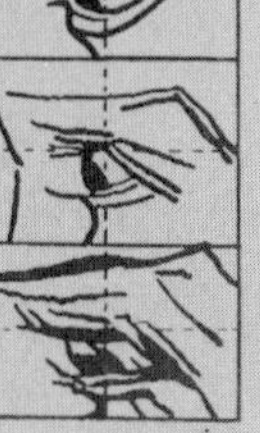

9. **Blick der physischen Liebe.** Der Augapfel liegt etwas unter der Achse. Das untere Augenlid ist stark hochgezogen.

10. **Blick der physischen Ernährung.** Der Augapfel liegt stark unter der Achse. Das untere Augenlid ist normal.

11. **Ordinärer Blick.** Der Augapfel liegt sehr stark unter der Achse, von unten wie gierig hervortretend.

12. **Gemeingefährlicher Blick.** Der Augapfel steht ebenfalls sehr stark unter der Achse und ist von unten hervorgespannt.

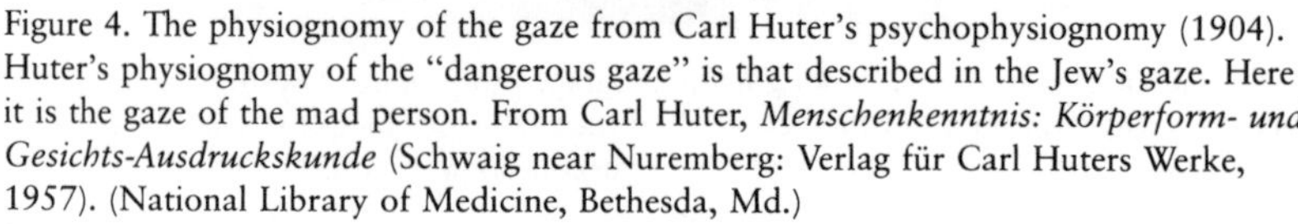

Mein System der Augensprache, wie ich es seit 22 Jahren in öffentlichen Experimentalvorträgen und bei privaten Untersuchungen erfolgreich anwende.

Figure 4. The physiognomy of the gaze from Carl Huter's psychophysiognomy (1904). Huter's physiognomy of the "dangerous gaze" is that described in the Jew's gaze. Here it is the gaze of the mad person. From Carl Huter, *Menschenkenntnis: Körperform- und Gesichts-Ausdruckskunde* (Schwaig near Nuremberg: Verlag für Carl Huters Werke, 1957). (National Library of Medicine, Bethesda, Md.)

and bulging, and it seems to be the main characteristic of the Jewish eye that the upper lid covers a larger proportion of the pupil than among other persons. This may serve to give a sort of nervous, furtive look to the eyes, which, when the pupils are small and set close together with semistrabismus, gives keenness to some Jewish eyes."[142] Anatole Leroy-Beaulieu, citing Galton's composite photographs of Jews in 1893, writes of "the pensiveness of the Jewish face; it is one of the characteristics of the race."[143] And among the markers of that face are the "large and sometimes blinking eyes, with heavy lids, that give the eyes a half-closed appearance" (113). The Jewish eye appears different and sees the world differently. With Freud's evocation of the Galtonian photographs, this image of the Jew is evoked. Hidden within those claims for universality are the images of race that Galton produces parallel to his other composites, in which the eyes and gaze of the Jew are pathologized.

This view reappears within the medical literature in the work of Jewish physicians, such as Moses Julius Gutmann, who writes of the structure of the Jewish face, of its typical form, as being the result of a combination of features that produces "the melancholy, pained expression (the 'nebbish' face)" that is associated with the Jew. For Gutmann and others this results from the "psychological history of the Jew."[144] The Viennese Jewish physician-anthropologist Ignaz Zollschan, in a text read by Freud, wrote that one "cannot deny that the Jews have a certain expression [that] one can imagine represented by that untranslatable word 'nebbish.'"[145] For Zollschan it is a reflection of the uniform nature of the Jewish race that he wishes to preserve through the instrument of political Zionism.

Sigmund Freud's own fantasy about the Jew also reflects the question of the meaning of the Jew's eyes. Freud tells of dreaming about Theodor Herzl sometime between 1905 and 1907: "A majestic figure, with a pale, dark-toned face framed by a beautiful, raven-black beard, with infinitely sad eyes. The apparition strove to explain to . . . [Freud] the necessity of immediate action if the Jewish people was to be saved."[146] Here the reversal of the image of the "nebbish" face reflects the reversal of the classical, negative visual image of the Jew with his Assyrian beard. Parallel images can be found at the fin de siècle in the work of the Viennese-Jewish artist Ephraim Moses Lilien, whose idealized images of the Jews were all modeled on Eastern Jews (often in historical settings). Indeed, when the Austrian Jewish artist Hermann Struck (well known for his portraits of Eastern Jews) made a lithograph of Freud, Freud immediately saw it as both familiar and uncanny: "Whatever is Jewish about the head has my full agreement, but something else has struck me as alien. I have come to the conclusion that it is the exaggerated opening of the mouth, the stretching forward of the beard, and the prominence of its outer contour. In trying to discover where these features could come from, I remembered the beautiful, malicious orchid, the *Orchibestia karlsbadiensis,* which we shared. This would produce a composite figure (as it is called in *The Interpretation of Dreams*) of Jew and orchid!" (fig. 5).[147] Struck had given Freud a picture of an orchid on their last meeting. But the enigma of what looks Jewish remains in Freud's evaluation of this portrait. Could it not be the Jewish eyes? They are strikingly different from those of the engraving Freud praised. Freud "sees" this Struck engraving as a Galtonian composite, echoing his use of Galton's technique as the model for dream formation, as will be discussed below.

Herzl's Jewish gaze with his "infinitely sad eyes"—the "nebbish" look—is quite the opposite of Freud's terrifying Professor Ernst Brücke, whose "terrible blue eyes . . . reduced [Freud] to nothing" when he was late in unlocking the door to the laboratory (*SE* 5:422). The "annihilating gaze" of the blue eyes of the Aryan professor reflects the difference between the dark eyes of the Jew, with their reference to the difference and pathology of the Jew, and the powerful, healthy gaze of the Aryan.[148] Little wonder that when Freud translated this experience of being seen as different into the symbolic world of his dreams, he transformed Brücke's "terrible" gaze into that of "sickly blue eyes" that could be dismissed: "It seemed to me quite possible that people of that kind existed as long as one liked and could be got rid of if someone else wished it" (*SE* 5:422). But Freud makes this powerlessness understandable in his world of dreams by linking this image of the now marginalized and powerless Aryan with that of one of his dead fellow Jewish medical students. Jews and Aryans are truly alike only when they are dead. It is at that moment that their gaze becomes equal.

The clinical gaze of the Jewish physician now becomes the object of the gaze of study. The Canadian physician William Osler returned to Berlin in 1884, a decade after undertaking postgraduate medical work in Germany. He commented on the "number of professors and docents of Hebrew extraction in the German Medical Faculties. . . . The number is very great, and of those I know their positions have been won by hard and honorable work; but I fear that, as I hear has already been the case, the present agitation will help to make the attainment of university professorships additionally difficult. One cannot but notice here, in any assembly of doctors, the strong Semitic elements; at the local societies and at the German Congress of Physicians it was particularly noticeable, and the same holds good in any collection of students. All honor to them!"[149] With all of Osler's good intent, the Jewish physician, who wants to see himself as a scientist, is visible to the Aryan scientist in a

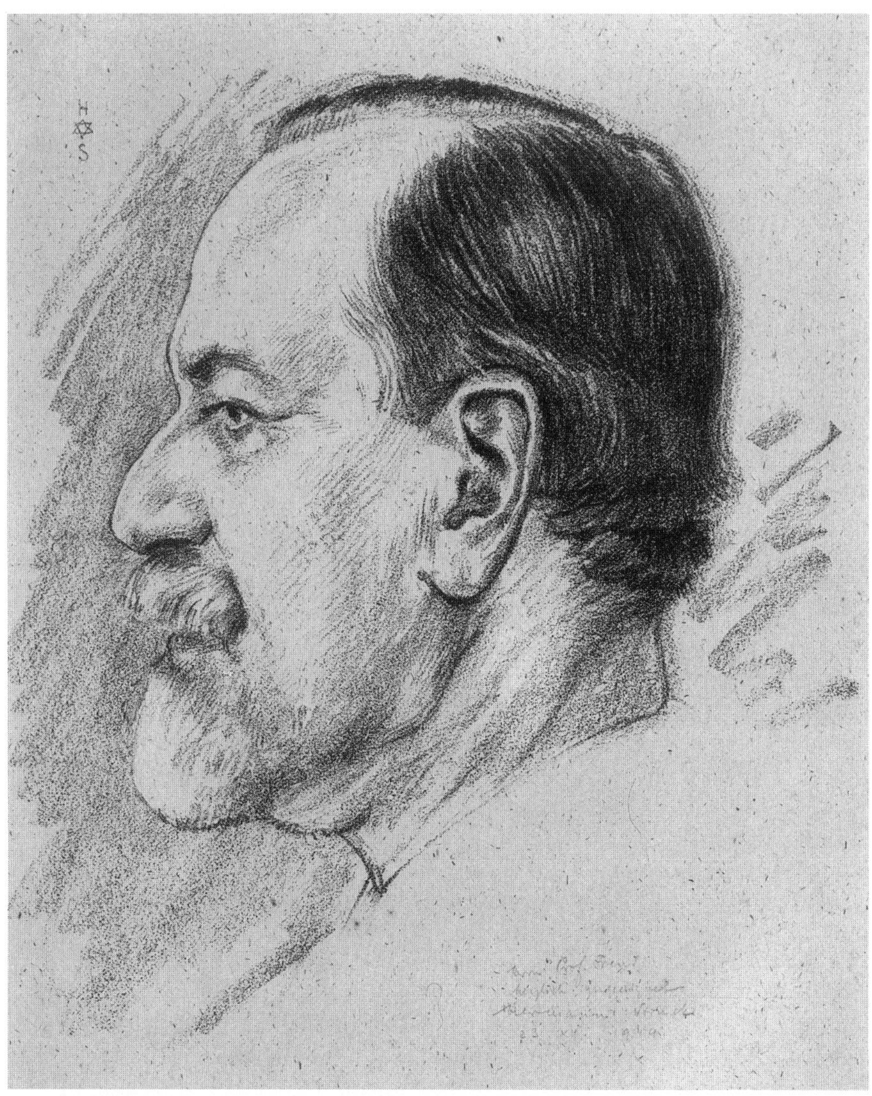

Figure 5. Hermann Struck's lithograph of Freud of December 23, 1914. Freud was moved by the Jewish nature of his appearance. (Freud Museum, London.)

direct and unmediated manner. The image of the eyes attributed to the Jew reappears in the context of the science of race. When the Jewish physician looks in the mirror he sees the person at risk, he sees the Jew; he also sees the physician, the healer. How can the image of the healer be the same as the image of the patient? How can the gaze that is pathological also be the gaze that diagnoses in order to cure? It is the biological definition of all aspects of the Jew that helps form the idea of the Jew at the fin de siècle. The scientific gaze should be neutral. The scientific gaze should be beyond or above all the vagaries of individual difference.[150] As George Herbert Mead put it: "Knowledge is never a mere contact of our organisms with other objects. It always takes on a universal character. If we know a thing, explain it, we always put it into a texture of uniformities. There must be some reason for it, some law expressed in it. That is the fundamental assumption of science."[151] Freud defines this view in his praise of Leonardo's "research not based on presuppositions," which isolated him and contemporaries such as Bacon and Copernicus from medieval science (*SE* 9:65). This is the birth of modern, neutral science as opposed to the "authority of the Church."

It is the striving of the neutral, the universal, for the overarching explanation that provides the rationale for the scientist-physician's gaze, especially in the world of Viennese academic medicine. Central to Freud's formulation of this idea of science is the work of the British eugenicist Karl Pearson, whose *Grammar of Science* Freud read closely before World War I. Pearson stated (and Freud underlined the words in his copy): "Nobody believes now that science explains anything; we all look upon it as a shorthand description, as an economy of thought."[152] Modern science trains "the mind to an exact and impartial analysis of facts." "Scientific law is a description, not a prescription." But it also demands that all scientists be equal and "civilized": "The universal validity of science depends upon the similarity to the perceptive and reasoning faculties in normal, civilized men." But are Jews, "normal, civilized men"? Science and the "'universality' of natural law, the 'absolute validity' of the scientific method, depends on the resemblance between the perceptive and reflective faculties of one human mind and those of a second." Even if the second is a Jew? The positivistic aspects of science, its claims to universality, lie in "the fact that all knowledge is concise description, all cause is routine" (9, 87, 47, 101, 133). Can even a Jew undertake such description, since the Jew truly possesses a different mental construction, a different manner of seeing the world?

Freud, who initially denies the difference of the Jew's gaze, seeing himself as the neutral analyst of his patients' psychopathologies, transvalues the difference of the gaze into a quality of therapy. For the special gaze of the Jew, with its cold and scanning qualities, becomes precisely not the gaze of the psychoanalyst. This is the gaze ascribed by Freud to his French patron Jean-Martin Charcot, whose view of the special risk of the Jew for mental illness reflected the late nineteenth-century presuppositions about the risk associated with being Jewish (*SE* 3:12). By 1910 Freud acknowledges the existence of countertransference, the affective response of the analyst to his patient, the "result of the patient's influence on his unconscious feelings" that needs to be overcome (*SE* 11:144–45).

But for the Aryan, even the sympathetic Aryan, the Jew, even the Jew as psychotherapist in Vienna, remained the exemplar of the particular, not of the universal. As H.D. said of Freud, he had the "precise Jewish instinct for the particular in the general, for the personal in the impersonal or universal, for the *material* in the abstract."[153] (In the Western vocabulary of difference, from Paul on, the Jew traditionally represents the material while the Aryan/Christian represents the spiritual.) It was this quality that set him apart for her, but it was the antithesis of the neutral gaze that marked the physician-healer. It is no wonder Freud consciously chose to place himself out of view of his patients: "I hold to the plan of getting the patient to lie on a sofa while I sit behind him out of his sight" (*SE* 12:133). Freud explains that such an arrangement has historical roots (as a tradition from hypnosis) but is also pragmatic. The patient is "anxious not to be deprived of a view of the doctor" (*SE* 12:139). Such an approach could be understood as a "scientific" one. And yet the question of being seen, of being observed—even by the patient—had an intense affective dimension for Freud. When he was asked about it by Hanns Sachs, Freud responded "abruptly: I cannot let myself be stared at (*anstarren*) for eight hours a day."[154] He could not tolerate being observed in such detail, much as Galton observed the pupils at the Jews' Free School.

The act of being observed is tied to the act of observing. The scientist, such as Galton, reduced the gaze of the Jew to an object of study. The Jews' gaze is never neutral. It is transformed within the discourse of psychoanalysis into a positive and productive factor, but only as a metaphor. It is a gaze that structures psychoanalysis. The Croatian Jew Victor Tausk, one of the earliest followers of Freud, commented to Lou Andreas-Salomé "on the nearly exclusive involvement of Jews in the progress of psychoanalysis. It was understandable, he said, that we could see the fabric more clearly in ancient and dilapidated palaces through their crumbling walls and could gain insights which remain hidden in fine new houses with smooth façades revealing only their color and their outward shape."[155] Tausk also firmly believed that the Jews had a disposition toward neurosis.[156] For him, it was this "common mental construction" that made them better psychotherapists. The Jew's gaze was that of the extraordinary physician; this simple reversal of the "cold, scanning gaze" of the Jew made into a diagnostic virtue precisely what the eugenicist labeled as pathology.

The meaning of the scientific model of the scientist's gaze reappears within the rhetoric of psychoanalysis. For Freud, Galton's photographs became the central model for visualizing how the unseen processes of the psyche work. He evokes the photographs of Galton as his model for how the dream works. Freud was well aware of the use of such composite photographs by Houston Stewart Chamberlain as one of the salient proofs for the immutability of race.[157]

It is in one specific context that the Galtonian model is first evoked.[158] Freud recounts a dream in which the face of his Uncle Josef was superimposed on that of his friend R. and "was like one of Galton's composite photographs. In order to bring out family likeness, Galton used to photograph several faces on the same plate" (*SE* 4:139). Freud evokes this technique in the most neutral manner possible. But Freud's Jewish uncle was in disgrace because he had been imprisoned for trading in counterfeit rubles in 1866, an act that could well have involved Freud's father and older half brothers (who then emigrated to England). Such a procedure, in this dream of his "uncle with the yellow beard" (February 1897), "adopt[ed] the procedure by means of which Galton produced family portraits: namely by projecting two images on to a single plate, so that certain features common to both are emphasized, while those which fail to fit in with one another cancel one another out and are indistinct in the picture."[159] This dream was evoked by a specific anti-Semitic incident. Freud's friend R., the ophthalmologist Leopold Königstein, had been turned down for an academic appointment in the medical faculty because he was Jewish. (Freud was also in line for a promotion at the same time and was certain it would be rejected for the same reason.)

In the Galtonian condensation of the images, what vanishes is the Jewishness of Freud's uncle and of Freud's friend, exemplified by the black beard. The "yellow" beard is at once the sign of the aging Jew (according to Freud the Jew's hair turns reddish, then yellowish, and then gray), but it is also the sign of the hidden Aryan within the Jew. The black beard is traditionally a sign of the Jew: "The hair of the ancient Hebrews was generally black. . . . Black hair was in any case considered beautiful, black being the general color, while light or blond hair was exceptional. . . . Among Jews the color of the hair has attracted special attention because, while the majority have dark hair, there is found a considerable proportion with blond and red hair. . . . Some believe that it is due to climate and environment . . . , while others attribute it to racial admixture, particularly to the admission of Aryan blood into modern Jewry."[160] For anti-Semites of the period, the "black-haired Jewish youth lurks . . . with satanic joy in his face . . . for the unsuspecting girl whom he defiles with his blood, thus stealing her from her people."[161] And Freud sees himself as a "black haired Jew": "It appears that I came into the world with such a tangle of black hair that my young mother declared that I was a little Moor" (*SE* 4:337). Freud sees himself as both Jewish and black, racially marked like the protagonist of Friedrich Schiller's drama *Fiesco,* which he quotes in the same context.[162] For the turn-of-the-century Viennese Jew it was possible to understand oneself as black but not as inferior. Ignaz Zollschan accepts the blackness of the Jew. Following Thomas Huxley, he divided all races into the "xanthochroe" (light) and the "melanchhroe" (dark). The Jews belong to the latter, but so do the Swiss.[163] It is a sign that cuts across the barrier traditionally separating the Jew from the Aryan.

In the 1940s Otto Fenichel, one of Freud's most orthodox Jewish supporters, characterized the anti-Semite's view of the Jew as stressing "their cultural or physical 'racial' peculiarities. Their hair frequently is black, even if their skin is not; moreover, they are foreign in their customs and habits, in their language, in their divine service. This foreignness they share with the Armenians, the Negroes, and the Gypsies."[164] This denial of the "blackness" of the Jews reflects the power, especially in American exile, of the meaning of the color of the Jews' skin and the central question of their visibility and transmutability. What is quite remarkable is that in the very same essay Fenichel could comment that the "anti-Semite can project onto the Jews, because the actual peculiarities of Jewish life, the strangeness of their mental culture, their bodily (black) and religious (God of the oppressed peoples) peculiarities, and their old customs make them suitable for such a projection" (31). The power of the "blackness" of the Jew can deform the very understanding of the scientist when he looks at the representation of his own body within the world of the anti-Semite.

The ability to be transformed into the hidden Aryan is both negative and positive. It is positive in that it means one would get an academic appointment; it is negative because it is a violation of the racial difference of the Jew. Freud's dream of the blond hair of his uncle is paralleled by a dream recounted by Ludwig Wittgenstein, the Viennese philosopher who was only of partial Jewish descent, in December 1929, in which a Jewish character (according to Wittgenstein himself) "has an angry face, slightly reddish fair hair and a similarly colored moustache (he does not look Jewish)."[165] Wittgenstein's incorporation of the rhetoric of anti-Semitism to articulate the anxiety about his own identity in this dream reveals how deeply the question of "appearing Jewish" was inscribed on the Viennese mentality of the period, and how the encoding of color triggers the sense of what is and what is not Jewish.

Freud evokes an earlier memory, the memory of being taken to the park at the age of eleven and having his fortune told by an old woman who foretells that he will become a great man, a cabinet minister. This evokes a period of Austrian history following the establishment of the new constitution in 1867, when it seemed that Jews would attain civil equality (*SE* 4:191–93). But even in this time of liberal treatment of the Jews, no Jew who had been even suspected of an illegal activity could be appointed to the faculty of the university. Indeed, his other colleague N. had once been the subject of legal proceedings, which had been dismissed. Here Freud's image of his father, whose hair turned gray with anxiety when his brother was convicted, merges with the image of the renegade uncle and the Jewish friend. And Freud's father is for Freud the internalized image of the Eastern Jew, whose response to the torment of the anti-Semite was to step into the gutter. (It is striking, and not at all incidental, that the heavy "Jewish" representation among the early psychoanalysts was in fact an eastern European Jewish presence: Franz Alexander, A. A. Brill, Joseph Breuer, Sándor Ferenczi, Ludwig Jekels, Hans Kelsen, Herman Nunberg, Theodor Reik, Hanns Sachs, Isidor Sadger, Sabina Spielrein, and Viktor Tausk all were either born in the East or were the children of eastern European Jews who had moved to Vienna.) Freud recounts his memory of a discussion with his father when he was ten or twelve, as they were walking the streets of Vienna, in which his father told about having his new fur cap knocked into the street by a Christian and how he stooped and picked it up out of the gutter. "This struck me as unheroic conduct on the part of the big, strong man who was holding the little boy by the hand" (*SE* 4:197). Being forced off the pavement with the accompanying cry of "hep! hep!" was part of the experience of many Jews of Freud's father's generation in both eastern and western Europe. It is clear that Freud's father did not automatically move into the gutter. His act of defiance and its subsequent punishment is read by his son as an act of cowardice. Jacob Freud's mentality, according to Freud, was a sign, like the appearance of the Jew, of the Jew's inferiority.

All Jews appear the same through the image of the "yellow" beard, which in turn evokes the liberal past, when Jews were seen like Aryans, at least in Freud's childish fantasy. "Seeing" the Jew is marked by the anthropology of race, which also had a sociological dimension. For it is the question of the Jew as "white-collar criminal" that also haunts the forensic literature of the time, as I shall discuss in chapter 4. The uncle shares Freud's racial identity and could never be a civil servant. This racial quality, the Jew as criminal, must be masked in order to free Freud the scientist to see as clearly as Francis Galton. Freud's use of Galton's method of seeing the commonality of features also reflects on the assumption that there are communal features (such as race) that define the process of seeing. It is precisely this process of seeing that is denied to the eye of the Jewish scientist. And the evocation of Galton and his photographs represents this denial of a Jewish manner of seeing, a Jewish epistemology. Galton is the gaze of "science" even in his evocation of the meaning of the Jew's gaze.

Such a denial of the act of the Jew seeing the Jew can be observed in a footnote to *The Interpretation of Dreams* (added in 1919) (*SE* 4:181–82). There Freud excerpted a recent essay by Otto Pötzl, who worked in Julius Wagner-Jauregg's psychiatric-neurological clinic at the University of Vienna. Freud, who did not think much of Pötzl's appropriation of psychoanalysis, had used his interest in psychoanalysis to provide a link with the academic psychiatrists in Vienna.[166] He had even intended to review the essay for one of the psychoanalytic journals.[167] Returning to Vienna in 1922 from Prague, Pötzl succeeded Wagner-Jauregg in the chair of psychiatry at the university. Pötzl remained on the fringes of the psychoanalytic community in Vienna because of his empirical research, but he felt himself indebted to Freud in "the teaching I do . . . ; in it I and my students are your enthusiastic followers."[168] Freud registered a "session" with Pötzl on May 9, 1931, in his daily chronicle, where he recorded only the most salient events of the day.[169] Pötzl's politics, at least according to the non-Jewish Viennese psychoanalyst Richard Sterba, became pro-Nazi after the Anschluss, but he continued to be loyal to Freud, to whom he offered assistance.[170]

In the paper cited by Freud in the note to *The Interpretation of Dreams,* Pötzl used a combination of the empirical approach to the psychology of the senses and psychoanalytic theory to illustrate how daytime residue was transformed into the stuff of dreams. Pötzl exposed his subjects briefly to a photograph and then asked them to draw an image. He was able to show (from the patients' self-reports) how the "unseen" aspects of the original photograph appeared within their dreams. As Freud noted: "The material that was taken over by the dream-work was modified by it for the purposes of dream-construction in its familiar 'arbitrary' (or, more properly, 'autocratic') manner." When one closely examines what Freud would have seen when he read Pötzl's paper, one is struck by what was not "seen."

The second subject of Pötzl's experiment was shown an image of the Wailing Wall, the sole remnant of the destruction of the second temple and the most holy place of the Jews (figs. 6–14).[171] The image comprised the wall and several male Jews praying. What the subject registered in the high-speed exposure of 1/100 of a second was a series of black and white stripes. In the subsequent dream the subject reported "seeing" a high sea with a tiny black ship. Eventually the subject reported that there were also figures on the deck of the ship with their arms held in front of them.

Pötzl interrogated his subject, who remembered seeing in the dream "a picture. I still know that many people stood at a wall; but I can't remember how they were dressed." The subject is sure, however, that the experimenter had shown him or her pictures of the boat before the

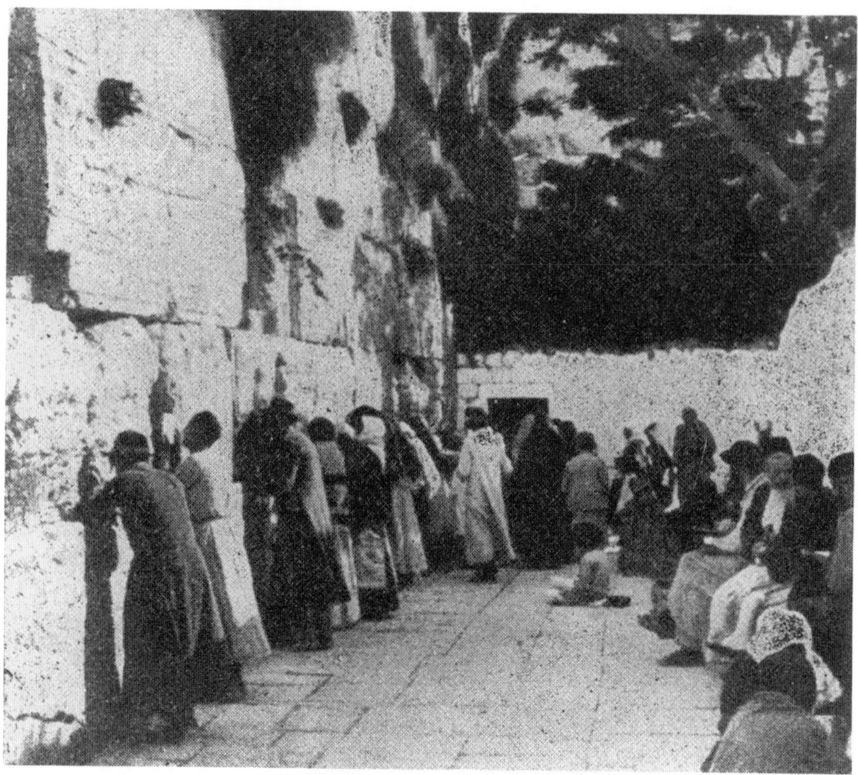

Figure 6. Otto Pötzl's original photograph of the Wailing Wall. Its subject matter was unstated in the experiment. The subject was exposed to this photograph for 1/100 of a second. This and the following images are from Otto Pötzl, "Experimental erregte Traumbild in ihren Beziehung zum indirekten Sehen," *Zeitschrift für die Gesamte Neurologie und Psychiatrie* 37(1917):278–339, here 300. (National Library of Medicine, Bethesda, Md.)

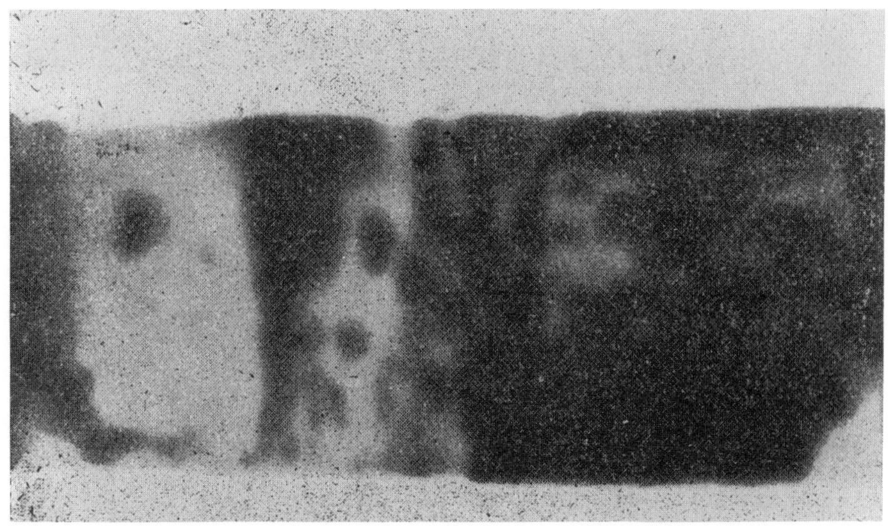

Figure 7. This image is a "reconstruction" of what the subject informed Pötzl he or she had seen. In reality it is a blurred reproduction of the upper half of Figure 6.

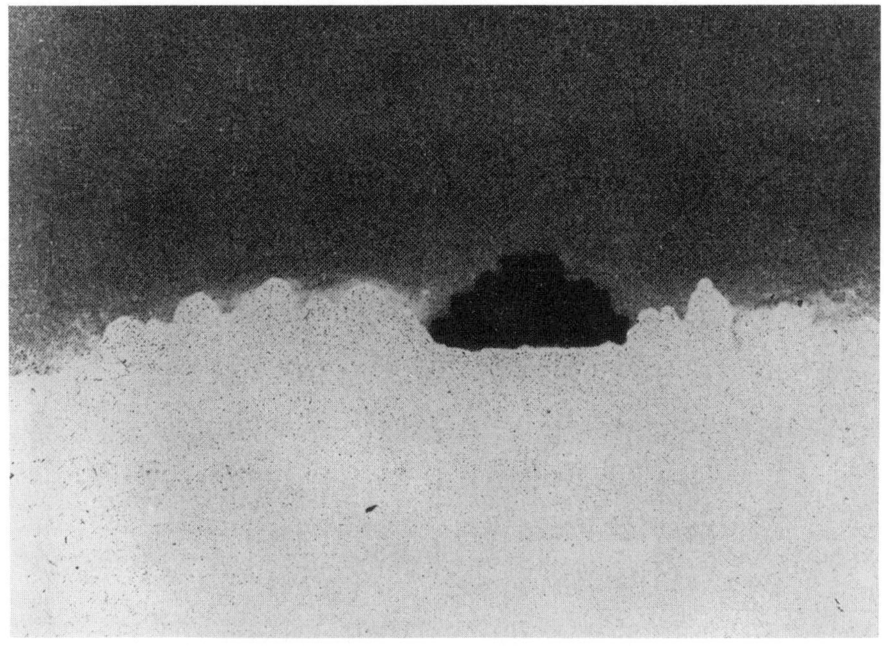

Figure 8. The first of the "dream images." The subject remembered that in the dream "there were high seas, water, white waves; the ship was very black."

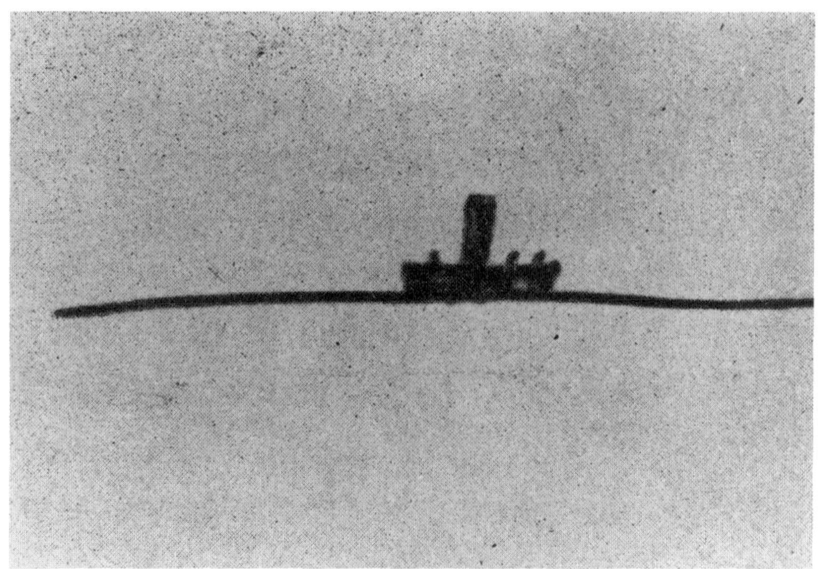

Figure 9. The subject's original drawing of the dream ship.

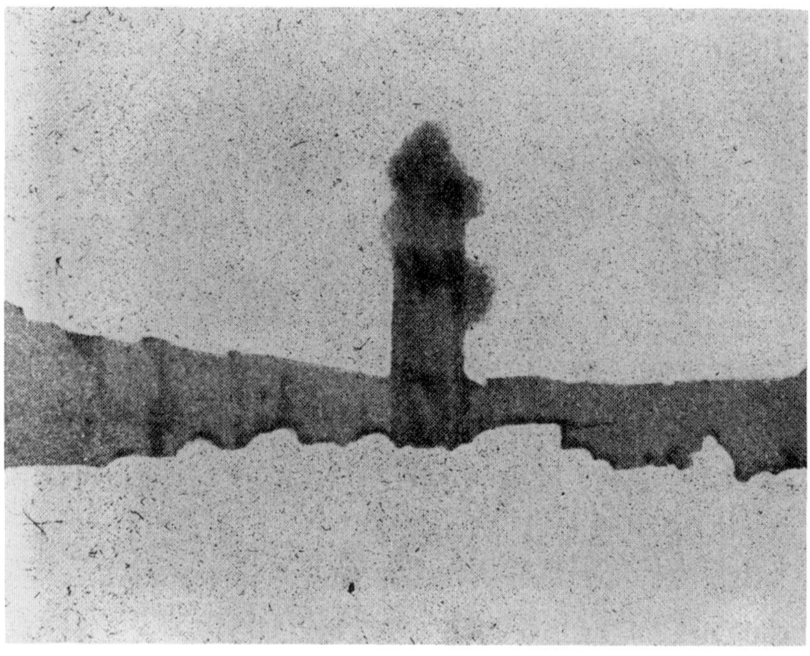

Figure 10. Second stage of the dream: "The ship is bigger and seen from the side; all white, no one aboard."

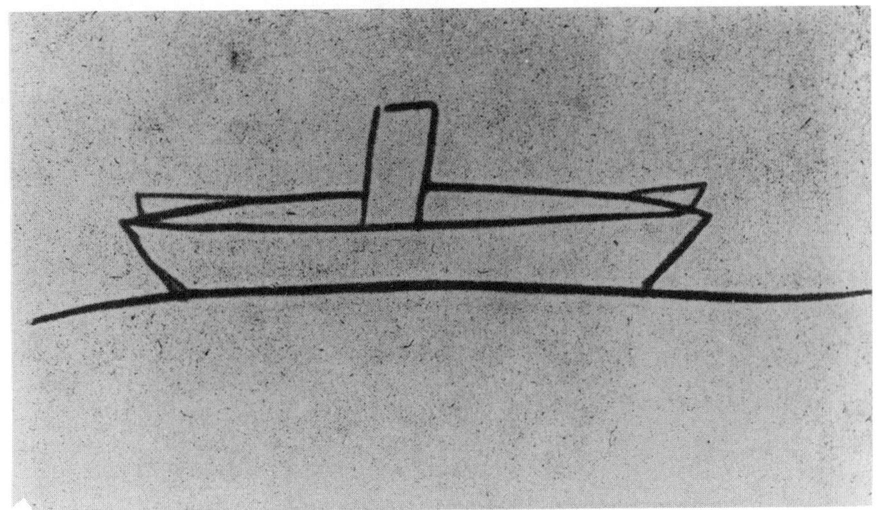

Figure 11. The subject's drawing of this phase.

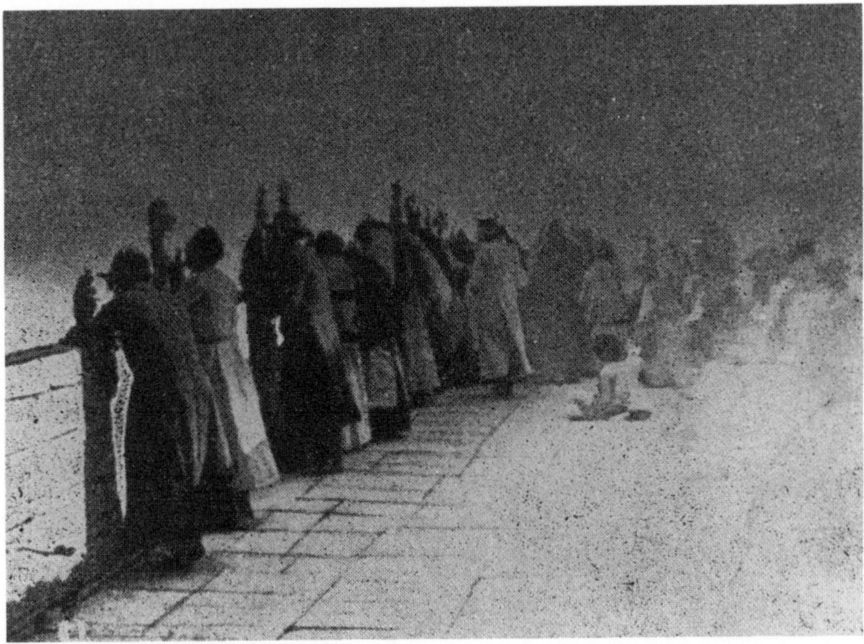

Figure 12. The narrative existing between dream and exposition: On board the ship, the subject dreamed of "many people, tiny like dots; moving about in a lively manner; they moved their arms as if they were waving cloths." This is the bottom of the original photograph in Figure 6, masked and reproduced as the dream image.

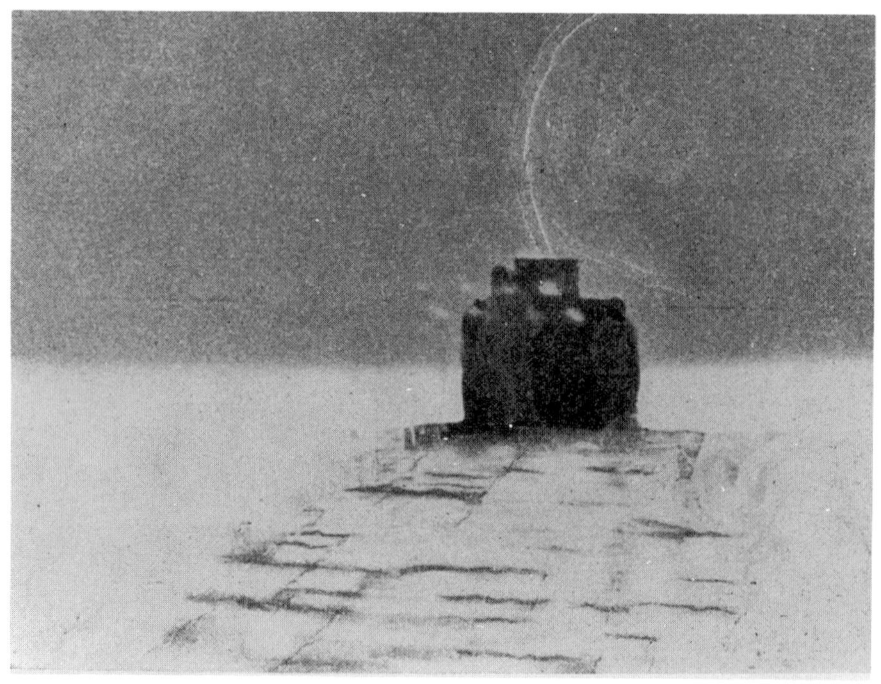

Figure 13. The isolation of elements perceived in the dream: the ship as seen in the distance.

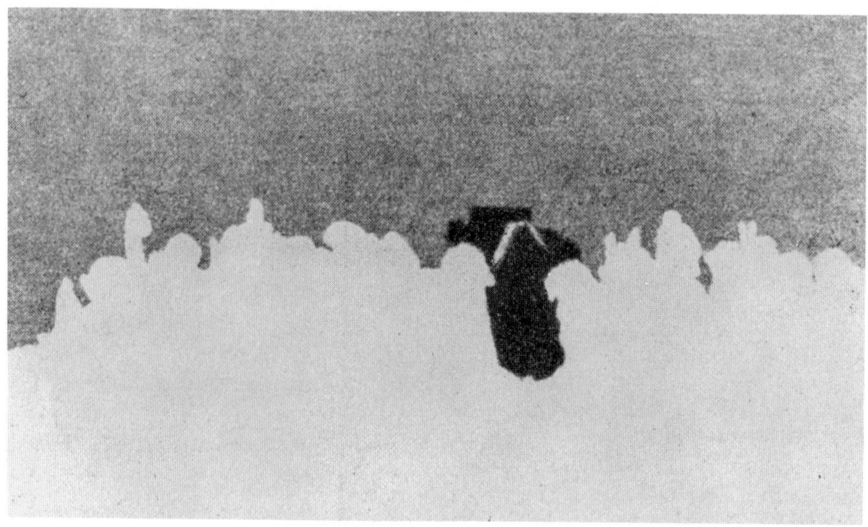

Figure 14. The ship as a space in the crowd scene in the original.

experiment. Pötzl cites this act of remembering as a form of the "fausse reconnaissance," false memories or déjà vu, that Freud also found in the course of psychoanalytic treatment (*SE* 13:201–77). The central anecdotes of Freud's paper, referred to by Pötzl, concerned castration anxiety. (Freud evokes the case of the "Wolf Man" here for the first time.) Freud links castration to the meaning of circumcision in Western culture.[172] The photograph of male Jews evoked for Pötzl Freud's account of the false memories associated with the anxiety of castration. What strikes one in reading Pötzl's account of Freud's summary of it is that the manifest content of the photograph and the dream—the eastern European Jews moving through Vienna on their way west across the ocean on ships—completely vanishes. And this even though Pötzl noted the power that exposure to this photograph had in shaping the dreams of his subject. The associations are reduced to the retention of retinal images by the interpreter, or as the false memories of such cognitive acts, rather than reflections of the social realities beyond the clinic door. We can never know whether the subject Pötzl used was a Jew or not, but Freud's citing this bit of empirical science as a means of providing the validity of his dream theory shows how selectively he saw. He "saw" these images not as a Jew but as a scientist and was quite content with Pötzl's empirical experiments and his claims for them. For the importance of Pötzl's experiment was its cool, calm, dispassionate account of the act of seeing and of remembering. It was the evocation of the science of the experimental psychology of Wilhelm Wundt, rather than his ethnopsychology. The use of the Wailing Wall and all its associations with the historical memories of the Jews is obliterated in Pötzl's experiment and in Freud's reading. Pötzl, however, provided a clue that it was present, if only in nuce. He argued that the symmetry between the cognitive processing of sensory experiences and their reappearance within the dream is shaped by the experience of the organism. He cites Lafcadio Hearn, the extraordinarily popular Anglo-Greek writer of the fin de siècle, saying that the occurrence of anxiety or ghosts in dreams is the "appearance of phylogenetic experiences." Here the memory of the Jews reappears as a force that provided one of the structures shaping the dream. The "Jewish" gaze reappears here. Jews do see differently from everyone else, and they register images such as pictures of Jews in a different, anxiety-provoking way. Freud suppresses the act of the Jew seeing the Jew. He claims a neutral, scientific appraisal of the act of seeing that would counter his own particularistic manner of remembering. Freud ends his paper on déjà vu with the claim of the psychoanalyst's success: "After he has succeeded in forcing the repressed event (whether it was a real or of a physical nature) upon the patient's acceptance in the teeth of all resistances, and has succeeded, as it were in rehabilitating it—the patient may say: 'Now I feel as though I had known it all the time.' With this the work of the analysis has been completed" (*SE* 13:207). In Pötzl's experiment there is never the moment of acknowledgment; for Freud to acknowledge this as though he had known it all the time would be to evoke his own Jewish phylogenetic memory.

Jews in the Medicine of Nineteenth-Century Vienna

For the Jewish physician in late nineteenth-century Germany and Austria, the ability to enter the sphere of "science" meant acknowledging the truth of the scientific project and its rhetoric. But entering the field of medicine did not meaning shedding one's identity as a Jew. As early as 1842 the conservative ophthalmologist Anton Edler von Rosas, in a long piece published in one of the major medical journals in Austria, had lamented the decay of the medical establishment in Vienna because of the "annually greater increase of Israelites into the study of medicine."[173] (The figures he gave were that in 1842 there were seventy-one "Christians" and nineteen "Jews" studying medicine in Vienna—that is, a full quarter of the students were Jews.) For Rosas these Jews were ill fit to practice medicine because they were "so identified with the spirit of capitalism" and because they had a "much greater tendency to be quacks" (18–19). That Jewish physicians were quacks, that they practiced within a medical tradition that ran counter to the prevailing one in the German-speaking lands, and that they used secret Jewish treatments as a means of hurting rather than helping their Christian patients was a commonplace of the medical literature from at least the sixteenth century (fig. 15).[174]

Rosas's cure is to exclude Jews "as long as they continue exclusively to trade and as long as they remain subservient to the laws of Moses."[175] Isaac Noah Mannheimer, the rabbi of the Seitenstettengasse synagogue

---

Figure 15. The contrast between the "Christian" body, that of Christ as healer, and the body of the Jewish quack, taken from a 1698 tractate against Jewish physicians. All of the Jew's physical attributes point toward his dishonesty. From Christian Trewmundt, *Gewissenloser Juden-Doctor In Welchem Erstlich Das wahre Conterfeit eines Christlichen Medici, und dessen nothwendige Wissenschafften / wie auch gewissenhaffte Praxis, zweytens Die hingegen Abscheuliche Gestalt dess Juden-Doctors Wie auch dessen Unfehigkeit zur Lehr und Doctors-Würde / und die schad-volle Bedienung der Krancken Aus geist- und weltlichen Rechten / mit unumstösslichen Gründen vorgestellt wird* (Freiburg, 1698). (National Library of Medicine, Bethesda, Md.)

IHS

Auxilium meum â Domino. *Psalm. 120.*

Ni Deus adfuerit, Viresq; infuderit herbis

Nil tibi Dictamnus, nil panacæa iuvat.

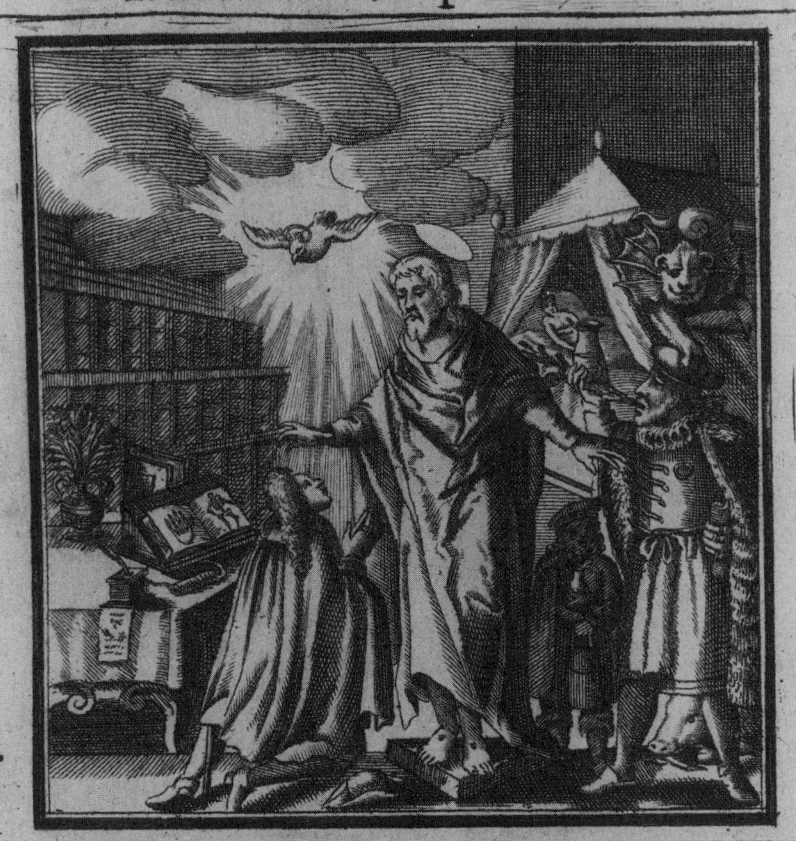

IESU. IEHOVA IUVA

Erranti, pereunti, ægro, via, vita, Salusq;

Christe, tuum rege, duc, et benedic Medicum.

Auxilioq; tuo pereat Medicaster Apella;

unica cui, Christi, est cura, necare genus.

and the de facto "chief rabbi" of Vienna (although this title did not officially exist), offered a long rebuttal of Rosas's comments in another medical journal.[176] He contradicts all of Rosas's claims but also makes it clear to his medical public that the purpose of training Jewish physicians was to serve the Jewish population of the empire.[177] These Jewish physicians will not be competing with his Christian readers for patients. Rosas's own rejoinder to Mannheimer also agrees with his assumptions.[178] Jewish physicians serviced Jews and were Jews and thus were different in all respects from other physicians.

The Jewish physician had a special status in Vienna during the nineteenth century. As fine an observer of European Jewry as Leopold von Sacher-Masoch makes this the centerpiece of his tale of Austrian Jewry included in his "ethnographic" account of European Jewry.[179] In his story of "two physicians" the reader observes the confrontation between the "scientifically trained" Jewish physician and his primitive, miracle-working counterpart. Only science can win, and religion must bow gracefully to its preeminence. Sacher-Masoch's tale of science and the Jews reflects the siren song of the Haskalah (the Jewish Enlightenment), which perhaps even more than the general Enlightenment saw science as the path of escape from the darkness of the ghetto into the bright light of modern culture. It was a modern culture defined very much by d'Alembert's assessment of science and technology as the tools for the improvement of the common man. But science, especially applied science such as medicine, implied the ability to enter into the mainstream of the "free" professions.[180] It implied a type of social mobility increasingly available to Jews, especially in Austria, over the course of the nineteenth century.[181] But even with this social mobility, Jewish doctors remained labeled as Jews because they were understood as part of an immutable or at least identifiable racial category.

And Jewish medical scientists were understood as being different. On the one hand, they were condemned as mechanical and impersonal. This was in light of the general sense that medicine was becoming more "scientific." The development of nineteenth-century medicine from its focus on bacteriology in the 1880s to its focus on biochemistry at the turn of the century meant a real shift of interest from the "organic" to the "inert" on the part of the medical scientist. This argument is to be found elsewhere in the medical debates of the period. Emil Du Bois-Reymond, for example, excoriates the direction of modern medicines as "too utilitarian, too materialistic, and . . . in the process of being destroyed by the very industries to which it gives rise." This he labels as "Americanization" of medicine. John S. Billings, founder of the Johns Hopkins University Hospital, defends this "dreadful permeation of European civilization by realism" as merely the natural progress of science.[182] For the Viennese Jew Otto Weininger, the author of the essential fin-de-siècle work of self-hatred, this "Americanization" was the result of the "Jewification" of modern medicine. Jews are natural chemists, which explains why medicine has become biochemistry: "The present turn of medical science is largely due to the influence of the Jews, who in such numbers have embraced the medical profession. From the earliest times, until the dominance of the Jews, medicine was closely allied with religion. But now they make it a matter of drugs, a mere administration of chemicals. . . . The chemical interpretation of organisms sets these on a level with their own dead ashes."[183] The Jews focus on the dead, the inert. This view is seconded by Hermann Schneider, in a volume Freud knew and used, who remarks that the Jew today "as a physician adopts those natural laws and material experiences that he could have created; once he acquires them, he knows how to apply them to expand them logically and empirically, but only in details."[184] Jewish doctors are in no way original; they merely follow in the path of true medical genius that lies beyond their ability.

On the other hand, Jewish physicians were condemned because they "only know how to 'schmus' [gossip] [with their patients]. With their 'Oriental shrewdness,' they quickly determine what the patient wants to know and hear." Julius Moses, the Jewish physician and Social Democratic politician, translated this attack into a productive mode of therapy. "We would only wish," he wrote in 1932, "that all good physicians could know how to 'schmus,' that they could develop a true rapport with their patients and thus supplement the purely mechanical mode of treatment through psychotherapy."[185] Jewish physicians are either too materialistic or too unscientific, too distant or too familiar. In both cases they violate the German and Austrian cultural icon of the ideal physician. This image continues, in the rhetoric of the late ninteenth and early twentieth centuries, a European tradition of labeling the Jewish physician as dangerous and corrupting.

For late nineteenth-century Jewish scientists, especially those in the biological sciences, the path of social and cultural acceptance was complex. It entailed, more than in any other arena of endeavor, the acceptance of the contradiction between being "subject" and being "object." One of the basic premises of nineteenth-century biological science was the primacy of racial difference. For the physician-scientist the case became even more complex. It was not merely that there was a hierarchy of race, with each race higher (or lower) on a "great chain of being"; the very pattern of illness varied from group to group and marked the risk each group faced in confronting life, especially "modern" civilized life.[186] The Jewish physician was the "observer" of this form of disease, but because he (and the Jewish physician was almost always male until the very late nineteenth century), also entered into the competition of civilized society (i.e., the public sphere of medicine), he was precisely the potential "victim" of exactly these illnesses. The demands of "scientific objectivity" could therefore not be met by Jewish physicians, and they were forced to undertake complex psychological strategies to provide themselves with an "objective" observing voice. Certainly one of the most telling is the construction of a closely defined "subject" with a clearly delineated causality for the subject's exposure to risk. The complexity of Sigmund Freud's construction of his own subject and the shift in his sense of what causes psychic illness is in no small part the result of his need to avoid the arguments of race.[187]

No arena in the science of race is more contested for the Jewish scientists of this period than the mutability or immutability of the very signs (and/or symptoms) that define the Jew. The question is not whether such signs exist, but whether they are alterable or are permanent qualities of the Jewish mind and body. This problem focuses the definition of the subject on the mutability of "Jewishness." The reinterpretation and universalization of the meaning of these signs within the rhetoric of psychoanalysis can be examined within the debates about the meaning of conversion and its relation to the nature of the Jew.

2
CONVERSION, CIRCUMCISION, AND DISCOURSE

Conversion as a Biological Act

How can one become whole and healthy? How can one shed the trauma of one's Jewishness? The answer is clearly that one cannot—the Jewishness of the body and the psyche is indelible. But the hatred of the Jewish body is also a disease. What if one could become totally different and thus stop being the cause of the Other's illness? An older model, the model of religious conversion, which had haunted the Jews for almost two millennia, had been consistently present in European society since the early church. Conversion was a central theme of the Jews of the nineteenth century. In the period following the Jewish Enlightenment of the late eighteenth century, the Haskalah conversion seemed to be a civil (rather than religious) alternative. Heine could speak of conversion as the "entrance ticket into European culture."[1] However, by the end of the nineteenth century conversion was no longer seen as a viable alternative. This earlier model permitted converts to acquire social and institutional status. Indeed, Sigmund Freud's uncle by marriage, Michael Bernays, the famous professor of German at the University of Munich, converted in order to be granted a chair.[2] At the close of the century such status was not sufficient to mask the essence of the Jew for scientific anti-Semites. Older views, such as those of Theodor Mommsen[3] and Heinrich Treitschke,[4] which demanded that the Jew become a Christian in order to become a full-fledged German, ring strange in fin-de-siècle scientific ears accustomed to hearing the Jew contrasted with the "Aryan" rather than the "Christian." Indeed, by the end of the century the call for converts, such as the anonymous author of a pamphlet published in 1880, that "there is only one solution for the Jewish question, the turning of the Jews to their true king, Jesus Christ," sounds hopelessly antiquated.[5] Rather, it is clear that conversion was understood as an illusion, a claim for the cure of something that could not be cured.

As A. A. Brill, the pioneer English translator of Freud, noted, conversion occurred as a result of a "special emotional state": "Some like Heinrich Heine—a most sensitive poet—accepted baptism as a salvation for his Jewish disabilities."[6] It is the transformation of conversion from a religious to a medical category that has significance for Jewish scientists at the fin de siècle.

What must be understood is that the promise of conversion also presented a complex model that combined images of cultural and biological integration. The assumption was that eliminating all the social barriers between Jews and Christians would eliminate the mutually exclusive sexual selectivity of both groups. Thus in a letter of November 12, 1861, the Polish Jewish sociologist Ludwig Gumplowicz wrote about civil emancipation to his friend the Galician Jewish nationalist Philipp Mansch:

> *Civil marriage!* My reply: that is supposed to be part of our striving—that has to come. You have read the motion of the Commission for Religion—decided by Smolka. You are finding that "religion is no obstacle to matrimony!" . . . Give me your word that we shall marry the most beautiful Christian girls—alias *shikses*—in case that motion becomes law! I am joking and yet the matter is no joke. The day is not far where even this last wall of separation is bound to fall—and we are compelled to take leave from this shadow of our nationality which is long decayed but which for centuries keeps creeping after us like a vampire, sucks our blood and destroys our vitality.[7]

Diseased Jews can be cured only by removing *themselves* from the source of disease, their Jewishness, and this can be finally undertaken only with complete biological integration. But Gumplowicz's first point for the regeneration of the Jews, the means by which the final goal—intermarriage—can be accomplished, is the "acceptance of the language of the people among whom one lives." The abandonment of the language of the Jews, a language that defined the limitation of the Jew's psyche, was closely associated with the abandonment of the sexual selectivity of Jewish marital practices. For the Jewish liberals of the mid-nineteenth century, all roads led to acculturation, and the ultimate form of acculturation was sexual symbiosis.

Converts, the society in which they lived had seemed to say—stop being Jews—and you will become full-fledged members of the majority society (fig. 16). Traditionally, Jews were no more accepted as Christians then than seen as "Aryans" at the close of the nineteenth century. Indeed, one of the pamphlets written against the very idea of Jewish political emancipation in Vienna in 1782 was entitled: "The Baptized Jew: Nei-

SCHLEMIEL

Darwinistisches.

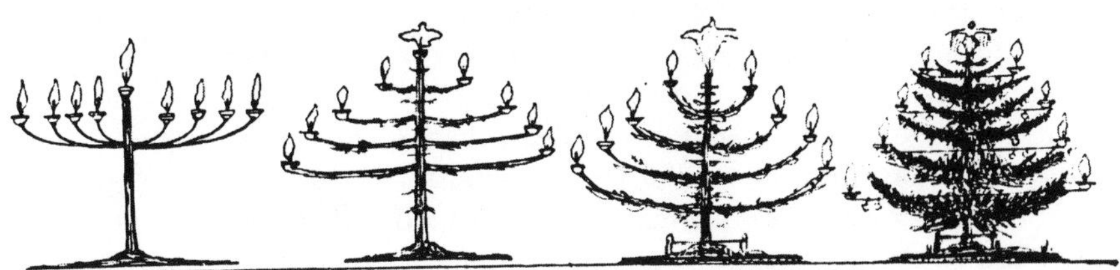

Wie sich der Chanukaleuchter des Ziegenfellhändlers **Cohn** in Pinne zum Christbaum des Kommerzienrats **Conrad** in der Tiergartenstraße (Berlin W.) entwickelte.

Figure 16. A "Darwinian" model for conversion, or "How the Hanukkah menorah of the leather dealer *Cohn* in Pinne evolves into the Christmas tree of commercial councilor *Conrad*," from *Der Schlemiel* 2 (1904). The desired potential for the biological change is translated into a satire on this theme once the impossibility of such transformation is acknowledged. (National Library of Medicine, Bethesda, Md.)

ther Jew nor Christian."[8] But the promise still existed. What then does conversion mean by the end of the century in the culture in which Freud finds himself? It has been claimed that "the stern voice of Freud's conscience . . . prevented him from taking the assimilationist path" and that he, "like every Jew who has been set apart, yearned unconsciously to become part of . . . [the Christian] world."[9] Even Ernest Jones, who dismissed such speculation, noted that Freud "for five minutes toyed with [the] idea" of converting to Protestantism as such a conversion would have enabled him to avoid a religious marriage ceremony.[10] Protestantism was the preferable religion for Jewish converts in Vienna, since one was legally considered a Christian while not being a Catholic. Such a conversion was understood as not demanding the same sense of religious conviction as becoming a Catholic in apostolic Vienna. As Moritz Saphir, the mid-nineteenth-century Hungarian Jewish newspaperman (himself a double convert), observed: "When I was a Jew, God could see me, but I could not see Him, then I became a Catholic and I could see Him, but He could not see me. Now I am a Protestant and I don't see Him or He me."[11] But this was a midcentury view. By the turn of the century Sigmund Freud avoided converting, even in this most superficial manner, for by the fin de siècle even this mode of conversion becomes a pathological sign.

The view that a Jew could "convert," that is, could cease being a Jew, assumed that by the close of the nineteenth century Jews had a true option to "assimilate." Conversion to Christianity of whatever form would have meant integrating biologically into the greater society. And this was, as we have seen, understood as an impossibility. Jews could not convert out of their race. Jacob Wassermann's quintessential anti-Semite speculates, "Whether, after conversion, they cease to be Jews in the deeper sense we do not know, and have no way of finding out. I believe that the ancient influences continue to operate. Jewishness is like a concentrated dye: a minute quantity suffices to give a specific character—or, at least, some traces of it—to an incomparably greater mass."[12] Or to put it in the form of a "Jewish joke," as Theodor Reik did, "Jewish . . . wit denies the possibility of a change of this kind and asserts: Once a Jew, always a Jew. The story is told in New York of the banker Otto Kahn and of the humorist Marshall P. Wilder who was a hunchback. Strolling along Fifth Avenue, Kahn pointed to a church and said: 'Marshall, that's the church I belong to. Did you know that I was once a Jew?' Wilder answered: 'Yes, Otto, and once I was a hunchback.' The conviction that there is an unalterability about being Jewish is expressed better in this dry sentence than in many treatises."[13] Reik's view is based on the acceptance of the idea of the racial identity of the Jew at the close of the nineteenth century. It echoes the views of the fin-de-siècle Viennese Jewish poet Fritz Löhner, who described an entertainer who performed routines in a Jewish accent: "The man understood his art well / He was a baptized Jew, / And when he spoke as he usually spoke, / he mimicked the Jews." ("Und wenn er sprach, wie er eben sprach, / So machte der den Juden nach!")[14]

As long as "Jew" was primarily a religious or national label, it could be changed; once it became primarily a racial label, the question of conversion—at least in one generation—became moot. And yet the Jews of Europe were converting. Indeed, the general consensus of statisticians during the late nineteenth century was that the Jews would totally disappear within a few generations. Indeed, there had been a long history of "voluntary" as well as forced conversion in Austria from the Middle Ages into the nineteenth century.[15] For example, until 1867 it was impossible for a Jewish child to be left at the orphanage founded by the liberal Austrian monarch Joseph II without undergoing baptism. Until 1861 mothers who left a child there were not told the child's new name so that they "would not interfere in the child's Christian education."[16] By the beginning of the twentieth century, while there was an ongoing, and ever increasing, sense that Viennese Jews were converting in even greater numbers, the realities were quite different. In 1904, with a total Jewish population of about 130,000, only 617 Jews either converted or left the religious community. But this was an extraordinary increase over time: in 1868 only 2 converted; in 1870, 24; in 1880, 113; in 1890, 318; in

1900, 607.[17] Indeed, the highest rate of conversion among German-speaking Jews seemed to be in Freud's Vienna.[18] At exactly the moment when it was felt that Jewish integration into the Aryan world was impossible, the reality was that there was a sense that this biological integration was occurring and that the hope of the mid-nineteenth-century assimilationists, such as Ludwig Gumplowicz, would be realized.[19]

The greater the potential reality became, the more intensely the theoretical possibility was denied. Change could take place, other characteristics could be acquired to alter the mind or body that had become Jewish or was so fixed within the race—but only over time. Werner Sombart, the non-Jewish economist whose study of the Jews and capitalism had set the tone for much of the anti-Semitic social science of the opening decades of this century, stated the matter quite clearly in 1912:

> If you ask me about the economic impact of assimilation, we must make it clear what the immediate impact of conversion to Christianity and mixed marriages would be. It is clear that the Jewish religion would be destroyed, evidently also the Jewish essence, that means the specificity of the Jewish *Volk*-character. . . . Not because (as those who believe in the geographic situation determining race) a human being can become another when he desires. No one "can leave the race" as one can leave a religious community. It will come about because the two most powerful qualities which define the essence of the group will vanish: religion and inbreeding.[20]

For Sombart it is the Jews' endogamous marriage or, in terms of nineteenth-century biology, the Jews' inbreeding that determines their nature.[21] Sombart's argument, most clearly outlined in *The Jews and Modern Capitalism* (1911), assumes "that Jewish characteristics are rooted in the blood of the race, and are not in any wise due to educative processes."[22] Sombart draws extensively from the anthropological and biological literature of his day. The Jewish mind is a fixed cognitive structure. Thus all attempts at conversion are fruitless: "Again and again men appear on the scene as Christians, who in reality are Jews. They or their fathers were baptized, that is all" (7). This view becomes a commonplace in the ethnological literature of the period. Relying on Sombart, Hans F. K. Günther commented that "one hears said about a Jew who has left the Hebrew faith for another one or who is now 'without religion,' that he is no longer a Jew. . . . Judaism, at first both race and religion, can now encompass (like other people) many religions. There are today Catholic and Protestant or even 'free-thinking' Jews just as there are Catholic, Protestant, and non-religious Englishmen, Frenchmen, Germans, Russians, etc."[23] Conversion out of the race is impossible, since being a Jew is immutable.

Even the philo-Semitic writers of the period, such as Anatole Leroy-Beaulieu, saw the Jews as a biological unit, albeit a unit that has been created by pressures from outside itself: "Imagine animals, horses or dogs, shut up for four or five hundred years in an enclosed park, strictly isolated from all their fellow animals, and condemned to a uniform diet. It is in some such fashion that the Jews have been treated. A human species was created, in the same way as breeders create an animal species."[24] It is the special qualities of this new species of human beings that are of interest to the social and biological scientist of the fin de siècle. And one of the central categories is the "psychology of the Jew" or "how, from a moral point of view, his extreme suppleness [of mind] becomes a defect" (175). Liberal Jewish thinkers, such as Theodor Gomperz, counter this argument in subtle ways. Gomperz, in a text Freud owned and knew well, evokes the rhetoric of a positive racial mixing from contemporary biology in his image of Thales: "This extraordinary man was a product of racial crossing."[25] (Freud underscored this line and none other in this section of the text.) For liberals such as Gomperz, the end result of racial crossing could be the overall improvement of the human species. This counterview was possible, but usually only if it were projected, as by Gomperz, into distant times and cultures.

But one of the important qualities of the Jewish type is its extraordinary mutability. Jews can literarily mimic the physical nature of the people they live with: "He is able to give himself the personal appearance he most desires. As in days of old through simulating death he was able to defend himself, so now by color adaptation of other forms of mimicry. The best illustrations may be drawn from the United States, where the Jew of the second or third generation is with difficulty distinguished from the non-Jew. You can tell the German after no matter how many generations; so with the Irish, the Swede, the Slav. But the Jew, in so far as his racial physical features allow it, has been successful in imitating the Yankee type, especially in regard to outward marks such as clothing, bearing and the peculiar method of hairdressing."[26] Here the very mutability of the Jew is a sign of the Jews' difference. The Jews' culture remains unchanged even as their physiology seems to alter.

For the famous Jewish literary historian Ludwig Geiger in Berlin the answer is acculturation: "If one desires assimilation—and that can only mean becoming German in morals, language, actions, feelings—one needs neither mixed marriages nor baptism. No serious person would suggest an assimilation that demanded that all Jews had straight noses and blond hair." It is still the biology of the Jew that remains immutable even though his culture may shift. Geiger emphasizes the acculturation of the Jew—the loss of any Jewish qualities of language that reflects the internal moral and emotional definition of the German. It is the curse of difference in the form of the Jew's *Mauscheln* that Geiger wishes to escape. This is mutable even if the biological exterior of the Jew is fixed. But biology defines personhood, as the liberal, non-Jewish German dramatist Frank Wedekind noted: "The difference between Jew and non-Jew rests on the racial uniqueness of the Jew. The meaning of this difference appears to me to be one, which like the difference between male and female, demands further, mutually useful cross-fertilization. Jew and non-Jew are the two souls in the breast of humankind, eternally antithetical and eternally necessary. . . . The Jew has the ability to maintain his Jewish essence against lower cultural contexts as well as to assimilate into higher cultural contexts."[27] Jews can escape the curse of difference by becoming like those above them on the *scala naturae.* And they accomplish this by sounding like those who are better, not by looking like them. Assimilation becomes the mirroring of the better qualities of the Germans, their language and culture.

But baptism did not make the Jews vanish, even in the eyes of their new coreligionists. They became no less visible as Jews. As the German Jewish Berlin language philosopher and journalist Fritz Mauthner noted in 1912: "What speaks against any assimilation through baptism is the mockery of the Christians and the resistance of those Jews who retain their religion. Not without reason. It is inherently impossible for an adult and educated Jew to become a Christian out of conviction."[28] This impossibility was because of the "common mental construction" that makes them into the ultimate rationalists and thus enables them to reject the irrationality of such religious practices as conversion. As Ludwig Braun stated in 1926 at the B'nai B'rith celebration of Freud's seventieth birthday: "We Jews, dear Brothers, stand more open to the world, that is the metaphysical world, than do the Christians, especially the Catholics. This is a result of our education, especially our religious education, and the atmosphere in which we are raised. We are not constrained by dogma. . . . In his inner being the Jew, the true Jew, feels only one eternal guide, one lawgiver, one law. That is morality."[29] This image of the Jews as following only "natural law," rather than the complicated rules and rituals of traditional Judaism, imagines them as the ultimate rationalists, at one with God and nature.

There is a debate about whether Freud toyed with the idea of converting to Christianity at points in his early life.[30] It seems clear that, as an adult, he understood the temptation to convert as a form of seduction, quite analogous to the seduction he initially saw at the heart of the neurotic's problem. In October 1897 Freud's self-analysis led to his explication of the Oedipus theory, the fearful domination of the fantasy life of the male child by the father. The basis for this theory lies in the "universal even in early childhood . . . of being in love with my mother and jealous of my father."[31] Freud labeled these structures of attraction and repulsion the "Oedipus" complex. He wrote to Wilhelm Fliess on October 15, 1897: "I have found love of the mother and jealousy of the father in my case too, and now believe it to be a general phenomenon of early childhood. . . . If that is the case, the gripping power of Oedipus Rex . . . becomes intelligible, the Greek myth seizes on a compulsion which everyone recognizes because he has felt traces of it himself. Every member of the audience was once a budding Oedipus in fantasy, and this dream-fulfillment played out in reality causes everyone to recoil in horror with the full measure of repression which separates his infantile from his present state."[32] The image of the audience at the play, the play being the Greek tragedy, provides a universal context for the assumption that incest and inbreeding are phylogenetic desires (reflecting earlier historical practices) that must be overcome in order to acquire the veneer of civilized behavior. Freud evoked all the power of European culture to frame his view of the primeval forces that are played out within the psyche of the infant.

The actual origin of the Oedipus complex, according to Freud, was much more pedestrian. It was shaped by the tales of Freud's nursemaid, "an ugly, elderly, but clever woman" named Theresa Wittek, who introduced him, at the age of two, to stories "about God Almighty and hell," to Catholicism.[33] She is the "prime originator" of Freud's fantasies: "She was my teacher in sexual matters and complained because I was clumsy and unable to do anything." And it was this woman who "washes [him] in the reddish water in which she had previously washed herself" (269). It is the menstrual blood, the very proof that the woman's genitalia had been wounded that he sees in their joint bathwater. Freud's association with this individual is not only in terms of the sexual seduction he imagined her undertaking, but also in terms of her religious seduction. Freud's mother remembers the woman as "an elderly person, very clever, she was always carrying you off to some church, when you returned home you preached and told us all about God Almighty" (271). Freud's statements about her attempts to "seduce" him through the attractions of Christianity were formulated within a month (October 1897) of the abandonment of the seduction theory. And Freud converted this experience, his own fantasy about the body and soul of the Christian Other, into the universal language of the Oedipus theory. The Oedipus myth has its origin in the tale of the seduction (through conversion) of the male Jewish child by the old Catholic servant rather than in the seduction of the mother by the male child. This simple reversal of Freud's own story about the fantasy (or reality) that formed his own initial sexual experience stressed the problem of conversion and his own mother's response. In retelling the tale of his seduction as the tale of Oedipus, Freud repressed one of the salient elements of the Greek legend, the religious motivation for Oedipus's exposure, the primitive belief in the oracle that warned Laius either to have no children or to expose the child lest he be killed by him, whereupon (in a later version used by Sophocles) the child would marry his mother.[34] It is the power of blind religious faith seeking vengeance for the brutal acts of Laius's mother. The Oedipus story, as we shall see in chapter 3, is multifaceted. Its location in Freud's self-analysis is vital to understanding the significance the myth held for him. The expected sense of abandonment that Freud reported he felt when his nanny was incarcerated because of the charge that she had pilfered some coins is echoed here. The real question that has been raised is whether the successful attempt to get rid of the nursemaid may have had to do with her attempts to convert the child.[35]

The rhetoric of conversion that Freud employed in discussing the origins of the Oedipus complex is taken from the discourse on infant baptism of the mid-nineteenth century. The baptism of a Jewish child by a Christian nursemaid is a topos in the conversion literature of the period. Case after case is reported in the popular press. Without a doubt the most famous was the case of Edgardo Mortara, who was secretly baptized by one of his parents' servants and in 1858 was forcibly removed from his parents' home at the age of six to be raised as a Catholic in Rome.[36] Such kidnappings following secret baptism were unusual, but they showed the risk of having a Christian servant. (In the Papal States it was against the law.) This case was still being fought in the courts a decade later and was widely reported in the newspapers of the day. In the mid-1860s another such incident was widely reported in the European press. Joseph Coen, in Rome, was kidnapped by a priest to whom he delivered mended shoes and was raised as a Roman Catholic. It is one of the anxieties of the Jewish parent in the 1850s and 1860s, especially in those lands, such as the Austro-Hungarian empire, that were dominated by the Roman church. Freud's parents may well have had the nursemaid "locked up" for stealing.[37] But Martin Freud, Sigmund's oldest son, comments on his father's having been taken to church, "possibly with the idea of laying the early foundations of a conversion."[38]

By the 1890s this specter was part of the legend of Jewish social instability—parents feared for their children even though the social reality at the fin de siècle had become quite different. One eastern European Jewish woman commented: "Nannies" took their charges "to church every morning. I would love the scent of the incense, and when I was lost, and I would walk off, my mother was sure that I was somewhere in church. . . . I loved the quiet, the coolness, the darkness, the smell of it, it did something to me. I don't know, maybe I should have been born a Catholic—it lured me."[39] Yet it was not children but adults who were converting to Christianity.

In 1897 Freud rejected any sense that such a seduction was possible. The abandonment of the actual seduction as the primary etiology of hysteria was paralleled by an abandonment of the notion that conversion was a possibility. Here one can see that Freud's rejection of conversion (*Konversion*), the pathological transference of one's emotions from one religious system to another, is paralleled by his rejection of conversion (*Konversion*) as the translation of "real" traumatic experiences into neurotic symptoms.[40] But even within Freud's representation of the origin of hysteria as primarily an intrapsychic process there is the echo of the question of conversion. In *The Interpretation of Dreams,* Freud's view is that the identification of the hysteric with what is desired is the mechanism by which hysterical symptoms are produced. Hysterical symptoms represent not merely the experiences of the individual "but those of a large number of other people. It enables them, as it were, to suffer on behalf of a whole crowd of people and to act all the parts in a play singlehanded." Although Charcot had already postulated a link between the psychopathology of the crowd and that of the hysteric, Freud stressed the mimetic representation of this relationship. It is an "assimilation" (*Aneignung*) that "expresses a resemblance and is derived from a common element which remains in the unconscious" (*ein im Unbewußten verbleibendes Gemeinsames*) (*SE* 4:149–50; *GW* 2/3:155–56). The hysteric is thus much like the Jewish convert who psychopathologically mimics the reality of the Christian. The convert's desire to be Christian is a powerful shaping force, as is the desire of the hysteric. This desire shapes the "common mental construction" of the convert.

The meaning of conversion is thus both culturally and personally contextualized. The "old woman" became an archetypal figure within the family romance that Freud comes to designate by the classical term "Oedipus complex." Seduction becomes part of the fantasy life of the child, and that only within sexual terms. By the close of the nineteenth century, the debate about conversion had shifted substantially. It is the question of whether, not how, one converts that takes up the interest of medical science.

By the time Freud entered the world of science, his fascination with Christianity, especially in its Catholic form, had clearly turned to disgust. He symbolized the conflict between Judaism (and himself as a Jew) and Catholicism (the religion of the imperial monarchy) within his dream interpretation in the detailed interpretation given of Hannibal, the Semitic general, and the anxiety Freud associates with his trip to northern Italy in 1897 (and his articulation of the resultant "Rome neurosis").[41] (It was only in 1901, after the break with Fliess, that Freud actually visited Rome and confronted the medieval Catholic city that haunted his dreams, as well as the classical one he idealized.) Freud rejected the possibility of conversion as early as his marriage in 1886 to Martha Bernays (with its mandatory religious ceremony), and he translated the attraction this would have had for him into its opposite, an antagonism to Catholicism and to organized religion in general. Religion became, for Freud, one of the means through which civilization repressed instinctual drives: this religion was thus interchangeable with specific forms of mental illness, such as obsessive neurosis (*SE* 9:124). Indeed, by the time Freud wrote his most telling critique of religion, *The Future of an Illusion* (1927), his rejection of religion had become a paean to science. As Freud concluded the volume: "No, our science is no illusion. But an illusion it would be to suppose that what science cannot give us we can get elsewhere" (*SE* 21:56). Science is the antithesis of religion and exposes its devices just as the science of race exposes the hidden nature of the Jew. That Freud's distaste for religion also extended to Judaism as a ritual practice is not surprising. All religion suppresses the universal essence of the human being. Freud's identity as a Jew is set; it is the "common mental construction" of the Jew. For being Jewish—in the terms of Freud and his scientific contemporaries—had little or nothing to do with religion. It was a category that reflected racial rather than religious identity.

Conversion as Madness

Conversion thus becomes, for the scientific mind of the late nineteenth century, not only an impossibility but, even more markedly, a sign of pathology.[42] The logic is clear. If you try to work against nature—and race and its qualities, no matter how defined, are natural categories—then what result are pathologies. Thus conversion becomes itself a sign of psychopathology. This view had already entered the discussion of the nature of religious enthusiasm in the eighteenth century. William Hogarth's images of the Methodists were parallel to his images of Bedlam. In Germany it is Christian Heinrich Spiess, who in 1795–96 presents the descent into insanity of the "beautiful Jewess Esther L." One central aspect of her madness was her assumption of the role of a Christian noble, which totally obscured her Jewish identity. It was her peculiar accent that gave her away, to the careful reader of her case study. In the course of unraveling her identity, her voluntary conversion to Catholicism proved her ultimate undoing and the act that led her down the slope to madness and destruction.[43] This view of religion as the causative factor in the madness of the Jews is also found in the medical literature of the eighteenth century. The Jewish physician Elcan Isaac Wolf accounts for the "sensitivity of the nerves" of Jews by their "religious services, because we pray and worship with all our powers, our bodies, as well as our soul, the highest, infinite being. Our unnecessary mortification, our holy laws, present for the ignorant occasions for misuse, and these then result in the horrible grounds for many illnesses."[44] Indeed, specific Jewish religious practices, such as the *mikva* (the ritual baths), are seen by physicians such as Peter Joseph Schneider as leading to the pathological intensification of the emotions, and as a result to hysteria as well as other organic diseases.[45] Within the German medical tradition, it was the German Romantic psychiatrist Karl Ideler who in 1847 depicted a series of nineteen case studies of religious mania, many of them representing conversion—but from one Christian group to another.[46] All these figures, literary and medical alike, were described as enthusiasts, and all presented what was read as a sexual aspect to their pathology.

In the high science of the nineteenth century, medicine linked enthusiasm (with its hidden text about sexuality) and psychopathology when it came to discussing the meaning of conversion. This condemnation of an enthusiasm that would lead to conversion had its strongest statement in the work of one of William James's students at Harvard, the Stanford psychologist Edwin Diller Starbuck. Translated into German in 1909, Starbuck's views had also been broadly circulated in the work of the educational psychologist Ernst Meumann.[47] Starbuck, who is in general very sympathetic to religious conversion, provides a chapter full of counterexamples of the "abnormal aspect of conversion."[48] What would make conversion into a pathological state or at least into a sign of an underlying pathology? For him the core of conversion as a pathological sign lies in "*the emotionalism and excitement of religious revivals*." Starbuck is careful to note that the "alienist thinks in terms of psychiatry. . . . Religionists, on the other hand, are liable to have an apperceptive faculty which colors whatever happens in connection with the nominally religious as a divine manifestation." It is the impact of emotionalism on the "mob mind" that is seen as pathological. It is a "contagion," he notes, quoting Gustave Le Bon. It takes the form of a "state of ecstasy, with the tendency to produce a slight obsessional climax." These are "beyond the limits of the normal and . . . [are] pathological" (165, 164, 167, 167, 168, 179). It is this type of conversion experience, limited in Starbuck's work to conversions within and to Christianity, that marks the pathological convert.

The psychological literature of the fin de siècle has relatively few examples of Jewish conversions to Christianity, even though the Christian literature of the age was full of them. One of them was well known to Freud. William James draws on Starbuck's work extensively in his Gifford Lectures at the University of Edinburgh, published as *The Varieties of Religious Experience* (1902). James, like Starbuck, saw the process of conversion in pathological terms. He traced in "religious phenomena" qualities such as "religious melancholy, [which] whatever peculiarities it may have *qua* religious, is at any rate melancholy."[49] What is striking is that one of James's examples of conversion is the case of Alphonse Ratisbonne, "a freethinking French Jew" who converted to Catholicism in 1842. This is one of the exemplary cases of conversion in the religious literature of the nineteenth century. James quotes Ratisbonne's own account of the process of conversion, in which he abandons his "attachment to the Jewish people." He is suddenly like "one born blind who should suddenly open his eyes to the day" (183–84). James, as Philip Rieff noted, "passed over evidence of the conversion experiences of intellectuals, or conversions based on doctrinal grounds, in favor of the experiences of untutored or disturbed minds swayed by revivalist fervor."[50] Religious conversion, even among Jews, is a problem of a specific form of pathology as understood by non-Jewish psychologists. For one of Freud's contemporaries, Sante de Sanctis, the professor of psychiatry in Rome, religious conversion is a symptom of adolescence. Freud read this study carefully, noting those passages and remarking that it was primarily females about the age of fourteen and males about the age of sixteen who convert.[51] For Sante de Sanctis conversion is one of the symptoms of puberty, as the sexual impulse is checked by social convention and diverted into religion. Conversion is thus a sign of repressed sexuality and is associated with a transitional stage of development.

The question of the nature of mass hysteria, of the conversion experience in groups as well as in individuals, underlies Freud's own reading of group psychology. His critique of Gustave Le Bon accepts Le Bon's view that the experience of the crowd is indeed a manifestation of "religious sentiment"[52] and that the experience of the individual in a crowd is analogous to the conversion experience—a disease that spreads as if it were a hypnotic "contagion" (30). Le Bon sees all the manifestations of the crowd, whether in the service of religious or political goals, as a type of religious "fanaticism." Such fanatical views can also be found among individuals across all cultures. People are marked by a "blind submission, fierce intolerance, and the need of violent propaganda" when they function in groups (74). But what of those individuals whose feelings swing from extreme to extreme and who experience such feelings on their own? Le Bon's example of the latter is the "case of educated Hindus brought up at our European universities," who can "present the most flagrant contradictions." The question then arises of what factors bring the individual to move within the crowd in certain specific ways. This is attributed to the contradictions that exist within specific types of individuals. Such contradictions can also be the result of crossbreeding: "It is only when, as the result of the intermingling of different races, a man is placed between different hereditary tendencies that his acts from one moment to another may be really entirely contradictory" (62–64). There are the models for the diseased individual, whose mental state is a reflex of either cultural or biological "mixing"—this is the madness attributed to the convert.

Havelock Ellis sees the mind of the convert as the source of this pathology of excess: "The comparatively rare cases in which individuals of more than average mental culture are attracted in any number to a religious movement of this kind seem to belong to periods of over strenuous intellectuality. . . . This is the most important key to the psychology of 'conversion.'"[53] In the medical literature of the late nineteenth century these "ecstatic states . . . may be plainly seen to bridge the gulf between the innocent fooleries of ordinary hypnotic patients and the degraded and repulsive phenomena of nymphomania and satyriasis."[54] Indeed, such religious phenomena were described by Francis Galton in 1883 as symptoms of hysteria.[55] The ecstasy of the convert becomes a diagnostic category of insanity. It is a "disease being used by dishonest or foolish people as a bond of union for religious sects."[56] The relationship, as Havelock Ellis notes, is a biological one: "The connection between spiritual exaltation and organic conditions [is] . . . plain."[57] And it is directly related to the psyche of the individual.

Freud is referring to this type of born-again Christian in his comment to James Jackson Putnam about C. G. Jung, in a letter of July 8, 1915, after his break with Jung: "What I have seen of religious-ethical conversion has not been inviting. Jung, for example, I found sympathetic as long as he lived blindly, as I did. Then came his religious ethical crisis with its higher morality, 'rebirth,' Bergson, and at the very same time, lies, brutality, and anti-Semitic condescension toward me. It has not been the first or the last experience to reinforce my disgust with saintly converts."[58] It is the Christian who is blinded by a religious mentality: "We Jews have an easier time," writes Freud, explaining why Jung was so difficult to accept, "having no mystical element."[59] ("Mysticism" is a quasi-clinical term. Max Nordau can write of it as "a cardinal mark of degeneration.")[60] For Christians can (and do) speak of religion. "It is an unfortunate fact that almost every Jew is distressed and discomfited because of his religion," writes A. A. Brill, "though he rarely speaks of it." He comments that the reason for this is that "religion has often been used as an excuse for persecution and brutality. . . . Moreover, experience teaches that emotions are suggestible, nay contagious."[61] This view certainly fits with Freud's claim (made to the British non-Jew Ernest Jones) in 1908 that "it has never been my fortune to know a Jew possessing religious belief, let alone an orthodox one."[62] Jews are rationalists; they are not susceptible to conversion, which is good, since one cannot truly ever stop being a Jew. Rationality, that "common mental construction" of the Jews, is the antithesis of the convert.

Yet this rationality is often understood as a symptom of biological degeneration. The Jew is certainly seen as "overintellectualized," and this overintellectualization is one of the sources of his pathological state. As the Heidelberg sociologist Alfred Weber notes about the Jews: "The longer a people undergoes the process of civilization, the more intellectualized it is—to speak in a specifically biological manner: its genetic substance is implanted with intellectual gemmules, so that it is born with the tendency to place all the aspects of its essence in the conscious, which already reflects its personal fate."[63] This view is to be found in the work of Heinrich Coudenhove-Kalergi, which Freud knew and used.[64] But Weber and other commentators on the question of conversion and its positive or negative qualities all reflect on the nervousness of the Jew as a predisposing factor in conversion. Jews are pathological in that they are susceptible to the pressures of civilization, such as the pressure to convert.

Conversion is a sign of underlying biological pathology. The comments by Freud's psychiatric colleague at the University of Vienna, Richard Krafft-Ebing, typify the general tenor of these observations:

> Statistics have been collected with great care to show the percentage of insanity in the various religious sects, and it has been shown that among the Jews and certain sects the percentage is decidedly higher. This fact stands in relation with religion only in so far as it constitutes a hindrance to marriage among those professing it; the more when its adherents are small in number, and there is consequent insufficient crossing of the race and increased inbreeding. This is a phenomenon similar to that observed in certain highly aristocratic and wealthy families, whose members, whether from motives of honor or money, constantly intermarry, and thus have many insane relatives. In such cases the cause is not moral, but anthropologic.[65]

This parallels the views of French historian Anatole Leroy-Beaulieu, who sees among the religious and political revivalism of the fin de siècle "signs of racial decline and degeneracy . . . in Palestine perhaps more than elsewhere. Those anaemic German Jews who, after a lapse of eighteen centuries, have returned to the home of their robust ancestors, reminded me of the enfeebled sons of old houses, who come back to die in the dilapidated castles of their fathers."[66] The source of such insanity is the deviant sexuality associated with certain forms of religious experience, such as conversion: "Very often excessive religious inclination is itself a symptom of an originally abnormal character or actual disease, and, not infrequently, concealed under a veil of religious enthusiasm there is abnormally intensified sensuality and sexual excitement that lead to sexual errors that are of etiological significance."[67]

For Krafft-Ebing the "anthropological" cause of the greater incidence of insanity among the Jews is their endogamous marriages, which, as a liberal, he compares to the degeneracy found in the inbred upper class. But it is mysticism, inherent in the image of the Eastern Jew, that he contrasts with the rationality of the Western religion. Here Krafft-Ebing stands in a long tradition of "liberal" anti-Semitism. Nietzsche's bête noire, David Friedrich Strauss, for example, labeled biblical miracles, such as the Resurrection, as the product of a hysterical fantasy, "fantastic," "oriental," "especially female," of the Jews.[68] (Freud read this text as a young man and it made a considerable impression on him.)[69] The result of this stress on inbreeding and mysticism is a focus on the exclusivity of the Jews. And mysticism is a sign of the Jew from the East, not of the Western Jew.

Jewish Converts

The rejection of "conversion" by even "godless" Jews such as Sigmund Freud seems to be a sign of the need to comprehend the separateness of the Jew as having a positive valence. Being centered within one's race came to have a positive quality, since escaping one's racial fate was impossible. Labeling converts as "sick" becomes a widely used trope of the fin de siècle. Indeed, there is a large literature discussing the question of conversion and the resulting mixed marriages in purely medical/disease terms.[70] Conversion is rarely if ever understood as an act of belief.[71]

It was Fritz Wittels, later to become the first biographer of Freud, who wrote a study of the "baptized Jew" in 1904. Wittels stressed that the Jew's desire for baptism was a neurosis, rejecting conversion as a matter of convenience.[72] The German Jewish novelist Ernst Lissauer commented that "baptism, following the bureaucratic rules that declare the Jewish faith an obstacle to promotion, is merely joining the state church; it is an official, not a confessional, act."[73] For Wittels such a "baptized Jew" was a congenital liar who showed a form of "ethical insanity." Or as Anatole Leroy-Beaulieu wrote in 1893, "The de-judaised Jews are, in too many cases, lacking in moral feeling."[74] The implications of the Jew's *Mauscheln,* the corrosive and corroding nature of the Jew's discourse, comes here to have pathological significance as a sign of the "diseased" Jew, the Jewish convert. But for Wittels is was not enthusiasm that marked the psychopathology of conversion, but rather the highly manipulative, self-serving rational psyche of the convert. Thus he excluded only artists and lovers from the psychopathological category of the convert (since they are irrational anyhow) and saw all other converts as suffering from a form of mental illness.

For Wittels the "baptized Jews" are similar to Lombroso's born criminals. They show an innate pathology. "He lies without having the feeling that it is something dishonest" (*Taufjude,* 6). Wittels does believe in the abstract that a Jew can convert for reasons of belief, but he attests to knowing none of this type personally. True believers are usually the ill, women, and children. The ultimate form of the convert is the self-hating Jew, the outsider, who hates the duplicity of his fellow Jews. The self-hating Jew internalizes the "sense of the slave" that stigmatizes the Jew in Christian society. "Such rabble only poisons the well" (7, 9, 10, 40). This view is echoed in the image evoked by the German American psychiatrist Ernst Harms, who reports the case of a Jew he saw in an asylum "in the state of almost total amnesia, who kept crossing himself. I was assured that he was not Catholic but had great difficulties in socialization." For Harms this image of the demented Jew crossing himself is proof of the "impossibility of adapting to a new system, as the conscious mind is still bound to the older life-forms."[75] The conflict that results in the self-hating or mad Jew is the conflict between the innate "common mental construction" of the Jew and the desire to submit to the societal pressure to convert and stop being a Jew. Since this is impossible, given the innate nature of the Jew, the sole resolution is madness.

At the meeting of the Viennese Psychoanalytic Society on December 9, 1908, Wittels recounted a case of a patient who had come to him specifically because of the publication of his work on baptized Jews, Jews trying to pass as Christians. It was a young man of about thirty who suffered from "anti-Semitic persecution, for which he holds his inconspicuously Semitic nose responsible. He therefore plans to have the shape of his nose changed by plastic surgery."[76] Wittels and his patient lived in an age of the semiotics of the nose, according to their contempo-

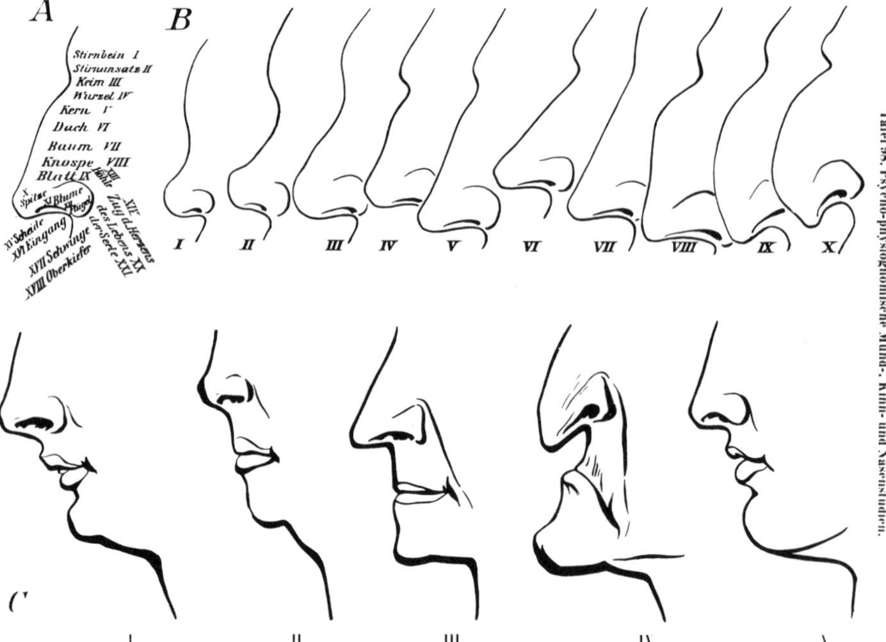

Figure 17. The physiognomy of the nose and its relation to character and to beauty in a physiognomy of the fin de siècle. Carl Huter compiled his physiognomy in 1904, and it reflects the fantasies of the period about the body. The scale runs from the child's nose (I) to the nose of the Jew (X). The "German" nose (IV) is the norm. From Carl Huter, *Menschenkenntnis: Körperform- und Gesichts-Ausdruckskunde* (1904; Schwaig near Nuremberg: Verlag für Carl Huters Werke, 1957). (National Library of Medicine, Bethesda, Md.)

rary Rudolf Kleinpaul. Every race could be read in the nose, including the "Jewish ram's nose" (fig. 17).[77] Wittels attempted to persuade him that his anxiety about his nose was merely a displacement of anxiety about his sexual identity. "This the patient declared to be a good joke." The evident analogy of Wittels's suggestions did not occur to him. If a patient comes to him expressly because of his writing about the neurosis of conversion, if he wishes to have his nose rebuilt to hide his Jewishness, then the question of his own "paranoid" relationship to his circumcised penis, that invisible but omnipresent sign of the male's Jewishness, is evident. Freud picks up on this directly and notes that "the man is evidently unhappy about being a Jew and wants to be baptized." "At this point Wittels remarks that the patient is an ardent Jew. Nevertheless, he does not undergo baptism. In this fact lies the conflict that has absorbed the meaning of other conflicts." To be a Jew and to be so intensely fixated on the public visibility of that identity is to be ill. Then Wittels revealed the name of the patient to the group, and Freud recognized that the patient's father was an engaged Zionist. Freud then read the patient's desire to unmake himself as a Jew as a sign of the rejection of the father. Freud, however, did not comment on the link between the strong Jewish identity and the rejection of the visibility that particular identity entailed. There was a real sense that the Jewish body, represented by the nose, could never truly be changed.

Conversion becomes a sign of pathology that has its roots in the "common mental construction" of the Jews. This view is seconded by the physician Felix Goldmann in Oppeln, who in 1912 provides a historical study of the pathology of conversion among the Jews.[78] Goldmann not only lists in great detail the infamous history of baptized Jews, who were active in attacks on Jews and their religious and social institutions, but also attributes the reappearance of the "blood libel" in the nineteenth century to two baptized Jews, Paulus Meyer and "Dr. Justus," that is, Aaron Brimann. (The association of the blood libel and the discourse about the nature of racial mixing is discussed in chapter 4.) Goldmann raises the question of the pathology of these actions and points to a series of such figures who were active in the anti-Semitic movement of the times, such as Robert Jaffé (co-worker of Theodor Fritsch, editor of the most notorious anti-Semitic newspaper of the fin de siècle) and Maximilian Harden (born Isidor Witkowski), editor of the muckraking journal *The Future*. Goldmann sees these converts not only as unethical and immoral but as diseased.

This creation of a pathologized, lying Jew, a Jew whose diseased psyche is exposed in words as well as actions, is reflected in Freud's image of the Eastern Jew. And it is, of course, the enthusiastic Eastern Jew who forms the basis for the general Christian image of the convert. In a letter written to Wilhelm Fliess during April 1898 Freud refers to his brother-in-law Moriz Freud (a distant cousin who married his sister Marie) as a "half-Asian" who suffers from "pseudologica fantastica."[79] He is "half-Asian" because he is from Bucharest, and the disease he is said to suffer from is the psychiatric diagnosis for those mythomanic patients who lie in order to gain status. "Pseudologia fantastica" is a syndrome in which "an extraordinary vanity forms the motor, the need for the extraordinary, the need to appear more than one is, to have experienced more than one has, more than one can experience in the course of daily life. . . . The pleasure that accompanies such vacillation is so great that it cannot be controlled, even when the substance of the lie is immediately evident; it is simply impossible for such characters to stay with the truth."[80] They commit acts such as stock fraud, confidence games, "lying and swindling," traditionally associated with Jews in the forensic literature of the period.[81] The sign of this form of madness can already be found early in the developmental cycle, "when teenagers and high-school students send themselves anonymous love letters, correspond with one another with pompous-sounding pseudonyms, indulge in secret societies, etc." Such a diagnosis "in ethically inferior individuals . . . predestines the individual to the speciality of a common criminal, as an international confidence man." It is such an individual who can be converted to Christianity.

But such a description—from the scientific claims of psychoanalysis to the youthful correspondence between Freud and Silberstein (with their highly literary pseudonyms, often written in schoolboy Spanish) to the "scientific congresses" of Freud and Wilhelm Fliess—seems to take the hidden measure of another eastern European Jew, Sigmund Freud. Indeed, the proposal at the turn of the century that there was a typical "Jewish psychosis" was couched in terms redolent of Freud's representation of his brother-in-law. This psychosis consisted of a markedly "Jewish argumentativeness" as well as an overly critical rationality that "calls everything into question."[82] Equally important, Freud diagnoses the three daughters (his cousins) as "hysterical": "The youngest, a rather gifted child, severely so. I doubt the father is innocent in this case either." The "guilt" of the father, as in the guilt he attributed to his own father, lies in his Eastern Jewish identity, in the taint of Jewishness passed on from one generation to another.[83] Hysteria is a potential reflex of being an eastern European Jew (like Freud and his cousins), and it manifests itself in hysterical actions—such as conversion.

Freud rejects conversion, even though he is tempted by its promise. The fascination with conversion—as a personal as well as professional choice—follows him his entire life. He notes this in his own interpretation of his Hannibal dream.[84] But Freud never converts, and indeed he stresses this in his autobiography. What does conversion mean for Freud? In a letter to Max Graf, the father of "Little Hans," Freud argues that having Graf's son baptized will not change his essential "Jewishness": "If you do not let your son grow up as a Jew, you will deprive him of those sources of energy which cannot be replaced by anything else. He will have to struggle as a Jew, and you ought to develop in him all the energy he will need for that struggle. Do not deprive him of that advantage."[85] Being a Jew is being a member of a race, possessing a "common mental construction." In a powerful letter to his fiancée Martha from Paris in 1886, Freud recounted that he found himself confronted with his own Jewish identity, as an inheritance of "all the obstinate defiance and all the passions with which our ancestors defended their temple." He saw himself as a "Jew, who is neither German nor Austrian."[86] If anything the pressures he perceived in the world of science made it clear to him that conversion was neither a practical nor a realistic alternative to remaining a "godless Jew."

Freud's own most detailed analysis of the meaning of conversion appears in an analytic response to a letter received from an American colleague upon the publication of his interview with the German-American newspaperman George Sylvester Viereck in 1926. The letter, as Freud describes it, recounted a conversion episode in which the American physician as a young medical student was first confronted with a corpse in the dissecting room and then overcame his horror of death and accepted the truth of Christianity. Such tales were typical of the conversion literature of the period. What made this story unique was its medical setting.

Freud answered this missive by stating that he had never heard such an "inner voice" and that, at his advanced age, if God did not hurry "it would not be my fault if I remained to the end of my life what I now was—'an infidel Jew.'"[87] (The last phrase Freud cited in English from his letter. Freud's own sense of a lack of religious mission is echoed in the opening of his *Civilization and Its Discontents* [1930].[88]) The tone of Freud's own summary is ironic, but his correspondent's response is anything but: "In the course of a friendly reply, my colleague gave me an assurance that being a Jew was not an obstacle in the pathway to true faith and proved this by several instances. His letter culminated in the information that prayers were being earnestly addressed to God that he might grant me 'faith to believe'" (*SE* 21:170). Here we have the conflict outlined: the Jew who saw his Judaism not as a religion but as a "common mental construction" was confronted by a Christian who not only wished him to convert but presented him with cases of Jews who had converted. Here we have an answer to the immutability of the racial definition of the Jew—Jews who can truly become Christians in spite of their Jewish mind-set.

Freud's response to this call for conversion was to examine the conversion episode as a neurotic break and to relate it to the Oedipus complex. As we have seen, the medical literature of the fin de siècle saw the convert as a psychopath. The American physician's faith had been cast into doubt when he saw the body of a "sweet-faced dear old woman" brought into the dissecting room. Freud read his response to "the sight of a woman's dead body, naked or on the point of being stripped" as a "longing for his mother which sprang from his Oedipus complex." (One sees here also Freud's own childhood experience with his family servant and his belief that she attempted to convert him.) This triggered anger and fear of the father, which was translated into rejection of the deity. This displacement into the discourse of religion, according to Freud, had nothing to do with the rational mind: "The conflict seems to have been unfolded in the form of a hallucinatory psychosis: inner voices were heard which uttered warnings against resistance to God" (*SE* 21:171). Conversion becomes a psychosis, reflecting the universal model of the Oedipus complex and resolves itself in the "complete submission to the will of God the Father" (*SE* 21:171).[89]

Here the tensions concerning the nature of the Jew's conversion are laid out in detail. True conversion as advocated by enthusiasts is at best a neurosis; Jewish converts who dissimulate conversion are pathological. It is a symptom of psychopathology, to follow Freud's rhetoric. His own experience, his own attraction to the prospect of conversion, at least as a child, was itself tied to the image of an old woman seen naked. In his reading of Freud's paper, Theodor Reik stressed the "intimate connection between the peeping impulse and desire for knowledge, the investigatory impulse."[90] But we can also evoke the special status of both Freud and Reik seeing as scientists rather than as children or as Jews. Here the motif of the seeing of the gaze is replicated—but in this context it is the Jewish scientist seeing the Christian convert gazing.

The scenario Freud evokes is not only a personal one but, given his own identification with the dissecting room (as I shall discuss in chapter 3), one that reflects on his own sense of professional identity and the anti-Semitism he associated with his medical career.[91] Freud's response not only rejected religious faith—this was to be expected—but cast the very idea of conversion in the pathological terms of the medical literature of his day. The image of the psychopathological convert was evoked by the serious claim of his correspondent that his racial identity as a Jew would not stand in the way of his conversion. The "common mental construction" of the Jew appeared in the most direct manner unaffected by the argument. Freud was quite prepared to turn this claim into material for analysis of the neurotic text.

Freud's discomfort in the intellectual presence of a Jew who is equally drawn to Christianity and to Judaism can be judged in this response to Franz Werfel. In 1926 the two had met, and Werfel had given Freud a copy of his new drama *Paul among the Jews,* which turns on the question and meaning of Paul's conversion.[92] The public response in Vienna to the publication of the drama was a consistent rumor that Werfel had converted to Catholicism. Freud was very distant in his reception of the play, and Werfel wrote him a passionate letter in which he defended his role "as a Jew" writing about conversion at a moment in time when one could still be both Christian and Jew. Freud's answer to this letter stressed the arrogant tone of the afterword to Werfel's drama as well as his sense that Werfel's confusion about the meaning of conversion reflected a deep distrust of his own Jewish identity.

Freud's reading during this period linked the question of conversion and that of the pathological Jew. In his library there is to be found the German translation of the documentary study by the Soviet Slavist Leonid Grossmann of the relationship of Fyodor Mikhaylovich Dostoyevsky to Abraham Urija Kowner, also known as Albert Kowner.[93] (This volume was part of the series of Dostoyevsky translations in which Freud's own "Dostoyevsky and Parricide" had served as introduction to an earlier volume [*SE* 21:175–89].) Kowner was an eastern European Jew, born in Vilnius, who was raised within the strict tradition of Eastern Jewish orthodoxy. Like many eastern European Jews for whom the Enlightenment ideal of acculturation still existed in the mid-nineteenth century, he painstakingly (and against the wishes of his family and community) acquired a Russian education. He became a journalist, one of the few professions open to (and strongly associated with) the Jews. In 1871 he moved to Saint Petersburg, where he became extremely well known as an advocate of liberal causes. In 1875 he was arrested and convicted of passing a bad check for 160,000 rubles; he was sent to prison, and then into Siberian exile. From Siberia he wrote to Dostoyevsky, whose powerful anti-Semitic views had been echoed in his own journalism. Given the nature of Kowner's crime and the length, detail, and intensity of his correspondence, he would have fitted into the contemporary clinical definition of the individual suffering from "pseudologica fantastica." He was a "mad" Jew and showed it in all of his actions and statements.

Dostoyevsky entered into a public exchange of letters with Kowner, who became converted to Dostoyevsky's political and also religious views. Kowner was dismissed by his Jewish contemporaries as a "convert, a braggart, and an apostate," but he remained a presence in Russian intellectual life until the beginning of the new century (Grossmann, *Die Beichte,* 233). He served the Russian intelligentsia as an example of the Jew who achieves insight into his own Jewishness yet still remains a Jew in all his qualities. The editor of this volume, Leonid Grossmann, labels him the Russian equivalent of Otto Weininger, who also had acquired true insight into the "common mental construction" of the Jew (230). Freud would have read this case quite differently, as an example of the impossibility of conversion. For him Kowner would have been the self-destructive, self-hating, insane Jew. But he would have also sensed the interchangeability of Kowner for all Jews. Not only does he come to represent the intellectual Jew in Dostoyevsky's text, but "when Kowner's portrait was published in a widely circulated German magazine [*Klad-*

derdatsch (May 23, 1875)], a totally innocent Jew was arrested in Berlin" (75–76). All Jews come to be "seen" as criminals. Their criminality is written on their physiognomy.

Freud was not the only Jewish psychoanalyst who was confronted by the psychic conflicts arising from conversion. In Theodor Reik's 1914 version of the case of "Dora," his pseudonym for his fiancée, the question of the nature of religious interest and psychopathology were linked. Dora's father was a "fanatical anti-Semite" and her mother "an apostate from Judaism."[94] Both opposed any relationship of their daughter with the Jewish psychoanalyst Reik. Reik needed to understand their feelings, "hypothesizing that the anti-Semitism of persons with neurotic tendencies is due in large measure to a transference of hostile feelings from their closest relatives (father, wife, etc.)." In other words, the father's all-consuming hatred of him is the result of his own relationship with his father or his converted Jewish wife, as Reik later surmises in his autobiography.[95] This is the origin of the neurosis that is labeled anti-Semitism. Unlike such neurotic anti-Semites, Jews themselves have split the "ambivalent attitude meant for the father. The deprecatory and antagonistic tendency now is directed against the religion, which is regarded as obsolete and superfluous, while the affectionate and delicate current flows toward the Jewish people to which the young Jewish generation in Western countries adheres with great pride (Zionism, Jewish nationalism)." Reik sees the rejection of religious identity as part of the splitting of the healthy from the unhealthy self. The healthy Jew is the national rather than the religious Jew. Religion in all forms is unhealthy. But the example Reik brings is one in which the hatred caused by the wife, a convert, is transferred to the Jews as a group. Anti-Semitism is a disease within the world of the Aryan. The cause here, unlike in Freud's comment, is the convert, the "apostate." She becomes the source of the hatred of the anti-Semite. It is the failure of the woman that causes the rejection of the Jew. According to Reik the Jew's religious identity (always the male Jew) is shaped by this "relationship with his father." Reik's view of the convert is that her presence has destroyed his relationship with his potential father-in-law.

Freud's own views echoed this position. In a discussion with Professor S. Ehrmann after a meeting of the "Vienna" Lodge of B'nai B'rith, Freud got into an intense discussion with a lodge brother who advocated conversion as a personal act if it enabled one to "fulfill life's goal, one that would otherwise have to be abandoned," such as "assuming a leadership function in the arts, sciences, or politics." Freud dismissed this out of hand, noting that such an act was never a private one, since it "endangered the common interest." It was unfair for the state to demand "that a member of a specific confession of a tribal community . . . deny his origin and his belief" without demanding this action from everyone. Such a demand would create "a common right *via facti* that would be a denial of the rights of everyone."[96] Freud's refusal to permit any type of conversion was an acknowledgment of the strengths of the Jews' "tribal community" as a collective. He was not opposed to mixed marriages, but they should not lead to conversion: "A Jew ought not to get himself baptized and attempt to turn Christian because it is essentially dishonest, and the Christian religion is every bit as bad as the Jewish. Jew and Christian ought to meet on the common ground of irreligion and humanity. Jews who are ashamed of their Jewishness have simply reacted to the mass suggestion of their society."[97] Freud's rejection of Judaism as a religion is made at the same moment when he saw the immutability of the "common mental construction" of the Jews. Intermarriage could no more obliterate this than could conversion.

Penises and Noses

The question of conversion plays a subtle role in articulating one further aspect of the ideology concerning sexuality and the male genitalia in Freud's work. Let us turn for a moment to the relationship of Freud with Wilhelm Fliess. Fliess (1858–1928) was an ear, nose, and throat specialist in Berlin who came to know Freud beginning in 1887, when Freud's work on the sexual etiology of neurosis was leading to the break with Josef Breuer. In Freud's correspondence with Fliess, the nature of the scientific endeavor of psychiatry and neurology and the definition of the medical practitioner were drawn into question.[98] Traditionally Fliess is represented as a marginal figure in the history of medicine. He is seen as the mute sounding board for Freud's views. It has been accepted that Fliess was a quack—he put forth absolutely mad views such as the intimate relationship between the nasal passages and the genitalia as well as the idea that male as well as female physiology reflected rigid periodic cycles. But quackery implies a misappropriation of the status of scientific medicine, and the implication of this misappropriation can help us clarify Freud's gradual redefinition of the science of medicine.

Given the Viennese discussion of who could be treated by Jewish physicians that began in the 1840s, it was no accident that Fliess's patients, Sigmund Freud included, were Jewish. The isolation still felt by the Jewish health care practitioner at the fin de siècle formed both Freud and Fliess. Both saw in the social status of medicine a chance to establish themselves in a society that rejected Jews but acclaimed academic physicians. Freud and Fliess both sought out specialties that were open to Jews, but they conceptually restructured these areas to reflect the higher sense of status of other medical specialties.

Sexual questions were dealt with by the physicians in the role of forensic specialist on deviant behavior as well as the syphilologist, who, as a dermatologist, occupied the lowest rung in Viennese medicine. Indeed, when Ferdinand Hebra assumed the chair in dermatology (a field nicknamed *Judenhaut,* "Jewskin") in Vienna, he was able to recruit only Jewish assistants! And psychiatry, with its transitional status between administration and practice, had an equivalently heavy and early Jewish representation. Thus Freud and Fliess sought out two areas, psychopathology and sexuality, where Jews were permitted to function on the level of the academician. Their meetings, which they dubbed "congresses," were mock academic events. Fliess's friendship with Freud was cast in the form of a professional association. They created imitations of the institutions of science: "After each of our Congresses I was strengthened anew for weeks, ideas kept crowding in thereafter, the pleasure in hard work was re-established, and the flickering hope that the way through the underbrush will be found burned quietly and radiantly for a while. Instructive it is not for me, this privation; I always knew what our meeting meant to me."[99] And their desire was to move the study of psycho- and sexual pathologies into a new area—that of neurology.

Freud and Fliess both needed the status of the higher academic specialties. Both sought this status in the area of neurology and addressed their need for prestige through their attempt to ask traditionally (in Viennese medicine) "Jewish" questions about sexuality and psychopathology through the higher-profile subspecialty of neurology. For Wilhelm Fliess, it was the movement from a concentration on the ear, nose, and throat to the interconnection of all human experience through the nervous system. Now, Fliess was clearly marginal to the Berlin medical community, as was Freud to that of Vienna. But being "marginal" means relating in a direct manner to the center. Both Freud and Fliess oriented themselves to the center of German medicine; both sought (and Freud obtained) the status of the medical academic. Both functioned in relation to a discourse—medicine—that was critical of marginality, and that defined marginality in racial terms.

Fliess's theories reflect a fascination with the link between human anatomy and psychology. His work centers on the relation between the periodic cycle he claimed to discern in men and women as well as the relation between the anatomy of the genitalia and that of the nose. Fliess focused on the nose and its relation to the female menstrual cycle. He observed a swelling of the turbinate bone of the nose during menstruation and claimed to have discovered "genital spots" on the inside of the nose. In 1897 he evolved the relation between menstruation and periodicity. While the menstrual cycle was twenty-eight days, other cycles of twenty-three days were also present. These views had analogies within mainstream medicine of the late nineteenth century, as in the work of Moritz Benedikt in Vienna and John Noland Mackensie at Johns Hopkins.[100] Fliess's theories, based on the best of late nineteenth-century endocrinological and neurological theory, appear to us as more than slightly mad, but they fulfilled a function for Fliess, as well as for Freud, in creating a sense of the new pathway that medicine could take.

Let us look at two of Fliess's "mad" ideas—the relation between the nose and the genitalia as well as his "proof" of male periodicity—in the light of the science of medicine, with all its racist overtones in late nineteenth-century Germany and Austria. It is precisely the implications of even the higher medical specialties, such as neurology, that colored Freud's and Fliess's sense of the status of medicine and the medical practitioner.

The idea that the nasal cavities were anatomically parallel to the genitalia grew out of the study of human embryology during the nineteenth century. As early as G. Valentin's 1835 handbook of human development, the parallels in the development of soft-tissue areas and cavities of the fetus had been noted.[101] By the publication of the standard physiological atlas of human embryological development by Wilhelm His in 1885, the assumption of such parallels was at the center of European embryology.[102] But the history of embryology, and His's very creation of "standard developmental stages," is rooted in the ideology of recapitulation. Nineteenth-century biologists believed that in the development of the human fetus into the "highest" form of life they could see the repetition of all the evolutionary stages. Central to this biological reworking of the *scala naturae* was the innate superiority of the human as the end of a teleological development of evolution. Biology placed humanity at the epitome of this development and saw in Ernst Haeckel's commonplace that "ontogeny recapitulates phylogeny" a statement of human superiority. But in late nineteenth-century Germany some humans were better than other humans. And the implied sense of this hierarchy was present in German embryology. Embryology also proved that the nasal passages and the incipient genitalia developed very early in the growth of the fetus. Fliess, by making this association overt, showed that the "head," as the source of the rational, and the "genitalia," as the source of the irrational, were related on an atavistic level and that the manipulation of one could affect the other.

The presumption of a primitive relation between sexuality and the nose is not only bad embryology but bad medicine. It points, however, to a necessary preoccupation by two Jewish scientists of fin-de-siècle Europe with the significance of this relationship between the "nose" and the "genitalia." For Fliess and Freud it served as a sign of universal development rather than as a specific sign of an "inferior" racial identity. The association between the Jewish nose and the circumcised penis was made in the crudest and most revolting manner during the 1880s. In the streets of Berlin and Vienna, in penny papers or on the newly installed *Litfassäulen,* or advertising columns, caricatures of Jews could be seen.[103] These extraordinary caricatures stressed one central aspect of the physiognomy of the Jewish male—his nose—which represented that hidden sign of his sexual difference, his circumcised penis. For the Jews' sign of sexual difference, their sexual selectivity, as an indicator of their identity was, as Friedrich Nietzsche strikingly observed in *Beyond Good and Evil,* the focus of the Germans' fear of the superficiality of their recently created national identity.[104] This fear was represented in caricatures by the elongated nose. (The traditional folkloric association between the size of the nose and that of the male genitalia was made a pathological sign.)[105] It also permeated the discussions of the science of the time. The essence of the Jewish body could be reduced to the difference from the "straight noses and blond hair" of the Aryan body.[106] In the "anatomical-anthropological" study of the nose by the Viennese anatomist Oskar Hovorka (1893), the form of the nose comes to be a sign of racial difference as well as a sign of the "idiot and the insane."[107] Look at the nose and you will see the basic sign of humanity in all its variety! When Fliess attempted to alter the pathology of the genitalia by operating on the nose (in this age at the beginning of cosmetic surgery), he was drawing on an accepted sense of the implication of human development joined to the association of the nose and the genitalia in the German biology of race.

This association of the nose and the genitalia was not merely in the popular mind. The central sign of male periodicity for Fliess (and for Freud) was male menstruation.[108] And its representation, according to Freud in his July 20, 1897, letter to Fliess, was an "occasional bloody nasal secretion."[109] Later, in his letter of October 15, 1897, Freud traced the implications of male menstruation for himself as well as (one assumes) for Fliess:

> My self-analysis is in fact the most essential thing I have at present and promises to become of the greatest value to me if it reaches its end. In the middle of it, it suddenly ceased for three days, during which I had the feeling of being tied up inside (which patients complain of so much), and

> I was really disconsolate until I found that these same three days (twenty-eight days ago) were the bearers of identical somatic phenomena. Actually only two bad days with a remission in between. From this one should draw the conclusion that the female period is not conducive to work. Punctually on the fourth day, it started again. Naturally, the pause also had another determinant—the resistance to something surprisingly new. Since then I have been once again intensely preoccupied [with it], mentally fresh, though afflicted with all sorts of minor disturbances that come from the content of the analysis. (270)

Jeffrey Masson, the editor of the edition of the letters between Freud and Fliess, commented on Fliess's observations on male menstruation that it is "highly unlikely that these communications to Freud played any role in Freud's research at the time" (199). Quite to the contrary—had Masson researched the history of the concept of male menstruation a bit he would have found a lively nineteenth-century medical literature on this topic, by writers such as F. A. Forel and W. D. Halliburton. Also, the fascination with this question in regard to the problem of hermaphroditism as a sign of bisexuality was as prominent in the nineteenth century as it had been in the Middle Ages.[110] Professor Paul Albrecht in Hamburg argued for the existence of "male menstruation" that was periodic and that mimicked the menstrual cycle of the female through the release of white corpuscles into the urine.[111] In Freud's own sources, such as the writing of the sexologist Paul Näcke, there was a detailed discussion of the question of "male menstruation" and its relation to periodicity.[112] Näcke cited among others Havelock Ellis, who had been collecting material on this question for years. With the rise of modern sexology at the close of the nineteenth century, especially in the writings of Magnus Hirschfeld, male menstruation came to hold a very special place in the "proofs" for the continuum between male and female sexuality.[113] The hermaphrodite, the male who menstruated, became one of the central focuses of Hirschfeld's work. But all of this new "science" that used the existence of male menstruation still drew on the image of the marginality of those males who menstruated and thus pointed toward a much more ancient tradition.

The idea of male menstruation is part of a Christian tradition of seeing the Jew as inherently, biologically different.[114] Thomas de Cantimpré, a thirteenth-century anatomist, presented the first "scientific" statement of this phenomenon (calling on Saint Augustine as his authority).[115] Male Jews menstruated as a mark of the "Father's curse," their pathological difference. This image of the Jewish male as female was introduced to link the Jew with the corrupt nature of the woman (both marked as different by the same sign) and to stress the intransigence of the Jews.

Thomas de Cantimpré recounts the nature of the Jews' attempt to cure themselves. They are told by one of their prophets that they would be rid of this curse by "Christiano sanguine," the blood of a Christian, when in fact it was "Christi sanguine," the blood of Christ in the sacrament, that was required. Thus the libel of the blood guilt, the charge that Jews sacrifice Christian children to obtain their blood, is the result of the intransigence of the Jews in their rejection of the truth of Christianity and is intimately tied to the sign of Jewish male menstruation. The persistence of menstruation among Jewish males is thus not only a sign of the initial "curse of the Father" but of the inherent inability of the Jews to hear the truth of the Son. For the intrinsic "deafness" of the Jews does not let them hear the truth that will cure them. The belief in Jewish male menstruation continued through the seventeenth century. Heinrich Kormann repeated it in Germany in 1614, as did Thomas Calvert in England in 1649.[116] And the view that attributed to the Jews diseases for which the "sole cure was Christian blood" persisted into the late nineteenth century.[117] It was raised again at the turn of the century in a powerfully written pamphlet by the professor of Hebrew at the University of Saint Petersburg, D. Chwolson, as one of the rationales used to justify the blood libel. Chwolson noted that the blood of Christians was claimed to be used to "cure the diseases believed to be specifically those of the Jews," such as male menstruation.[118] This version of the blood accusation (which will be discussed in chapter 4) ties the meaning of the form of the circumcised genitalia to the Jew's diseased nature.

Franco da Piacenza, a Jewish convert to Christianity, repeated this view in his catalog of "Jewish maladies," published in 1630 and translated into German by 1634.[119] He claimed that the males (as well as the females) of the tribe of Simeon menstruated four days a year! These charges continued throughout the age of Enlightenment in slightly altered form. In the work of F. L. de La Fontaine we find a survey of the health of the Polish Jews, published in 1792, in which their sexual pathology is stressed.[120] Jews show their inherent difference through their damaged sexuality, and the sign of that, in the popular mind, is that their males menstruate. Piacenza's charges were repeated in the seventeenth-century work of Chrysostomus Dudulaeus on the Wandering Jew, which was reprinted in 1856.[121] Freud's contemporary, the archracist Theodor Fritsch—whose *Anti-Semite's Catechism,* first published in 1887, was the encyclopedia of German anti-Semitism—saw the sexuality of the Jew as inherently different from that of the German: "The Jew has a different sexuality than the Teuton; he will and cannot understand it. And if he attempts to understand it, then the destruction of the German soul can result."[122] The hidden sign, the link between the woman and the Jew, is the menstruation of the Jewish male.

Freud and Fliess attempt to move this sign from being a sign of difference to being one of universality. Just as Franco da Piacenza tried to remove himself from the "curse of Eve" by claiming that only ancient Jews menstruated (and those of one of the "Lost Ten Tribes" at that)—not of course he and his contemporaries—so too do Freud and Fliess distance this charge from the Jews by making it universal. Thus the public sign of Jewish identity (from the standpoint of the anti-Semitic society they live in) is the nose that "menstruates." Indeed, Jewish social scientists such as Joseph Jacobs spend a good deal of their time denying the meaning of "nostrility" as a sign of the racial cohesion of the Jews. It is clear that for Jacobs (as for Wilhelm Fliess in Germany) the nose is the displaced locus of anxiety associated with the marking of the male Jew's body through circumcision, given the debate about the "primitive" nature of circumcision and its reflection on the acculturation of the Western Jews during the late nineteenth century. But its significance for Freud and Fliess, who are desperately trying to escape classification as "Jews" in the racial sense and therefore as inferior and different, is as a universal sign, a sign of the universal law of male periodicity that links all human beings, males and females.

The implicit charge of pathological bisexuality, of hermaphroditism, had traditionally been lodged against the Jewish male. (Male Jews are like women, among other ways, because both menstruate as a sign of their pathological difference.) Freud and Fliess turn this into a universal sign of human nature in a successful form of resistance to the racist substructure of European medicine. Fliess is not simply a quack; his "quackery" is accepted by Freud, since it provides an alternative to the pathological image of the Jew in conventional medicine.

It is from the intellectual and emotional relationship with Fliess, as is generally acknowledged, that Freud began to evolve the basic theories of psychoanalysis. But this relationship was played out against the cultural context that medical science is always a part of. For Freud the idea of friendship is always unstable and is linked to the image of betrayal. In 1892 Freud was developing the first clinical procedures for the treatment of hysteria. He began to work out many of the theoretical presuppositions behind these approaches in his correspondence with Fliess. In an early letter of May 25, 1892, to Fliess, Freud appended a footnote: "By the way and since nothing more intelligent occurs to me, let me inform you that I was startled to read on your last card a W. Ch. I realized only later that you write your first name equivocally."[123] This is a classic remark—one of Freud's first accounts of his own misreading, accounts that will become more and more important as he collects materials for his work on dreams as well as on the errors of everyday life. And this misreading of "Wlhm." as "W. Ch." evokes the image of his new friend Wilhelm Fliess as a convert, since the signature is that of one who had been baptized and given the ubiquitous baptismal name "Christian." If Freud's own view of the meaningfulness of such misreadings is correct, what does this misreading mean?

Freud had rebelled, in 1882, against the "Christian views of a few *Hofräte* who have long forgotten what work is like"[124] dominating the medical society of which he was a member. These included a number of Jewish converts to Christianity, who had made major careers for themselves in the Viennese medical establishment. It is clear that Freud had been greatly concerned with the question of conversion: his own professional academic life, he believed, depended on his overcoming his Jewish identity. By June 1892 Freud's relationship with Fliess had developed substantially. This was indeed the last letter in which Freud addressed Fliess with the more formal *Sie*. By the end of June 1892 he was addressing him with the familiar *Du*. Thus Freud was clearly beginning to see Fliess as a close friend. Here, in the moment when he is deciding to see his new acquaintance as a friend, he misreads the signature as "W. Ch." rather than "Wlhm." Suddenly Freud sees in his acquaintance perhaps a potential convert, one who would betray his own reality. And this is in the same letter in which Freud acknowledges Fliess's new marriage. His conversion is related to the ostensible subject of this letter to Fliess—the first meeting with Fliess and his new bride Ida on holiday at Reichenau. Freud's sense of betrayal is manifest in this "slip." To this point he and his friend had created the illusion of a scientific academy, writing papers and holding regular congresses by themselves. All the illusion of science in its neutrality negates any sense of the powerful emotional bonds that link Freud (in his own later estimation) to Fliess. Freud's powerful cathexis now seems in danger of being revealed, for Fliess has introduced the question of sexuality into the equation. His honeymoon with his wife forces Freud to bring his own wife along. What had been a celebration of the discovery of the new science is converted into a social meeting. The only image powerful enough to evoke this betrayal of their scientific twinning is that of the convert who betrays his faith. Converts abandon their faith and the institutions that bear them. But conversion out of the race is impossible—and Freud knows that. So this misreading is double-edged. It is an acknowledgment of the betrayal of their intellectual relationship but a sign of the immutability of that relationship. Freud placed the onus of the misreading on Fliess.

He cannot read Fliess's bad handwriting. It is Fliess who is at fault, not Freud. This ambivalence is articulated in Freud's "slip," but the ambivalence seems to be repressed until some three years later.

Fliess actually acted on his medical theories of the relation between the nose and the genitalia, undertaking surgical procedures on the nose to relieve sexual problems. As is well known, his surgical ineptitude almost killed Freud's patient Emma Eckstein. He left a wad of surgical dressing in her nasal cavity, which caused massive bleeding and infection. Fliess operated on Freud's nose during the same stay in Vienna in February 1895 when he operated on Emma Eckstein. Fliess's action, as Max Schur stated when he first revealed this material, must have negatively influenced Freud's image of the implications of science, both in the ineptitude it revealed and in Freud's having placed Fliess on an intellectual plane that clearly paralleled the level he himself wished to attain. Fliess's assumed role as a "surgeon," the highest of the medical specialties, was disguised only by his label as a "nose" doctor. His actions were those of medical practitioners whose status was clearly higher than that permitted him by the society he lived in. This denial was based on Fliess's racial identity.

On July 23–24, 1895, while Freud was completing his work *Studies on Hysteria* with Josef Breuer, he had the "dream of Irma's injection" on the night of July 24, 1895, which served him as the central, exemplary dream for his 1900 *Interpretation of Dreams*.[125] This dream, to which Freud gave extraordinary importance, came in the midst of his struggle with Fliess's role as scientist and friend. It recounts a medical consultation, an injection, the discovery of a botched medical procedure, and the scientific rationale for this. Freud retells the dream twice in his text. The first is his unbroken narrative of the dream; the second version stresses the central aspects of the dream. The first version is as follows:

> A large hall—numerous guests, whom we are receiving.—Among them was Irma. I at once took her on one side, as though to answer her letter and to reproach her for not having accepted my "solution" yet. I said to her: "If you still get pains, it's really only your fault." She replied: "If you only knew what pains I've got now in my throat and stomach and abdomen—it's choking me"—I was alarmed and looked at her. She looked pale and puffy. I thought to myself that after all I must be missing some organic trouble. I took her to the window and looked down her throat, and she showed signs of recalcitrance, like women with artificial dentures. I thought to myself that there was really no need for her to do that.—She opened her mouth properly and on the right I found a big white patch; at another place I saw extensive whitish grey scabs upon some remarkable curly structures which were evidently modelled on the turbinal bones of the nose.—I at once called

in Dr. M., and he repeated the examination and confirmed it. . . . Dr. M. looked quite different from usual; he was very pale, he walked with a limp and his chin was clean-shaven. . . . My friend Otto was now standing beside her as well, and my friend Leopold was percussing her through her bodice and saying: "She has a dull area low down on the left." He also indicated that a portion of the skin on the left shoulder was infiltrated. (I noticed this, just as he did, in spite of her dress.) . . . M. said: "There's no doubt it's an infection, but no matter; dysentery will supervene and the toxin will be eliminated." . . . We were directly aware, too, of the origin of the infection. Not long before, when she was feeling unwell, my friend Otto had given her an injection of a preparation of propyl, propyls . . . propionic acid . . . trimethylamin (and I saw before me the formula for this printed in heavy type). . . . Injections of that sort ought not to be made so thoughtlessly. . . . And probably the syringe had not been clean. (*SE* 4:107)

Let me give Freud's fragmentary retelling of the dream within Freud's explanation of the original dream narrative. At the beginning of the dream we find ourselves in

> the hall—numerous guests, whom we were receiving. . . . I reproached Irma for not having accepted my solution; I said: "If you still get pains, it's your own fault." . . . She looked pale and puffy. . . . I was alarmed at the idea that I had missed an organic illness. I took her to the window to look down her throat. . . . She showed some recalcitrance, like women with false teeth. I thought to myself that really there was no need for her to do that. What I saw in her throat: a white patch and turbinal bones with scabs on them. . . . I at once called in Dr. M., and he repeated the examination. . . . Dr. M. was pale, had a clean-shaven chin and walked with a limp. . . . My friend Otto was now standing beside the patient and my friend Leopold was examining her and indicated that there was a dull area low down on the left. . . . A portion of the skin on the left shoulder was infiltrated. . . . In spite of her dress. . . . Dr. M. said: "It's an infection, but no matter. Dysentery will supervene and the toxin will be eliminated." . . . Dysentery. . . . We were directly aware of the origin of the infection. . . . When she was feeling unwell, my friend Otto had given her an injection. . . . A preparation of proply . . . propyls . . . propionic acid. . . . Trimethylamin. . . . Injections of that sort ought not be made so thoughtlessly. . . . And probably the syringe had not been clean. (*SE* 4:108–17)

The day residue of the dream seems clear. Irma is a composite figure. On one level Irma, the patient depicted in the dream, is one of his favorite patients, Anna Lichtheim, the daughter of his religion teacher Samuel Hammerschlag, the woman after whom Freud will name his youngest child. Part of the character of Irma is also Emma Eckstein. But if this is the tale of Fliess and the botched operation, where is Fliess? The other actors in the dream are "Dr. M." = Josef Breuer; "my friend Otto" =

Oskar Rie, Freud's family pediatrician; and "Leopold" = Dr. Ludwig Rosenberg.[126] Wilhelm Fliess seems to have been completely repressed in Freud's dream-memory of the events.

The only mention of Fliess is in Freud's interpretation. His appearance is keyed in the second version of the dream by the word "trimethylamin . . . the chemical formula . . . [of which] was printed in heavy type, as though there had been a desire to lay emphasis on some part of the context as being of quite special importance."[127] In Freud's interpretation he is mentioned as "another friend" who had associated the genitalia and the nose, but who was at the time himself suffering from suppurative rhinitis, a disease of the nose. In the fragmentary retelling of the dream, which is selected so that Freud can interpret what seemed to him to be the most important aspects of the dream, the centrality of the disease and the chemical is stressed. What is the disease that Irma has, and what function does this chemical formula have in unraveling the story present in the dream?

Freud was quizzed on this aspect of his analysis by Karl Abraham, who queried whether what Irma suffered from was not syphilis: "I find that trimethylamine leads to the most important part, to sexual allusions which became more distinct in the last lines. After all, everything points to the suspicion of syphilitic infection in the patient; the spot in her mouth is the plaque representing the infection, the injection of trimethylamine which has been carelessly given, the dirty syringe (??) Is not this the organic illness for whose continued persistence you cannot be made responsible, because syphilis or a nervous disease originating from it cannot be influenced by psychological treatment."[128] Freud denied in his answer that the dream has anything to do with syphilis. Rather, he answers that hidden behind the dream is his own "sexual megalomania," his sexual cure for the anxiety neurosis that he diagnosed in three women patients (Mathilde Breuer, Sophie Paneth, Anna Lichtheim).[129] Freud's view at the time was that such anxiety neurosis was the product of the collection of sexual toxins such as trimethylamine in the body. But the true sexual anxiety in this case was Freud's in his intense relationship with Fliess. In his exchange with Abraham he stands as the "doctor" curing these female patients; in his dream, he is the feminized patient as well.

In the dream, Irma is given an injection of a preparation of propionic acid—proponesin, a clear, seemingly pleasant liquid. This narcotic is simply a "scientific place holder" according to Freud, but it leads us to the visualization of the formula. This is one of the basic means of symbolization in the dream, according to Freud's dream theory. We often see visual images rather than events, and these visual images have a symbolic value. "Dreams," according to Freud, "think predominantly in visual images" (*SE* 4:49). Now, it is clear that the power of seeing has a major component in Freud's awareness of the way science, as well as the mind, works. His training with Jean-Martin Charcot was a training in seeing the patient and the signs and symptoms the patient exhibited as the central key to diagnosis.[130] The nosology of the "categories" of difference is really quite analogous to Charcot's construction of the visual pattern of the actions of the hysteric. One can argue that Freud's intellectual as well as analytic development in the 1890s was a movement away from the "meaning" of visual signs (a skill he ascribes to Charcot in his obituary of 1893) and to the interpretation of verbal signs, from the "crudity" of seeing to the subtlety of hearing (*SE* 1:17). Charcot conceived the realism of the image to transcend the crudity of the spoken word. In a letter to Freud on November 23, 1891, he commented concerning the transcription of his famed Tuesday lectures that "the stenographer is not a photographer."[131] The assumption of the inherent validity of the gaze and its mechanical reproduction forms the image of the hysteric. The central argument that can be brought is that this vocabulary of seeing remains embedded in Freud's interpretation of the hysteric, who must be seen to be understood. This is not present in the earliest papers on hysteria written directly under Charcot's influence, such as Freud's differential diagnosis of organic and hysterical paralysis, written in 1886.[132] For Freud the rejection of Charcot's mode of "seeing" the hysteric is also a rejection of the special relationship the Jew has with the disease. The theme of the specific, inherited risk of the Jew for hysteria (and other forms of mental illness) was reflected in the work of Charcot that Freud translated.[133] But even more, this general claim about the hereditary risk of the Jew was linked to a diagnostic system rooted in the belief that external appearance was the source of knowledge about the pathological. For the "seeing" of the Jew as different was a topos of the world Freud lived in. Satirical caricatures were to be found throughout the German-speaking world that stressed the Jew's physical difference, and in the work of Charcot (and his contemporaries) these representations took on pathological significance. The model of seeing that Freud evokes in *The Interpretation of Dreams* is, however, not that of Jean-Martin Charcot, but that of the eugenicist Francis Galton. And the very idea of the composite central character, Irma, with specific qualities taken from a number of identifiable figures, is a Galtonian mode of seeing.

Yet Freud does not let the reader see what he sees in the dream. He describes in detail all the sights he "sees" in the dream except for one. Freud does not give us the visual image for the formula of trimethylamine **$(CH_3)_3N$**, which is found to be in vaginal secretions. According to Freud, the source of Irma's disease is thus in the sexuality of the Jewish female, the widowed Anna Lichtheim and Emma Eckstein. But hidden within the diseased nasal cavity, which has been shown by Fliess to be interchangeable with the vagina, is the symbolic reference to the person who betrayed Freud, to the "convert" who reveals himself by his action: It is **CH**, written bold for all to see, but unprinted in the text, a scientific text in which a formula could well have appeared. It is Wilhelm Fliess—hidden within the formula—the CH is the evocation of the earlier doubt about Fliess. It is the sign of "Christian," the convert, himself diseased. Freud refuses to print the formula, for it would have revealed more than he wanted. This violated one of the premises Freud presented in his mode of interpreting dreams, for visualization has a central role in creating the symbolic vocabulary of the dream. To deny the gaze of the Jew within the dream—a dream that is filled with the doctor's act of seeing and diagnosing, represses Freud's inability to deal with his own sense of betrayal and justified anxiety about Fliess's practices. It is the Jew Freud who would have been seeing the convert Fliess revealed in the visualized formula. This entire aspect vanishes as long as the formula remains unseen for the author and his reader. Just as the figures are robbed of any racial identity, so none is mentioned as a Jew, the "quack" Fliess vanishes, only to appear in the sign of the betrayer, the convert. Male sexuality becomes female sexuality, race is effaced only to reappear within the rules of interpretation that Freud outlines in his own text. The anxiety about Irma is a displacement of two fears. The first appears in the explanation—the death of Freud's patient Mathilde and the parallel Freud draws with Josef Breuer's agreement about her treatment with sulphonal, which led to her death, and Freud's consultation of him in the case of Irma. Unstated is the analogous role Fliess played in the treatment of Eckstein, which was all the more terrifying for Freud since he too had been Fliess's patient on that ill-fated trip to Vienna. To "see" Fliess, Freud must overcome his anxiety about his own body and its vulnerability. This is repressed and displaced onto the image of the woman and her sexuality. As readers, we must metamorphose the written word into the visual image Freud denies us, and this reveals to us the hidden "convert." It is at this moment that the relationship between Freud and Fliess becomes strained and finally dissolves over the work of another Jew, Otto Weininger, the convert and the neurotic. For it is indeed in a conflict about the work on bisexuality that Freud's friendship with Fliess ceased. But it is within the specimen dream, that central document in Freud's scientific life, the central text of *The Interpretation of Dreams*, that Fliess's betrayal is inscribed. In recording his memory of the dream, Freud repressed the visualization of the formula. These are the formulas of inscribed conversion that haunt Weininger's work, that haunt the pseudoscience of Freud's day and that Freud uses in his unpublished papers, such as those that accompanied his letters to Fliess. (The most notable of these is the "Project for a Scientific Psychology" [1895], which Freud quickly abandoned.)[134] For the type of visualization Weininger evoked was linked to the betrayal of the neurotic—the neurotic who was both convert and homosexual. And this is what vanished in *The Interpretation of Dreams* along with the figure of Wilhelm Fliess.

The model of "ontogeny recapitulating phylogeny" is central to Freud's assessment of the definition of the mentality of the Jew. In *Civilization and Its Discontents* (1930) Freud evokes a version of Haeckel's argument. Rather than positing a biological model of fixed, succeeding epochs or generations, Freud sees human psychological development as a variation on a theme. He notes that "the earlier phases of development are in no sense still preserved; they have been absorbed into the later phases for which they have supplied the material. . . . The fact remains that only in the mind is such a preservation of all the earlier stages along side of the final form possible, and that we are not in a position to represent this phenomenon in pictorial terms."[135] Here we have the abandonment of the Galtonian view of the visual representation of types. The abandonment of the image as fixed in the Galtonian sense is a return to the idea of the symbolic as Freud had outlined in *The Interpretation of Dreams.* It is a sign that could be understood in terms of nineteenth-century German Romantic hermeneutics, such as that of Samson Raphael Hirsch. Hirsch, one of the most important nineteenth-century German neo-Orthodox rabbinic authorities, argued that the symbolic conveyed to the inner eye information impossible to relay through logic.[136] It is a radical change in the meaning attached to the act of seeing. But it is also a model that evokes the idea of race as the universal—even if invisible—presence within the history of the individual. This model can be evoked to explain Freud's understanding of "common mental characteristics" that inscribe the Jew's psyche as thoroughly as circumcision marks the body of the male Jew.

Language and the Classical World

Freud created a new language for psychoanalysis that was intended to set it apart from the existing scientific discourse of the fin de siècle. Drawing on the status of science in Vienna, Freud also needed to distance himself from many of the presumptions of the language of science. One extended example must suffice. The cultural significance of Greek words and forms that Freud employed in creating a vocabulary for psychoanalysis has been little appreciated. Although it is certainly true that the medical vocabulary of nineteenth-century Europe (including the German-speaking countries) was "classical," that is, was composed of Latin- and Greek-based neologisms, the implication of such creations for the broader culture (in which the culture of the medical profession still played a part during this period of the rise of "international science," though to a less self-conscious level than in the eighteenth century) varied from cultural thought-collective to cultural thought-collective. When Freud uses Greek myth or even terms from Greek aesthetics (such as catharsis, which he takes from the highly popular study of Aristotle's poetics by Jakob Bernays, his wife's uncle), it is always in competition with the existing Latinate vocabulary of "high" science.[137] Latin was the language of the new Imperium, of the expansionist state. Germany, newly recreated in the 1870s, called itself the "New Rome." And Austria, the older, weaker "royal and imperial" state, felt itself threatened by the appearance of this new force in Europe. In opposition to the brutality ascribed to the image of Rome, to its anti-intellectualism, expansionism, and power, stood the European fantasy of Greece. E. M. Butler has amply shown that the German-speaking countries in the nineteenth century were under the domination of an Enlightenment image that characterized Greece as the primal culture and Greek as the language closest to the wellsprings of human experience.[138] But Greece was also the Greece of Byron—revolutionary Greece, in which an individual or a minority could challenge the domination of an imperial power. Thus Greece represented, in the nineteenth-century vocabulary of signs, not only the mind as opposed to the body, but individual action as opposed to entrenched power.

Freud's acceptance of the implications of Greek in the world of literature and myth was, at least in part, linked to his rejection of the Latinate technical vocabulary of "high sciences," biology and medicine, and the power this discourse represented. (He consciously uses Greek versions of classical myths even though it would have been more appropriate for a central European writer schooled in a German-language gymnasium to have used the Latin tradition in which he had read these myths.)[139] Thus the very evocation of Oedipus in the Oedipus complex recalled that it was from Sophocles' play that Freud had to translate as part of his high-school examinations. It was in that very high school, he remarked, that he first came to understand the label of "race" as it was applied to him (*SE* 20:9). It was the power to exclude him, on racial grounds, from the courts of power and to denigrate his undertaking on the ground that it was not "science" but "old wives' psychology." The association between the dominant position of the German political Imperium (with all its anti-Semitic overtones at the close of the nineteenth century) and the claims for centrality made by contemporary science was clear to Freud, and he rejected it through his use of Greek. This was, of course, a mode of distancing, since the intensity of anti-Semitism was as great in Vienna as it was in Berlin. But fin-de-siècle Austrian Jews saw anti-Semitism as a particularly "Prussian" problem.

Freud's creation of a new discourse for medical science, a science of healing that from its very inception focused on human sexuality, meant dealing with the question of the special discourse of Jewish sexuality, a discourse that dominated his age. And it demanded an awareness of the unique association between language (the matrix of discourse) and sexuality in the Austro-Hungarian empire. Language is the sign of discourse in a very special manner in the Austro-Hungarian empire, which had struggled with the recognition of Czech as an "official" language (in addition to German and Hungarian) during the late nineteenth century and did not even recognize the special language of the Jews, Yiddish, as a language at all. Indeed, the language of the Jews was a visible sign that their discourse was merely the biological reflex of their innate nature, and that nature, in terms of the late nineteenth century, was defined as sexualized and corrupt.

Thus it is vital to understand the personal significance for Freud of the evolution of a new manner of speaking about a series of questions in which aspects of his persona were closely implicated. The choice of the "liberating" language of the Greeks was closely tied to his sense of the link between the anti-Semitic rhetoric of the Imperium and his own ability to create a science that could transcend the limitations of this world, a world that made him (as a Jew) the object of its scientific interest. What must be noted is that Sigmund Freud, as a Viennese Jew of the late nineteenth century, was marked by the sign of his own sexual difference as embedded in the implications of his discourse. The Jew within would out no matter what attempts were made to disguise him. The convert is also unable to disguise his pathology. It is written on his tongue like the *Mauscheln* of the Jew. It is present in the form of the hidden Jew who must reveal himself. In an addition to *The Psychopathology of Everyday Life* (1901), Freud cites a case reported without commentary by Victor Tausk about a convert's experience:

> As my fiancée was a Christian and was unwilling to adopt the Jewish faith, I myself was obliged to be converted from Judaism to Christianity so that we could marry. I did not change my religion without some internal resis-

> tance, but I felt it was justified by the purpose behind it, the more so because it involved no more than an outward adherence to Judaism, not a religious conviction (which I never had). Notwithstanding this, I always continued later on to acknowledge the fact of my being a Jew, and few of my acquaintances know I am baptized. I have two sons by this marriage, who were given Christian baptism. When the boys were sufficiently old they were told of their Jewish background, so as to prevent them from being influenced by anti-Semitic views at their school and from turning against their father for such a superfluous reason. Some years ago I and my children, who were then at their primary school, were staying with the family of a teacher at the summer resort in D. One day while we were sitting at tea with our otherwise friendly hosts, the lady of the house, who had no inkling of her summer guests' Jewish ancestry, launched some very sharp attacks on the Jews. I ought to have made a bold declaration of the facts in order to set my sons the example of "having the courage of one's convictions," but I was afraid of the unpleasant exchanges that usually follow an avowal of this sort. Besides, I was alarmed at the possibility of having to leave the good lodgings we had found and thus spoiling my own and my children's limited holiday period, should our hosts' behavior towards us take an unfriendly turn because of the fact that we were Jews. As however I had reason to expect that my sons, in their candid and ingenuous way, would betray the momentous truth if they heard any more of the conversation, I tried to get them to leave the company by sending them into the garden. I said: "Go into the garden, *Juden* [Jews]," quickly correcting it to "*Jungen* [youngsters]." In this way I enabled the "courage of my convictions" to be expressed in a parapraxis. The others did not in fact draw any conclusions from my slip of the tongue, since they attached no significance to it; but I was obliged to learn the lesson that the "faith of our fathers" cannot be disavowed with impunity if one is a son and has sons of one's own. (*SE* 6:93)

This anecdote is recounted in extenso by Freud, who selects it to add to the 1919 edition of his work as a memorial to Tausk, who committed suicide in 1919.[140] His comment is that this is a "kind of self-betrayal, which did not lead to serious consequences." It is, of course, the Jew within speaking, the Jew who will not be denied. Conversion may mask the Jew, but it cannot efface him.

Freud projected aspects of his image of the immutability of the Jew within the world of Greek myth. The Jew hidden within, unchangeable, becomes the frightening exotic for the Aryan world. Just as the story of the Jewish child's conversion becomes the prototype of the story of Oedipus, so too is the Jew transformed into the Medusa. According to Freud, the fear of Medusa in Greek myth may arise because she is "a being who frightens and repels because she is castrated" and thus evokes the fear of castration in the male gaze by representing a "terror of castration that is linked to the sight of something" (*SE* 18:273). The act of seeing the Jew is tied to the epistemology of nineteenth-century science. And it is in the anthropological signs of the Jew, such as the Jew's hair, that this visibility can be read: "The hair upon Medusa's head is frequently represented in works of art in the form of snakes, and these once again are derived from the castration complex" (*SE* 18:273). The Jew is also the Medusa, for the very sight of the Jew's body evokes a hostile reaction from the Christian world. The genitalia of the Jew are just as sinister as the genitalia of the woman, since both evoke fear in the "normal" beholder—that is, the uncircumcised male. The sight of the Jew reminds the Aryan of what he can lose, what he could become.

Here is one of the reasons for Freud's flight into Greek. Greek, the language associated at the close of the nineteenth century with the image of Couperin and the Olympic movement, was the language of male bonding, of unabashed masculinity (with homoeroticism given positive value). Freud writes that "since the Greeks were in the main strongly homosexual, it was inevitable that we should find among them a representation of woman as a being who frightens and repels because she is castrated" (*SE* 18:274). Here the image of the romantic, Byronic Greece merged with the new cult of masculinity of the late nineteenth century. The "new" language is therefore a masculine language, but it is also an ambiguous one, as ambiguous as the "homoeroticism" Freud sees in his relationship with Wilhelm Fliess. Here the Jew vanishes completely. No Jew haunts the culture or literature of classical Greece. Oedipus and the Medusa may mask aspects of the Jewish body, but they are not identical with them. It is the masculine and the feminine that dominated this world. Only gender is present; race has been effaced through the adoption of this new neoclassical discourse.

Karl Abraham continued this approach in his analysis of the Prometheus legend. For Abraham, "the myth is a fragment of the repressed life of the infantile psyche of the race. It contains (in disguised form) the wishes of the childhood of the race."[141] Abraham relates to this ethnopsychological view not only classical myth, but also the myths and rituals of the Jews. Thus "the custom of the Jews rigidly required the clothing of the body," which he sees as a response to the anxiety of "the infantile wish to show ourselves naked before others" (37). Thus too he ascribes the Jew's "rigorous ethics . . . in regard to the sexual relation" to this desire to cover and hide their infantile nakedness. Abraham parallels Jewish myths with Greco-Roman and Indic legends, pointing out the similarities but also, as in the question of sexual ethics and the disclosing of the body, the great differences. The "common mental construction" of the Jews revolves about their sexuality and about their specific "wish fantasies from the childhood of the race. One thinks of the wish dream of the chosen people and of the promised land" (72). Jewish sexual activity and Jewish sexual selectivity set the mind of the Jew apart and are marked by the "symbolism of language." It is the rejection of such a negatively marked sense of difference that is echoed in Abraham's comment. Freud, in writing to Abraham in the winter of 1917, can echo this in ironically heralding the Balfour Declaration (which promised the establishment of a Jewish state in Palestine) as "the British experiment with the chosen people."[142] In Abraham's comment the negative associations with the language and sexuality of the Jews are transmuted into the atavism of their "common mental construction." Not the Jew today, at least not the acculturated Jew who has abandoned the pretensions of the biblical past, is the topic of Abraham's discussions, but the ancient Jew and his contemporary surrogate, the religious or political Jew. The acculturated Jew has abandoned the "wish fantasies from the childhood of the race" and has become capable of studying them as a scientist. The charges of a corrupt language and of a corrupt sexuality lodged against all the Jews are distanced by Karl Abraham in his use of the language of ethnopsychology.

The distancing of religious experience into the past, even the past ascribed to the herd, is one of the rhetorical strategies of these Jewish scientists. Theodor Reik, in a paper titled "The Uncanniness of Strange Gods and Cults" (1923), stated that even "Jews who were raised in religiously indifferent circumstances" feel a sense of the "uncanny" when confronted by Jewish rituals.[143] This sense of the uncanny is ascribed by Reik to an atavistic moment in their "common mental construction." But it is tempered by sensing these rituals as "grotesque" as well as "uncanny." Freud does not undertake anything similar until the very end of his life, in his writing of *Moses and Monotheism*. His focus in his early work, as Abraham notes, is the world of Greco-Roman myth and the symbolic language of European culture.

Freud's innovation of a new language of psychotherapy with its Greek myths can be seen as an alternative to the language of clinical psychiatry of his day. Freud pioneered a new nomenclature that drew on classical allusions. Here he was opposed to the innovations of his contemporary Richard Krafft-Ebing, who evoked contemporary culture with his linkage of "sadism" and "masochism" as terms for diagnostic categories. These labels were taken from the names of two writers who were either recovered during this period (the Marquis de Sade) or contemporary to it (Leopold Sacher-Masoch).[144] Freud's creation of this new language, indeed his entire creation of an abstract metapsychology, can be seen as "an effort to form an alternative language to German given the latter's built-in deprecation of and menace toward the Jew. . . . The assimilative Jew was thus essentially provided with another language. In a fashion, metapsychology replaced the void left by the loss of Yiddish and Hebrew; it allowed the Jew to transcend to some slight degree the German tongue's world view. In other ways, however, metapsychology represented a flight from meanings too painful to confront for the founding Jewish analysts."[145] Among these meanings were the readings given the Jewish body—not merely Jewish culture—within the world of medical science. For the Jew, especially the Jewish psychoanalyst, had to construct an entirely new web of meaning for the Jew's body as well as psyche. The focus of medicine remained on the intersection between mind and body. This reconstruction of a new body language needed to reinterpret every aspect of the body from the phallus to the foot.

3

THE DEGENERATE FOOT AND THE SEARCH FOR OEDIPUS

The History of the Jewish Foot

Freud's professor of biology, Carl Claus, provided a standard Aristotelian definition of "the human being" for the fin de siècle in his textbook on zoology: "With rationality and articulated language, with an upright posture, with hands and wide-soled, short-toed feet."[1] The humanity of the human being is circumscribed by the biological features Claus outlines. Humanity is defined in terms of the feet! This chapter will examine a "footnote" to the language of the Jew's pathophysiology: the reading of the Jewish foot in the culture of the late nineteenth century and Sigmund Freud's response to this vision. Carl Heinrich Stratz, whose fin-de-siècle pamphlet on the ethnology of the Jews Sigmund Freud owned, saw the Jew in no uncertain terms as defined by the form of his "flat feet." For him it was a commonplace that "European Jews have a greater percentage of physically handicapped individuals than the people among whom they live as well as non-European Jews. In addition to knock knees, flat feet, hunched backs, concave chest there are inherited constitutional illnesses. . . . One often sees *ill* and *ugly* Jews, but stupid ones hardly at all."[2] In another text from Freud's library, the stereotype of the Jew is understood as being "little, weak, knock-kneed and fat."[3] The assumption that the feet of the Jews are a sign of general physical degeneration leads to a complex response on Freud's part.

The idea that the Jew's foot is unique has analogies with the hidden sign of difference attributed to the cloven-footed devil of the Middle Ages. This is nowhere more evident than in the images illustrating the *Trophaeum Mariano-Cellense,* an account of the possession by devils of one Christoph Haizmann, a native of Bavaria, in 1677. This text served as the basis for Freud's reading (in 1923) of "a seventeenth-century demonological neurosis" (fig. 18).[4] At the turn of the century the images of the limping devil and the limping Jew are truly interchangeable. In

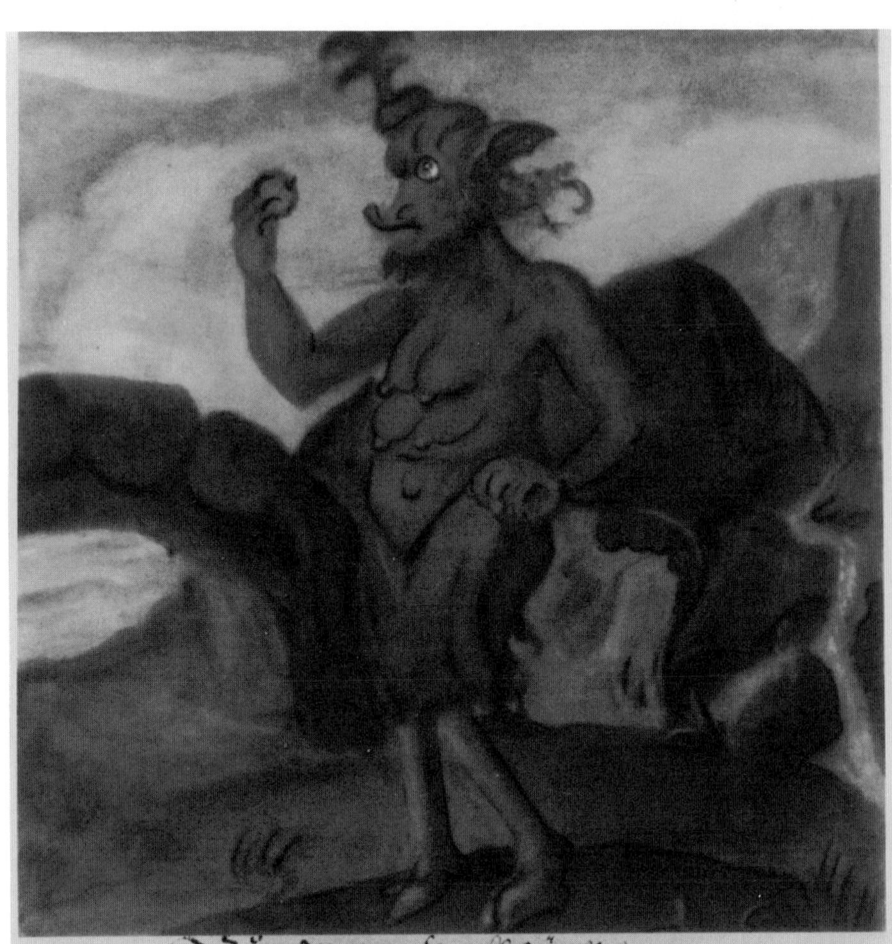

Zum Vierten; die abscheulichste gestalt, ist dise, in welcher er mir
vorkomen, vnd bey sich habent einen grossen gelben beitl, vnd mir einen grossen
Ducaten dargewisen, mit vermelden, disen
beitl voll ducaten wolte er mir iezt geben,
vnd sovill ich werde verlangen, oder
begehren, nach meinen wüntsch
solt ich es alzeit haben; aber
ich solliches gar nit an-
genomben.~

Oskar Panizza's *Council of Love* (1895), Freud's reading of which is discussed in chapter 1, the "Jewish" devil limps:

> The Devil turns on his right heel, smiles sardonically, and shrugs his shoulders. He feigns regret. Very much the Jewish merchant. A painful moment. . . .
>
> Mary . . . : By the way how is your foot?
>
> The Devil . . . : Oh, so-so! No better! But no worse, actually! Oh, god! (Hitting his shorter leg a blow.) There's no change any more! Blasted thing!
>
> Mary (in a lower voice): Your fall did that?
>
> (The Devil, not reacting, is silent for a while; then he nods gravely.)[5]

That the shape of the foot, hidden within the shoe (a sign of the primitive and corrupt masked by the cloak of civilization and higher culture), could reveal the difference of the devil was assumed in early modern European culture.

The association between the sign of the devil and the sign of disease was well established in the early modern era. Early evidence of the view that associates the faulty gait of the Jew with disease caused by demonic influence appears in Robert Burton's *Anatomy of Melancholy,* where Burton writes of the "pace" of the Jews as a sign of "their conditions and infirmities."[6] Johann Jakob Schudt, a seventeenth-century Orientalist, commented on the "crooked feet" of the Jews among other signs of their physical inferiority.[7] By the nineteenth century the relation between the image of the Jew and that of the hidden devil is to be found not in a religious but in a secularized scientific context. It still revolves in part about the particular nature of the Jew's foot—no longer the foot of the devil but now the pathognomonic foot of the "bad" citizen of the new national state. The political significance of the Jew's foot within the world of European medicine is thus closely related to the idea of the "foot," soldier, of the popular militia, which was the hallmark of all the liberal movements of the midcentury. In the 1770s the image of the Jew was of one who was physically handicapped. Johann Caspar Lavater commented on the physiognomy of Moses Mendelssohn (who was indeed round-shouldered) that he "was in no way born to be an athlete."[8] And that was the image all Jews bore. The Jew's foot marked him as congenitally unable and therefore unworthy of being completely integrated into the social fabric of the modern state.[9] This was stated, for example, in Johann David Michaelis's answer in 1783 to Christian Wil-

---

Figure 18. The goat-hooved devil from the seventeenth-century case of "demonical possession" of Christoph Haizmann analyzed by Freud in his 1923 paper. (From MS 14.084 of the Austrian National Library, Vienna.)

helm Dohm's call for the civil emancipation of the Jews. Michaelis argued that Jews could not become true citizens because they were worthless as soldiers owing to their physical stature.[10]

As early as 1804, in Joseph Rohrer's study of the Jews in the Austrian monarchy, the weak constitution of the Jews and its public sign, "weak feet," were cited as "the reason that most Jews called into military service were released, because most Jewish soldiers spent more time in the military hospitals than in military service."[11] This link of the weak feet of the Jews and their inability to be full citizens (at a time when citizenship was being extended piecemeal to the Jews) was for Rohrer merely one further sign of the inherent, intrinsic difference of the Jews. In Hermann Schaaffhausen's late nineteenth-century anthropological representation of the Jew, the gait of the Jew is related to the form of the foot: "Jews walk with their toes pointed forward and need to lift their flat feet more than do we, like the dragging gait of a lower-class individual."[12] What is of interest is how this theme of the weakness of the Jews' feet (in the form of flat feet or impaired gait) becomes part of the necessary discourse about Jewish difference in the latter half of the nineteenth century.[13]

There was an ongoing debate throughout the late nineteenth century and well into the twentieth that continued the basic theme Rohrer raised in 1804. The liberal novelist and journalist Theodor Fontane felt constrained to comment in 1870 on the false accusation that Jews were "unfitted" for war in his observations about the role Jewish soldiers played in the Seven Weeks' War of 1866 (which led to the creation of the dual monarchy and the liberal Austrian constitution). His example is telling to measure the power of the legend of the Jewish foot: "Three Jews had been drafted as part of the reserves into the first battalion of the Prince's Own Regiment. One, no longer young and corpulent, suffered horribly. His feet were open sores. And yet he fought in the burning sun from the beginning to the end of the battle of Gitschin. He could not be persuaded to go into hospital before the battle."[14] For Fontane, the Jewish foot serves as a sign of the suffering the Jew must overcome to become a good citizen. This becomes part of the liberal image of the Jew. Mark Twain finds it necessary to place special stress on the role of the Jew as soldier in his 1898 defense of the Jews, noting that the Jew had to overcome much greater difficulties in order to become a soldier than did the Christian.[15] This view of the innate cowardice of the Jew was even cited by Jewish physician-anthropologists, such as Cesare Lombroso, who saw the innate "fearfulness" of the Jews as a result of an "atavistic memory" impressed upon them as a result of the "persecutions of the Middle Ages."[16]

Jewish scientists, such as the cofounder of ethnopsychology Heinrich Steinthal, were constrained to see the cause of physical deformity, especially the deformity of gait, as a result of the pressures of civilization: "Our body is predetermined to have a specific gait because of our nature, that is, because of our anatomical construction."[17] Only "our artificial, self-consciously rehearsed patterns restore us to the natural." Only the soldier, who "is trained and schooled in his pattern of exercise walks naturally." It is the soldier who is "natural man" and is therefore also healthy, while civilization deforms the Jew's gait into a parody of the natural. Becoming a soldier also means being restored to health and natural form. Steinthal's comments are not, however, neutral—they come in a detailed review of Ernest Renan's study of the nature of the Jews and reflect a German Jewish universalization of Renan's very specific discussion of why Jews are not adequate soldiers.

In 1867 Austria institutionalized the Jews' ability to serve in the armed services as one of the basic rights of the new liberal constitution. This became not only one of the general goals of the Jews but also one of their most essential signs of acculturation. But, as in many other arenas of public service, being "Jewish" (here, espousing the Jewish religion) served as a barrier to status. Steven Beller points out that at least in Austria there was "in the army evidence [that there was] a definite link between conversion and promotion."[18] István Deák noted that of the twenty-three Jewish generals and colonels in the Austro-Hungarian army before 1911, fourteen had converted by the close of their service.[19] Indeed, one of the legends that grew up about the young, "liberal" monarch Franz Josef in the 1850s was that he promoted a highly decorated corporal from the ranks when he discovered that he had not been promoted because he was a Jew, with the remark: "In the Austrian army there are no Jews, only soldiers, and a soldier who deserves it becomes an officer."[20] Evidently it was difficult but not impossible to achieve the rank of officer. And the Jews wanted to be officers. Theodor Fontane observed that "it seemed as if the Jews had promised themselves to make an end of their old notions about their dislike for war and inability to engage in it."[21] The status associated with the role of the Jew as soldier was paralleled by the increasingly intense anti-Semitic critique of the Jewish body as inherently unfit for military service. This critique became more and more important as the barriers of Jewish entry into the armed services in Germany and Austria were lessened in the closing decades of the nineteenth century. What had been an objection based on the Jew's religion came to be pathologized as an objection to the Jewish body. Images of Jewish difference inherent within the sphere of religion become metamorphosed into images of the Jew within the sphere of public service.

The image of the Jew's foot became a central factor in the representation of Jewish difference in the late nineteenth century. The German artist and poet Wilhelm Busch, in his best-known work, *Pious Helene* (1872), actually listed the Jew's "heel" before he mentioned the Jew's nose in this often cited anti-Semitic image:

> Und der Jud mit krummer Ferse
> Krummer Nas' und krummer Hos',
> Schlängelt sich zur hohen Börse
> Tiefverderbt und seelenlos!
>
> [And the Hebrew, sly and craven,
> Round of shoulder, nose, and knee,
> Slinks to the Exchange, unshaven
> And intent on usury.][22]

(Sigmund Freud had a large volume of Wilhelm Busch's work placed in his waiting room in Vienna for the amusement of his patients.)[23] This image had a political dimension. In 1893 H. Nordmann published a pamphlet "Israel in the Army," in which the Jew's inherent unfittedness for military service is the central theme.[24] The title image stressed the Jew's badly formed, unmilitary body. One of the standard anti-Semitic catalogs of the physiology of the Jew at the fin de siècle presented the image of the Jew's foot as one of the salient markers of Jewish difference (fig. 19). This image was found on postcards from the period as well as in the leading Viennese anti-Semitic journals.[25] In each case it reflected the physical disfranchisement of the Jew. The foot became the hallmark of difference, of the Jewish body's being separate from the real "body politic." As Otto Fenichel commented in the mid-1940s:

> The physically inferior are a badly-treated minority, and, therefore, their revenge is feared. This fear is condensed with the deep feelings of uncanniness entertained toward the devil and the cripple-god, and increases when any physical disadvantage is combined with superiority in certain mental spheres (think of the uncanny, skillful, lame blacksmith of the sages). Such a combination is considered proof of a magic alliance with supernatural powers (particularly so if the bearers of such marks regard themselves as the "chosen people"). Like the Jewish language, the typical Jewish physical appearance is felt and cartooned as diabolically ugly.[26]

The association of the body and language of the Jew is clear; what is most interesting is the Jewish psychoanalyst's further association of this image with the world of Greco-Roman myth. The Jew becomes Hephaes-

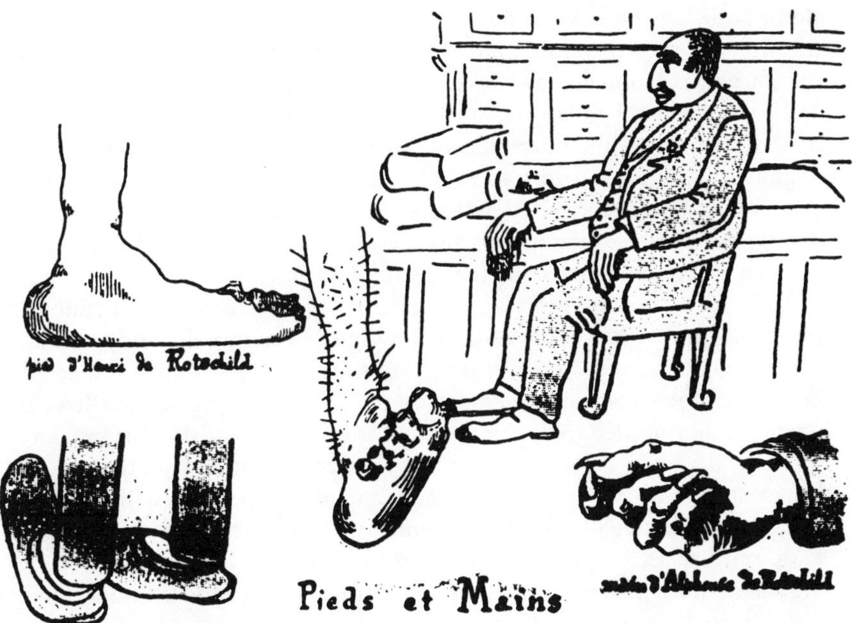

Figure 19. The image of the atavistic Jewish foot from the anti-Semitic physiological study of the Jew's body by "Docteur Celticus," *Les 19 tares corporelles visibles pour reconnaître un juif* (Paris: Librairie Antisémite, 1903). (National Library of Medicine, Bethesda, Md.)

tus. These images aimed at depicting the Jew as unable to function within the social institutions, such as the armed forces, that determined the quality of social acceptance. "Real" acceptance would be true integration into the world of the armed forces. For Fenichel, commenting on the universal nature of social stereotyping, such a move could be found within the world of myth, in which all evil is the same.

The Jewish response to the charge that Jews cannot become members of society because they cannot serve in the armed services becomes one of the foci of the Jewish response to turn-of-the-century anti-Semitism. The Defense Committee against Anti-Semitic Attacks in Berlin published its history of "Jews as soldiers" in 1897 in order to document the presence of Jews in the German army throughout the nineteenth century.[27] After the end of World War I, this view of Jewish nonparticipation became the central topos of political anti-Semitism. It took the form of the "Legend of the Stab in the Back" (*Dolchstosslegende*), which associated Jewish slackers (war profiteers who refused to serve at the front) with the loss of the war.[28] In 1919 a brochure with the title "The Jews in the War: A Statistical Study Using Official Sources" was published by Alfred

Roth, accusing the Jews of having systematically avoided service during the war in order to undermine the war effort of the home front.[29] On the part of the official Jewish community in Germany, Jacob Segall in 1922 provided a similar statistical survey to the 1897 study in which he defended Jewish soldiers during World War I against the charge of feigning inabilities in order to remain on the home front.[30] In the same year, Franz Oppenheimer drew on Segall's findings in order to provide an equally detailed critique of this charge, a charge that by 1922 had become a commonplace of anti-Semitic rhetoric.[31]

There were also attempts on the part of Jewish physicians to counter the argument of the weakness of the Jewish body within the body politic. Their arguments are, however, even more convoluted and complicated because of the constraints imposed by the rhetoric of science. As Jewish scientists they needed to accept the basic truth of the statistical arguments of medical science during this period. They could not dismiss these published statistical "facts" out of hand and thus operated within these categories. Like Segall and Oppenheimer, who answer one set of statistics with another set of statistics, the possibility of drawing the method of argument into disrepute did not exist for these scientists, since their status rested upon the validity of these positivistic methods. And their status as scientists provided a compensation for their status as Jews. As Jews, they were the object of the scientific gaze; as scientists, they were themselves the observing, neutral, universal eye.

In 1908 the eugenicist Dr. Elias Auerbach of Berlin undertook a medical rebuttal, in an essay on the "military qualifications of the Jew," of the "fact" of the predisposition of the Jew for certain disabilities that precluded military service.[32] Auerbach begins by attempting to "correct" the statistics that claimed that for every 1,000 Christians in the population there were 11.61 soldiers, but for 1,000 Jews in the population there were only 4.92 soldiers. His correction (based on the greater proportion of Jews entering the military who were volunteers and therefore did not appear in the statistics) still finds that a significant portion of Jewish soldiers were unfit for service (according to his revised statistics, of every 1,000 Christians there were 10.66 soldiers; of 1,000 Jews, 7.76). He accepts the physical differences of Jews as a given but questions whether there is a substantive reason that these anomalies should prevent them from serving in the military. He advocates the only true solution that will make the Jews of equal value as citizens: the introduction of "sport" and the resultant reshaping of the Jewish body.[33] Likewise, Heinrich Singer attributes the flat feet of the Jew to the "generally looser structure of the Jews' musculature."[34]

More directly related to the emblematic nature of the Jewish foot is the essay by Gustav Muskat, a Berlin orthopedist, which asks "whether flat feet are a racial marker of the Jew."[35] He refutes the false charge that "the clumsy, heavy-footed gait of the Semitic race made it difficult for Jews to undertake physical activity, so that their promotion within the military was impossible." While seeing flat feet as the "horror of all generals," he also refutes the charge that Jews as a group are particularly at risk for this malady. Like Auerbach, Muskat sees the problem of the weaknesses of the Jewish body as a "real" one. For him, it is incontrovertible that Jews have flat feet. Thus the question he addresses is whether this pathology is an inherent quality of the Jewish body that would preclude the Jew from becoming a full-fledged member of secular (i.e., military) society. For Muskat the real problem is the faulty development of the feet because of their misuse. The opinion that it is civilization and its impact on the otherwise "natural" body that mark the Jew becomes one of the major arguments against the sign value of the Jewish foot as a sign of racial difference.[36] The Jew is, for the medical literature of the nineteenth century, the ultimate example of the effect of civilization (the city and "modern life") on the individual.[37] Civilization in the form of the Jewish-dominated city "is the real center for the degeneration of the race and the reduction of military readiness."[38] The Jew is the city dweller par excellence as well as the most evident victim of the city.[39] And the occupation of the Jew in the city, the role as merchant, is the precipitating factor for the shape of the Jew's feet.[40]

For nineteenth-century medicine cities are places of disease, and the Jews are the quintessential city dwellers. It is the "citification" of the Jew, to use Karl Kautsky's term, that marks the Jewish foot. The diseases of civilization are the diseases of the Jew. In 1940 Leopold Boehmer can speak of the "foot as the helpless victim of civilization."[41] The shape of the Jew's foot is read in this context as the structure of the Jewish mind. The pathognomonic status of the Jew's body is a sign of the Jew's inherent difference. The Jew's body can be seen and measured in a manner that fulfills all the positivistic fantasies about the centrality of physical signs and symptoms for the definition of pathology. It can be measured as the mind cannot.

Muskat's argument is a vital one. He must shift the argument away from the inherited qualities of the Jewish body to the social anomalies inflicted on the body (and feet) of all "modern men" by their manner of living. He begins his essay with a refutation of the analogy present within the older literature, which speaks about the flat foot of the black (and by analogy of the Jew) as an atavistic sign, a sign of the earlier stage of development (in analogy to the infant, who lacks a well-formed arch). Muskat notes that flat feet have linked the black and the Jew as "throwbacks" to more primitive forms of life. He quotes a nineteenth-century ethnologist, Karl Hermann Burmeister, who in 1855 commented that "blacks and all of those with flat feet are closest to the animals." This view is seconded in one of the standard medical dictionaries of the period, one to which Sigmund Freud was asked to contribute and that helped shape his sense of professional identity.[42] There the statement is made that the "flat foot [*Pedes plani*] occurs in Jews and blacks, but perhaps here it is to be understood not as a pathological sign but as a racial one."[43]

Muskat begins his essay by denying that flat feet are a racial sign for any group, claiming they are, rather, a pathological sign of the misuse of the feet. (But he carefully avoids the implication that this misuse is the result of the urban location of the Jew or the Jew's inability to deal with the benefits of civilization.) He cites as his authorities a number of "modern" liberal commentators such as the famous Berlin physician and politician Rudolf Virchow, who had examined and commented on the feet of the black in order to refute the implication that flat feet were a sign of racial difference. Like other Jewish commentators, Muskat is constrained to acknowledge the "reality" of the "flat feet" of both the Jew and the black, but he cites the renowned Albert Hoffa[44] to the effect that only 4 percent of all flat feet are congenital. Flat feet are not a racial sign, they are "merely" a sign of the abuse of the foot. That 25 percent of all recruits in Austria and 30 percent in Switzerland were rejected for flat feet is a sign for Muskat that the Jewish recruit is no better nor worse than his Christian counterpart. (He never cites the rate of the rejection of Jewish recruits.) Muskat's rebuttal of the standard bias that sees the foot as a sign of the racial difference of the Jew still leaves the Jew's foot deformed. What Muskat has done is to adapt the view of the corruption of the Jew by civilization (and of civilization by the Jew) to create a space where the Jew's foot has neither more nor less significance as a pathological sign than does the flat foot in the general population. This attempt to universalize the quality ascribed to the Jewish foot does not, however, counter the prevailing sense of the specific meaning ascribed to the Jew's foot as a sign of difference.

Moses Julius Gutmann places the classical image of the flat foot into the new discussions of flat feet as a neurological syndrome in his 1920 dissertation, which attempted to survey the entire spectrum of charges concerning the nature of the Jewish body. Gutmann dismisses as excessive the common wisdom that "all Jews have flat feet."[45] He notes, as does Muskat, that Jews seem to have a more frequent occurrence of this malady (8 to 12 percent higher than the norm for the general population). And his source, like Muskat's, is the military statistics. But Gutmann accepts the notion that Jews have a peculiar pathological construction of the musculature of the lower extremities. Flat feet are one of the "diseases and weaknesses that make individuals inherently unfit for service." Another is the "loss or absence of the testicles."[46] Both make the male less than a full-fledged man.

In a standard handbook of eugenics published as late as 1940, the difference in the construction of the musculature of the foot is cited as the cause of the different gait of the Jew.[47] The German physician-writer Oskar Panizza, in his depiction of the Jewish body, observed that the Jew's body language was clearly marked: "When he walked, Itzig always raised both thighs almost to his mid-rift so that he bore some resemblance to a stork. At the same time he lowered his head deeply into his breast-plated tie and stared at the ground.—Similar disturbances can be noted in people with spinal diseases. However, Itzig did not have a spinal disease, for he was young and in good condition."[48] The Jew looks as if he is diseased, yet it is not the stigmata of degeneracy that the observer is seeing, but the Jew's natural stance.

This image of the pathological nature of the gait of the Jews is linked to their inherently different anatomical structure. Flat feet remain a significant sign of Jewish difference in German science through the Nazi period. The gait of the Jew is a salient sign of the Jew's essential physical difference in the most widely cited ethnological description of the Jews written in the 1930s.[49] And this view is always connected with the discourse about military service. According to Baur, Fischer, and Lenz's standard handbook of racial hygiene, first published in 1921: "Flat feet are especially frequent among the Jews. Salaman reports during the World War that about a sixth of the five thousand Jewish soldiers examined had flat feet, while in a similar sample of other English soldiers it occurred in about a fortieth."[50] In 1945 Otmar Freiherr von Verschuer can still comment without the need for any further substantiation that great numbers of cases of flat feet are to be found among the Jews.[51]

The debate about the special nature of the Jew's foot and gait enters into another sphere, that of neurology, which provides a series of links between the inherent nature of the Jew's body and psyche. This concept too has a specific political and social dimension. The assumption, even among those physicians who saw this as a positive quality, was that the Jews were innately unable to undertake physical labor:

> In no period in the history of this wonderful people since their dispersion, do we discover the faintest approach to any system amongst them tending to the studied development of physical capacity. Since they were conquered they have never from choice borne arms nor sought distinction in military

> prowess; they have been little inducted, during their pilgrimages, into the public games of the countries in which they have been located; their own ordinances and hygienic laws, perfect in other particulars, are indefinite in respect to special means for the development of great corporeal strength and stature; and the fact remains, that as a people they have never exhibited what is considered a high physical standard. To be plain, during their most severe persecutions nothing told so strongly against them as their apparent feebleness of body.[52]

It is within such a medical discourse about the relation between inability to serve as a citizen and the form of the Jew's body that the debate about Jews and sport can be located. Elias Auerbach's evocation of sport as the social force to reshape the Jewish body had its origins in the turn-of-the-century call of the physician and Zionist leader Max Nordau for a "new muscle Jew."[53] This view became a commonplace of the early Zionist literature, which called upon sport, as an activity, to be one of the central means of shaping the new Jewish body.[54] Nordau's desire was not merely for an improvement in the physical well-being of the Jew, but rather an acknowledgment of the older German tradition that saw an inherent relationship between the healthy political mind and the healthy body. It was not merely *mens sana in corpore sano,* but the sign that the true citizen had a healthy body that provided the ability to be a full-scale citizen, itself a sign of mental health. Nordau's cry that "we have killed our bodies in the stinking streets of the ghettos and we must now rebuild them on the playing fields of Berlin and Vienna" is picked up by the mainstream of German Jewish gymnastics. It is through the articulation of Nordau's views about the reconstitution of the Jewish body that the first Jewish gymnastic society, the Makkabi-Turnverein, was founded.[55]

In Vienna at the third Jewish Gymnastics Competition, all the lectures on the need for increased exercise among the Jews departed from the assumption of a statistically provable physical degeneration of contemporary Jewry.[56] The medicalization of this theme is continued in 1908 by M. Jastrowitz of Berlin in the *Jewish Gymnastics News,* the major Jewish newspaper devoted to gymnastics.[57] Jastrowitz accepts the basic premise of Nordau's conviction, that the Jewish body is at risk for specific diseases, and attempts to limit and focus this risk. For Jastrowitz the real disease of the Jews, what marks their bodies, is a neurological deficit that has been caused by the impact of civilization. Jastrowitz, like most of the Jewish physicians of the fin de siècle, accepts the general view that Jews are indeed at special risk for specific forms of mental and neurological disease. He warns that too great a reliance on sport as a remedy may exacerbate these illnesses. For Jastrowitz, the attempt to create the "new muscle Jew" works against the inherent neurological weaknesses of the Jew. This is the link to the general attitude of organic psychiatry of the latter half of the nineteenth century, which saw the mind as a product of the nervous system and assumed that "mind illness is brain illness." Thus the improvement of the nervous system through training the body would positively affect the mind (so Nordau). Jastrowitz's view also assumes a relationship, and he fears that, given the inherent weakness of the Jewish nervous system, any alteration of the precarious balance would negatively affect the one reservoir of Jewish strength, the Jewish mind. Jews could forfeit the qualities of mind that have made them successful in the world by robbing their brains of oxygen through overexercise. For Nordau and Jastrowitz the relationship between the healthy body, including the healthy foot and the healthy gait, and the healthy mind is an absolute one. The only question left is whether the degeneration of the Jewish foot is alterable. But this is not simply a problem for orthopedists; neurologists, such as Sigmund Freud, also become closely involved in this debate through the discussion of the new diagnostic category of intermittent claudication.

The diagnosis of *claudication intermittente* was created by Jean-Martin Charcot at the beginning of his medical career in 1858.[58] (Charcot not only taught Freud but also was Nordau's doctoral supervisor.) This diagnostic category was described by Charcot as the chronic recurrence of pain and tension in the lower leg, a growing sense of stiffness, and finally a total inability to move the leg, which causes a marked and noticeable inhibition of gait. This occurs between a few minutes and a half hour after beginning an activity such as walking. It spontaneously vanishes, only to be repeated at regular intervals. Charcot does not speculate on the etiology of this syndrome. Like flat feet, intermittent claudication is a "reality," that is, it exists in the real world, but like flat feet it was placed in a specific ideological context at the turn of the century.

Charcot determined that this syndrome seemed to result from reduction of blood flow through the arteries of the leg and led to the virtual disappearance of any pulse from the four arteries that provide the lower extremity with blood. The interruption of circulation to the feet leads to the initial symptoms and can eventually cause even more severe symptoms such as spontaneous gangrene. Charcot's diagnostic category was rooted in work done by veterinarians, such as Bouley and Rademacher, who observed similar alterations in the gait of dray horses.[59] Charcot does not speculate on any racial predisposition for this syndrome, unlike his feelings on the origin of hysteria and diabetes,[60] but the image of the

Jew's foot as an atavistic structure, similar to the flat feet of the horse (an argument refuted by Muskat) reappears at the very roots of this syndrome.

What is vital is that this diagnostic category soon became the marker in neurology for the difference between the Jewish foot and that of the "normal" European. This diagnostic category became part of the description of the pathological difference of the Jew, and it was itself differentiated from other "racially" marked categories that evoked the impairment of gait as part of their clinical presentation. Charcot clearly differentiated intermittent claudication from the chronic pain associated with the diabetic's foot (a diagnostic category so closely associated with Jews in nineteenth-century medicine that diabetes was commonly called the "Jewish disease").[61] In 1911 Joseph-Jules Déjerine also differentiated this syndrome from "spinal intermittent claudication."[62] This was one of the syndromes associated with syphilis, a disease that also had a special relationship to the representation of the Jew in nineteenth- and early twentieth-century medicine.[63] What is clear is that the sign of the "limping Jew" was read into a number of diagnostic categories of nineteenth-century neurology.

Very quickly, intermittent claudication became one of the specific diseases associated with eastern European Jews. H. Higier in Warsaw published a long paper in 1901 in which he summarized the state of the knowledge about intermittent claudication as a sign of the racial makeup of the Jew.[64] Most of the twenty-three patients he examined were Jews, and he found that the etiology of the disease was "the primary role of the neuropathic disposition [of the patients] and the inborn weakness of their peripheral circulatory system." By the time Higier published his paper at the turn of the century this was a given in the neurological literature. The debate about the flat feet of Jews as a marker of social stigma gave way to the creation of a scientific discourse about the difference of the Jew's feet that does not merely rely on the argument of atavism, which had been generally refuted in the neurological literature of the fin de siècle, but hinges on the question of the relation between the Jew's body and mind through the image of the deficits of the neurological system. Intermittent claudication became a sign of inherent constitutional weakness, so that it was also to be found as a sign for the male hysteric.[65] Hysteria was, of course, also a neurological deficit found among eastern European Jewish males. It was the male Jew from the East, from the provinces, who was at risk for hysteria. And the symptom of the hysteric that most characterizes the Eastern Jew was his impaired gait. The association of hysteria with the impairment of gait can be traced back to the eighteenth century.[66] It remained a truism of medical science through the decades. The hysterical and the limping Jew are related in the outward manifestation of their illness: both are represented by the inability of the limbs to function "normally," by the disruption of their gait, as we have seen in Freud's case of Dora (a pseudonym masking the identity of the eastern European Jew Ida Bauer).[67] Not only did Dora limp—the symptoms of her hysteria that represented the "false step" she had taken in her relationship to the man who attempted to seduce her—but her foot "had swelled up and had to be bandaged" (*SE* 7:103). The "swollen foot" of the Jew, as we shall see, takes on yet further significance in the context of the debate about the Jews' predisposition for specific forms of illness.

The link between the older discussion of "flat feet" and the new category of intermittent claudication was examined in a number of sources. H. Idelsohn in Riga made overt the association among the Jews, Charcot's category of intermittent claudication, and flat feet when he examined his Jewish patients to see whether there was any relation between the fabled Jewish flat feet and inherent muscular weakness.[68] He placed the discussion of the special nature of the Jewish foot into the context of a neurological deficit. Although he did not wish to overdetermine this relationship (according to his own statement), he did find that there was reason to grant flat feet a "specific importance as an etiological moment." He described the flat foot, citing Hoffa, as "tending to sweat, often blue colored and cold, with extended veins. . . . People with flat feet are often easily tired, and are incapable of greater exertion and marches" (300). He saw in this description a visual and structural analogy to Charcot's category of intermittent claudication. Heinrich Singer picked up Idelsohn's and Higier's views concerning the relation between intermittent claudication and flat feet and repeated them as proof of the "general nervous encumbrance borne by the Jewish race."[69] This conviction is echoed by Gustav Muskat in a paper of 1910, in which he made the link between the appearance of intermittent claudication and the preexisting pathology of flat feet.[70]

One of Idelsohn's major sources for his attitude was a paper by Samuel Goldflam in Warsaw.[71] Goldflam was one of the most notable neurologists of the first half of the century and the codiscoverer of "Goldflam-Oehler sign" (the paleness of the foot after active movement) in the diagnosis of intermittent claudication.[72] Goldflam stressed the evident predisposition of Jews for this syndrome. What was also noteworthy in Goldflam's discussion of his patients was not only that they were all Eastern Jews, but that almost all were very heavy smokers. He did attribute a role in the etiology of the disease to tobacco intoxication.[73] Idelsohn argued that since *all* of Goldflam's patients were Jews, it was clear that intermittent claudication was primarily a Jewish disease and that this was proved by the relationship between the evident sign of the difference of the Jewish foot, the flat foot, and its presence in a number of his own cases. He attributed its absence in the clinical description given by Goldflam (and others) to its relatively benign and usual occurrence, which was often overlooked because of the radical problems, such as gangrene, that occurred with intermittent claudication.

In a major review essay on the "nervous diseases" of the Jews, Toby Cohn, a noted Jewish neurologist (long the assistant of the noted Emanuel Mendel at the University of Berlin), included intermittent claudication as one of his categories of neurological deficits.[74] While commenting on the anecdotal nature of the evidence and calling on a review essay by the Jewish neurologist Kurt Mendel (who does not discuss the question of "race" at all),[75] he accepted the specific nature of the Jewish risk for this syndrome while leaving the etiology open. Two radically different etiologies had been proposed: the first, as we noted for Higier, Idelsohn, and Mendel, reflected on the neuropathic qualities of the Jewish body, especially in regard to diseases of the circulatory system. (Hemorrhoids, another vascular syndrome, are also cited as a "Jewish" disease.) The other potential etiology noted by Goldflam and Cohn did not reflect on the inherent qualities of the Jewish foot but focused on the misuse of tobacco and the resulting occlusion of the circulatory system of the extremities. Tobacco, according to Wilhelm Erb, played a major role in the etiology of intermittent claudication.[76] In a somewhat later study of forty-five cases of the syndrome, Erb found, to his own surprise, that at least thirty-five of his patients showed an excessive use of tobacco.[77] (This meant smoking forty to sixty cigarettes or ten to fifteen cigars a day.) Indeed, the social dimension the latter provide in their discussion of the evils of tobacco misuse is an answer to the image of the Jew's neurological predisposition to be unfit for military service.[78] But the misuse of tobacco is a sign of the Eastern Jew, not the Western Jew. Goldflam's patients were all seen in Warsaw. The noted Berlin neurologist Hermann Oppenheim observed that of the cases of intermittent claudication in his practice (forty-eight cases over five years) he found that the overwhelming majority, between thirty-five and thirty-eight, were Russian Jews.[79] The Eastern Jew's mind is that of a social misfit, and the body reifies this role, but this is not a problem of Western Jewry except by extension.

Certainly the most public discussion of intermittent claudication and its special relation to the Jewish foot came in August 1927, in a scandal concerning Otto Lubarsch, who succeeded Rudolf Virchow as professor of pathological anatomy at the Charité, the major teaching hospital in

Berlin. Lubarsch was reported in the popular press to have revealed the name of the person whose corpse he was publicly autopsying.[80] Although all deaths at the Charité resulted in autopsies (with no need for the consent of the family), the individuals' identities were kept strictly secret. Lubarsch, a converted Jew and a right-wing supporter of the monarchy (he had been involved in the 1920 attempt to topple the Weimar Republic), performed an autopsy on the body of Iwan Kutisker, a Russian Jew who had been convicted of embezzling some fourteen million marks from the Prussian State Bank. Kutisker's death following his conviction led to the accusation that his request for medical help had been ignored. The authorities, including the physicians who had examined him, claimed he had feigned his symptoms. Lubarsch's autopsy was meant to resolve this question once and for all.

In the autopsy, done before a classroom full of students, Lubarsch observed that "one normally finds intermittent limping among Eastern Jews because of their high consumption of cigarettes." In life Kutisker had shown no such symptoms. But Lubarsch continued and identified the patient by name to his audience, commenting that "he had been infected with syphilis twenty years ago and smoked daily, as it is the custom among Eastern Jews, twenty to thirty cigarettes." Lubarsch was quoted in the *Berlin Daily News* on August 1, 1927, and the newspaper attributed his comments to an attempt to conceal his own Jewish ancestry, since converts were felt to need to be even more anti-Semitic than the anti-Semites. This incident, which associated intermittent claudication with the limping foot of an Eastern Jew, a convert, syphilis, smoking, and the charge of dissimulation, became a major scandal. Lubarsch's right to teach was withdrawn by the authorities, and intermittent claudication became a public sign of the difference between Western Jews (such as Lubarsch felt himself to be) and Eastern Jews.

Here the parameters of the meaning ascribed to the Jewish foot are set: Jews walk oddly because of the form of their feet and legs. This unique gait represents the inability of the Jew to function as a citizen within a state that defines full participation as the ability to engage in military service. Jewish savants, who rely on the status of science as central to their own self-definition, cannot dismiss the statistical evidence of Jewish risk. They seek to "make sense" of it in a way that would enable them (as representatives of the authoritative voice of that very society) to see a way out. The "way out" is, in fact, to accept difference by attributing it to social rather than genetic causes and by projecting it onto a group labeled as inherently "different," the Eastern Jews. This is an important moment in the work of these scientists—for the risk they see lies in the East, in the "misuse" of tobacco by Eastern Jews. It is not accidental that the major reports on the nature of the Jew's gait come from eastern Europe and are cited as signs of the difference in social attitudes and practices among eastern European Jews. The rhetorical movement these scientists undertook implied an inherently different role for the Western Jew, serving in the armed forces of the empire, whether German or Austrian. This movement was important because the clean line between inheritance and environment was blurred in nineteenth-century medicine. The physician of the nineteenth and early twentieth centuries presumed that the appearance of signs of degeneration, such as flat feet, may have been triggered by aspects in the social environment but was, at its core, an indicator of the inherent weakness of the individual. The corollary to this is the inheritance of acquired characteristics—that the physiological changes that environment triggers become part of the biological inheritance of an individual. The damage rendered by environmental factors ("tobacco") to the Jewish foot thus marks subsequent generations. The loop is thus complete: whether hereditary or environmental, the qualities of "poor citizenship" are marked by the Jewish foot. For non-Jewish scientists of the late nineteenth century, this marker exists as a sign of the Jewish body. For Jewish scientists, whose orientation is Western (no matter what their actual geographic locus), these qualities are a sign of the atavistic nature of the Eastern Jews and serve as a boundary between the degenerated Jews in the East and the Western Jews.

Freud's Footwork

During 1879–80, Freud's academic career was interrupted for a year of compulsory military service. We know very little about what he did, but we do know that he marched, as all soldiers everywhere and at every time march. In a postcard to his friend Eduard Silberstein in January 1879 he notes that he has been marching with his unit throughout Bosnia.[81] He complains of lice and of fever, but he does not complain of sore feet. He was a good Jewish soldier except for being absent without leave on his twenty-fourth birthday, which led to a stiff punishment.[82] His reserve unit went on maneuvers in Olmütz in August and September 1887, where he literarily played at being a soldier, tagging "wounded" soldiers with descriptions of their "wounds." During this period he was promoted a full grade from *Oberarzt* to *Regimentsarzt*. "Rising at half-past three in the morning, they marched and marched until after noon" (1:193). To his mentor Josef Breuer he complained about the visibility of his status as an officer: "I detest the idea of having inscribed on my collar how much I am worth, as if I were the sample of some product." Freud's rejection of this type of visibility (an an officer) meant, however, that he acknowledged his own invisibility as a Jew in this role. But he also seemed to enjoy "playing at war," which fulfilled his childhood desire to become an officer.[83]

As a child, Freud recounted in *The Interpretation of Dreams,* he would play with wooden soldiers representing Napoleon's marshals. And his "declared favorite was already Masséna (or to give the name its Jewish form, Manasseh)" (*SE* 4:197–98). Napoleon's "Jewish" marshal was understood by the youthful Freud as his double, since he shared his birthday. And Freud had "dreams of becoming a great general himself."[84] Masséna was also very much the opposite, according to Freud's own account, of Freud's father. Freud saw in the "Jewish" soldier the pride in the power of the Jew as a member of the body politic. This feeling answered the humiliation he felt as a child when his father told him, while on a walk, that when he was assaulted by an anti-Semitic rowdy who tossed his hat into the street that he had simply moved into the gutter and picked up his hat.[85] (At the time this seemed such a "Jewish" response that Freud questioned whether his hero Masséna really was Jewish.)

Freud informs us that he compensated in fantasy for his father's perceived weakness and passivity by remembering the toughness of Hannibal's father, who pressed his son to swear vengeance on the Romans. No such demand for revenge against the non-Jews was forthcoming from Freud's father. Hannibal, the Semitic soldier, is thus but a "transference of an already formed emotional relation" of the association Freud had with the "Jewish" marshal Masséna and Jewish soldiers in general with their proud gait.[86] Jakob Freud revealed his weak, Eastern Jewish nature to his son during a walk. His timidity was shown to Sigmund by his father's stepping off the curb into the gutter to retrieve his hat. How very different from the account Sigmund Freud's eldest son Martin tells of his father's running, with his walking stick raised, into a crowd that had threatened his sons with anti-Semitic remarks![87]

Like Fontane's good soldiers, Freud did not complain about walking, because that would have been a sign of his unfitness for a role in the social structure of the empire. And the physical and psychological fitness of Jews for military service was a topic of public debate in Germany and Austria at the fin de siècle. One of the jokes Freud recounts in *Jokes and Their Relation to the Unconscious* (1905), which he collected in the mid-1890s, recounts the tale of a Jewish recruit: "Itzig had been declared fit for service in the artillery. He was clearly an intelligent lad, but intractable and without any interest in service. One of his superior officers, who was friendly disposed to him, took him on one side and said to him: 'Itzig, you're no use to us. I'll give you a piece of advice: buy yourself a cannon and make yourself independent!'" (*SE* 8:56). Freud explained that this joke revolved around the officer's showing Itzig how stupid he is by being even more stupid than the soldier. It also shows the importance Freud placed on Jews' being "declared fit for service." The question is raised here of whether Jews will be fit for the military. Freud's reading also excludes the clear reference to the alternative occupation suggested for Itzig—that of a "trading Jew." "Even if you are physically fit," the joke implied, "you are neither psychologically nor morally fit."

Freud's military service was also at a time when the question of the presence of Jews in the army, especially in the officer corps, was beginning to be raised. Given the great number of Jewish physicians, it is no wonder that Jewish doctors also were visible in the Austro-Hungarian army. In the 1870s Jewish physicians were a clear presence in the officer corps.[88] As early as 1855, there had been 157 Jewish officers in the imperial army; many of them were in the medical corps. By 1893 there were 40,344 Jews in the army, and 2,179 were officers. This was a much greater percentage than that of Jews (8 percent) in the general population.[89] The role of reserve officer, which gave the petite bourgeoisie in Vienna much of its class standing, was in general open to Jews as long as their numbers remained relatively small. In 1897, the first year that military statistics differentiated between career and reserve officers, the army had 1,993 Jewish reserve officers, or 18.7 percent of the total reserve officer corps.[90]

But as the numbers of Jews in the army officer corps increased, the general attitude toward Jews in the Austrian army worsened. Thus Arthur Schnitzler had his "royal and imperial" officer, *Leutnant* Gustl, in the 1901 novella of the same name, mull over the "nasty business" of what Jews were doing impinging on "his" world.[91] This was especially true for military physicians. In 1901 it became clear that while Jewish physicians had been appointed up through the ranks, even to the rank of general, the new imperial minister of war, Edmund Krieghammer, was refusing stipends to Jewish students who desired to become career medical officers.[92] By 1904 the official publication of Austrian Jewry noted a substantial decline in the number of Jewish medical officers and charged this decline to the rising tide of anti-Semitism within the army.[93]

One incident in Freud's life that turned on the social status of the reserve officer occurred at the beginning of 1885. He reports with great satisfaction to his fiancée Martha Bernays that his friend and scientific rival Carl Koller had clashed with a fellow surgeon who then turned on him and called him a *Saujud* ("Jewish swine"). Koller slapped the man, who was forced to accept this challenge to a duel with sabers, "as both were reserve officers."[94] (The credibility of the Jew as one socially able to present or accept challenges was one of the factors that marked the decline of Jewish social prestige in Germany and Austria during the latter half of the nineteenth century.) Officers were *satisfaktionsfähig,* worthy of being challenged to a duel, and this was a clear mark of social integration. Even Theodor Herzl found that he "relished the test and adventure of the duel, the so-called *Mensur,* which was considered manly and edifying."[95] On the same day as he wrote to Martha Bernays reporting this incident, Freud also wrote a moving letter to Koller congratulating him on his bravery and asking to address him with the familiar *Du.* Koller won the duel and was rewarded by his friends with a bottle of champagne. Koller's status as a reserve officer gave him a special relation to his society. Freud was quite aware of the importance of the army as a means of providing social status, of making the Jew officially acceptable. Thus the marching Freud undertook through Bosnia was itself a sign of belonging to the citizenry of the nation-state.

Freud's earliest confrontation with the theme of the Jew's foot is cast within the discourse of degeneracy theory. The mark of the criminal is written on the very body of the Jew for all to see. It is read in the stigmata of the degenerate, which reflect every aspect of the difference of the Jew and reveal his criminal nature. If the alteration of gait is a sign of degeneracy, a category Freud struggles against, it is a sign that is inscribed in Freud's paradigmatic text, the "dream of Irma's injection," the specimen dream in *The Interpretation of Dreams* (1900). There it is Josef Breuer, a transplanted Eastern Jew like Freud, who bears the mark of the Jew, the limping sign of difference. "Dr. M. looked quite different from usual; he was very pale, he walked with a limp and his chin was clean-shaven" (*SE* 4:107). This handicapped, ill individual is of course a very different Breuer from the heavily bearded, swarthy-skinned figure we know from the photographs of the mid-1890s. Freud provides an interpretation that ties the figure of Breuer to the figure of his older half brother, who had fled to England as a result of his uncle Josef's criminal acts: "I thought of my elder brother, who lives abroad, who is clean-shaven and whom, if I remembered right, the M. of the dream closely resembled. We had news a few days earlier that he was walking with a limp owing to an arthritic condition of his hip" (*SE* 4:112). Freud's own father as well as his older half brothers in England may well have been involved in trading in counterfeit rubles, a crime for which Freud's uncle Josef, whose figure haunted Freud's dreams, was jailed.

Freud sees Breuer and his half brother as aspects of the same composite image. But what are the similarities, the Galtonian qualities that shine through to create a composite of the two men? It clearly is nothing in their physiognomy, their occupation, or their location that makes them similar. What makes them alike is that they are older Jews, not quite Freud's father's age, but also not his contemporaries, who have "rejected a certain suggestion I had recently laid before them" (*SE* 4:112). Breuer's rejection of the theory of the sexual etiology of neurosis and Emmanuel Freud's rejection of an unspecified idea are linked. In Freud's dream it is the denying Jew who becomes the criminal Jew, limping as a sign of his difference. Hidden within the Jew is the sign of the degenerate, limping Jewish criminal. For it is the Jew who is three times more likely than other Austrians to commit economic crimes, such as "the counterfeiting of documents."[96] Jewish criminality in Freud's world as well as in his dreams is tied to the falsification and denial of the social "realities" of the world.

The diseased foot remained a sign of social affliction of the male Jew, and specifically of the Eastern Jew. In his scientific writings Freud transfers this image almost entirely into the realm of the female hysteric. The foot of the hysteric is in a real way at the core of her dilemma or at least represents this dilemma in the most visible manner. In a long note added in 1909 to *The Interpretation of Dreams,* Freud illustrated how the chronological reversal of events in dreams (where the end of a sequence of events comes at the beginning) is paralleled in the case of a hysterical patient:

> Hysterical attacks sometimes make use of the same kind of chronological reversal in order to disguise their meaning from observers. For instance, a hysterical girl needed to represent something in the nature of a brief romance in one of her attacks—a romance of which she had had a fantasy in her unconscious after an encounter with someone on the suburban railway. She imagined how the man had been attracted by the beauty of her foot and had spoken to her while she was reading; whereupon she had gone off with him and had had a passionate love-scene. Her attack *began* with a representation of this love-scene by convulsive twitching of her body, accompanied by movements of her lips to represent kissing and tightening of her arms to represent embracing. She then hurried into the next room, sat down on a chair, raised her skirt to show her foot, pretended to be reading a book and spoke to me (that is, answered me). (*SE* 4:328)

Freud's reading of the fantasy of seduction centers on the beauty of the foot. The beautiful foot is not the flat foot, at least according to Freud's professor of physiology, Ernst Brücke.[97] The flat foot does not reflect the aesthetic ideals of High Renaissance art but is a mark of the modern body. It is clearly not the mark of the exemplary Jewish woman, whether hysteric or historic, who limps. For if Freud's Dora suffered from a swollen foot and limped, so too did that figure who served the late nineteenth century as the exemplary Jewish woman, Rahel Varnhagen. Her "lame foot" became a sign of her difference, a difference like her Jewish identity, which she strove to overcome. It made her "ugly" in the eyes of the society she dwelled in, and she was constrained to internalize that sense of difference.[98]

It is the beautiful foot that is central to Freud's understanding of the young woman's fantasy about seduction. What is important is that she hurries into the next room. Her gait as well as her foot marks her as a sexualized being, fantasizing about the male's member. In another retelling of this case, also in 1909, Freud presents the material in slightly condensed fashion as a hypothetical case study: "Supposing, for instance, that a hysterical woman has a fantasy of seduction in which she is sitting reading in a park with her skirt slightly lifted so that her foot is visible; a gentleman approaches her and speaks to her; they then go somewhere and make love to one another" (*SE* 9:231). It is the exposed foot, naked and visible, that marks the self-absorption of the hysteric. The social act of exposing the foot to the gaze of the male, like the exposure of the Jew's foot to the gaze of the scientist, reveals the woman's desire to seduce the male. This is Freud's reading of Dora's misstep in her supposed attraction to and simultaneous repulsion by Herr K. The male Jew desires to disguise the Jewish foot, to maintain his manliness as an officer and a gentleman. But the racial sign of the Jewish foot becomes a substitute for the circumcised penis, the sexual center of Freud's concern. It becomes the sign of a pathology that transcends the category of race.

Freud stressed, in his studies of the development of human sexuality, the meaning of the foot fixation of the hysteric and tied it to a fantasy about smell (with its evocation of the *foetor judaicus,* the stench attributed to the Jew even in the medical literature of Freud's day).[99] He further tied it to that central marker of Jewish difference, the circumcised penis, in the form of the "castrated" genitalia of the female: "Both the feet and the hair are objects with a strong smell which have been exalted into fetishes after the olfactory sensation has become unpleasurable and been abandoned. Accordingly, in the perversion that corresponds to foot-fetishism, it is only dirty and evil-smelling feet that become sexual objects. Another factor that helps towards explaining the fetishistic preference for the foot is to be found among the sexual theories of children: the foot represents a woman's penis, the absence of which is deeply felt" (*SE* 7:155). The missing penis is the sign of the damaged genitalia, the sign of the inferiority of the Jew, at least according to Freud's reading. We know from the general discussions of this anxiety that it is the male

Jew who serves Freud as the example of the socially "castrated" member of society. The foot of the Other becomes analogous to the castrated/ circumcised penis, the missing member, for both the woman and the Jew.

Such a reading is further supported by Freud's clinical account of the patient who felt that a "young man whom she had met regularly near the doctor's house, and who used as a rule to look at her admiringly, had on the last occasion looked contemptuously at her feet" (*SE* 23:196). This contempt came from the patient's association of the young man with her elder brother and her attempt to micturate like him, during which she wet her shoes. Her brother "looked contemptuously at her shoes with the object of reminding her of her misfortune." The foot comes to represent the "envy for the penis" and forms part of the patient's psychological profile. Following that attempt she never tried to do anything a second time if she had failed at first. The missing penis is represented in her psychological makeup by the gaze at her foot. The patient had associated the young man with Freud (thinking that he was his son). The image of the Jewish male who looks contemptuously at the woman's foot (whether she is a Jew or not) certainly played a role in providing the symbolic and emotional associations for that episode. The interchangeability of the (Jewish) foot and the (circumcised) penis is possible only if both have the role of associating the castrated self (the woman) with the damaged Other (the Jewish male). This is a specifically Jewish reading of the foot.

The discussion of the castration complex is a central part of what Freud comes to call the Oedipus complex.[100] In reading the tale of Oedipus as a Greek transposition of his own "seduction" by the family's Catholic servant, Freud represses one of the salient elements of the legend. It is an element that is one of the most evident parts of the tale, since it is literally inscribed in the name of "Oedipus." Recently critics have pointed out that Freud eliminated the entire early history of Oedipus, whose name meant, even in the classical world, one with swollen feet. (The "swollen feet" of Freud's Dora thus reflect her own relationship to her syphilitic Jewish father.) Oedipus's father, Laius, exposed the child and pierced his ankles so that his ghost would not walk.[101] Polybus the shepherd found the child and named him Oedipus from the state of his feet. Freud knew this etymology from his primary reading of the Oedipus myth and closely marked much of the chapter in his source.[102] No mention of this is to be found in his discussion of the myth.

Much has been made of this concerning the repression of "child abuse" by Freud. More likely the central association with the damaged feet and impaired gait of Oedipus, given that Freud employs the myth to universalize the tale he tells of his own experience of seduction by the

Catholic servant, is to excise any reference to his own exposure to the temptation of conversion. Thus the damaged foot of the child of Greek legend points toward the foot of the Jew. Indeed, Karl Abraham understood the piercing of Oedipus's feet as an act of symbolic castration, and it is the overt association between circumcision (which marks the Jew) and castration that is evoked in this representation.[103] The very act Laius wishes to avoid, the incestuous marriage of his son, evoked the implications of Jewish sexual selection, which was understood as "dangerous inbreeding" in the science of the time.

But if the foot was a representation of the nature of the Jewish body within Freud's world, it also came to be a sign of the difference of the Jewish mind. The Eastern Jew was the Jew who spoke badly, with a marked accent. The limping of the Jew, the being on a poor footing, becomes a metaphor for Freud's language, his mode of reading. The Jew needs to be on "firm footing" when he reads as a scientist, and Freud fears that he is not. It is part of the discourse of interpretation based on "psychological probabilities and [that] lacked any objective proof" (*SE* 22:17), an interpretation about the nature of the Jewish body, and specifically the meaning of circumcision, as in his "historical novel" on Moses, that Freud fears may also not be on "firm footing": "The greater the importance of views arrived at in this way, the more strongly one feels the need to beware of exposing them without a secure basis to the critical assaults of the world around one—like a bronze statue with feet of clay" (*SE* 23:17). This view is repeated about his later *Moses,* the work that eventually appeared in its entirety only after he fled to England in 1938. He wrote to Arnold Zweig on November 1, 1934: "More important is the fact that this historical novel [the first part of his *Moses and Monotheism*] won't stand up to my own criticism. I need more certainty and I should not like to endanger the final formula of the whole book, which I regard as valuable, by founding it on a base of clay."[104] Freud's reading of Moses may well be like a Jewish statue, one that has feet of clay. This sense that the Jew's science is built on sand is an echo of the conclusion of *Beyond the Pleasure Principle* (1920), where Freud quotes Friedrich Rückert: "We may take comfort, too, for the slow advances of our scientific knowledge in the words of the poet:

> What we cannot reach flying we must reach limping. . . .
> The Book tells us it is no sin to limp.
>
> (*SE* 18:64)

It is of course not the Jew here who limps, but the progress of neutral, universal science, the new science of psychoanalysis. But Freud feared it would be regarded as a Jewish science, framed by the "common mental construction" of the Jews about him. Quoting a line from Rückert's "translations" from the Arabic (which were as popular in Germany as those of Edward FitzGerald were in England) evoked the "Orient" without directly evoking the Jew.

The analogy between the foot of the hysteric, which is revealed and reveals, and that of the Jew, which is hidden but still reveals, is echoed in Freud's own account of the Jewish foot. The clay feet of the Jewish reader in regard to the figure of the biblical Moses are mirrored in a strange omission in Freud's reading of another Moses. In this reading it is the position, the gait, that marks the Jewish foot as much as its form. This raised foot can be found in Freud's analysis of Michelangelo's statue of Moses, who "will spring to his feet—his left foot is already raised from the ground—[and] dash the Tables to the earth, and let loose his rage upon his faithless people" (fig. 20).[105] The statue has "his right foot rest[ing] on the ground and his left leg is raised so that only the toes touch the ground" (*SE* 13:221). Freud makes nothing of the placement of Moses' foot in these interpretations and descriptions that he quotes or paraphrases. There is an absence of any notice on his part of the feet of the statue, to such an extent that all the line drawings of the statue he provides cut the image off above the feet (fig. 21). As much as the fantasy of the "Jewish horns," reflected in Michelangelo's sculpture, it is vital to comprehend the significance of the feet for the image of the Jew as read by another Jew. The Jewishness of the image is repressed.

Freud's repressed image of the Jewishness of Moses echoes the underlined description of the statue from the guidebook Freud took with him to Rome.[106] That discussion turns that *Moses* into the hidden image of Michelangelo's patron, Pope Julius II, who shows a "manly anger at the idolatry of the Jews." Indeed, the power of the "ruler's face" is such that the "Jews of Rome come in droves every Saturday to hail their 'Capitano.'" Like Freud's Moses, who comes to be revealed as an Egyptian, Michelangelo's *Moses* is truly a Christian in disguise, whom the Jews worship.

Freud's critical approach to Michelangelo's *Moses* is itself a transvaluation of precisely that neurosis that he understands as underlying anti-Semitic attitudes. Anti-Semitism arises from the stress on "minor differences in people who are otherwise alike . . . [and that] form the basis of feelings of strangeness and hostility between them" (*SE* 11:199, 18:101, 21:114). This is the "narcissism of minor differences." To explain this concept Freud evokes the work of the famous Italian patriot and art critic Giovanni Morelli, who wrote under the pseudonym Ivan Lermolieff.[107] Morelli was able to distinguish "copies from originals" of works of art "by insisting that attention should be diverted from the general impres-

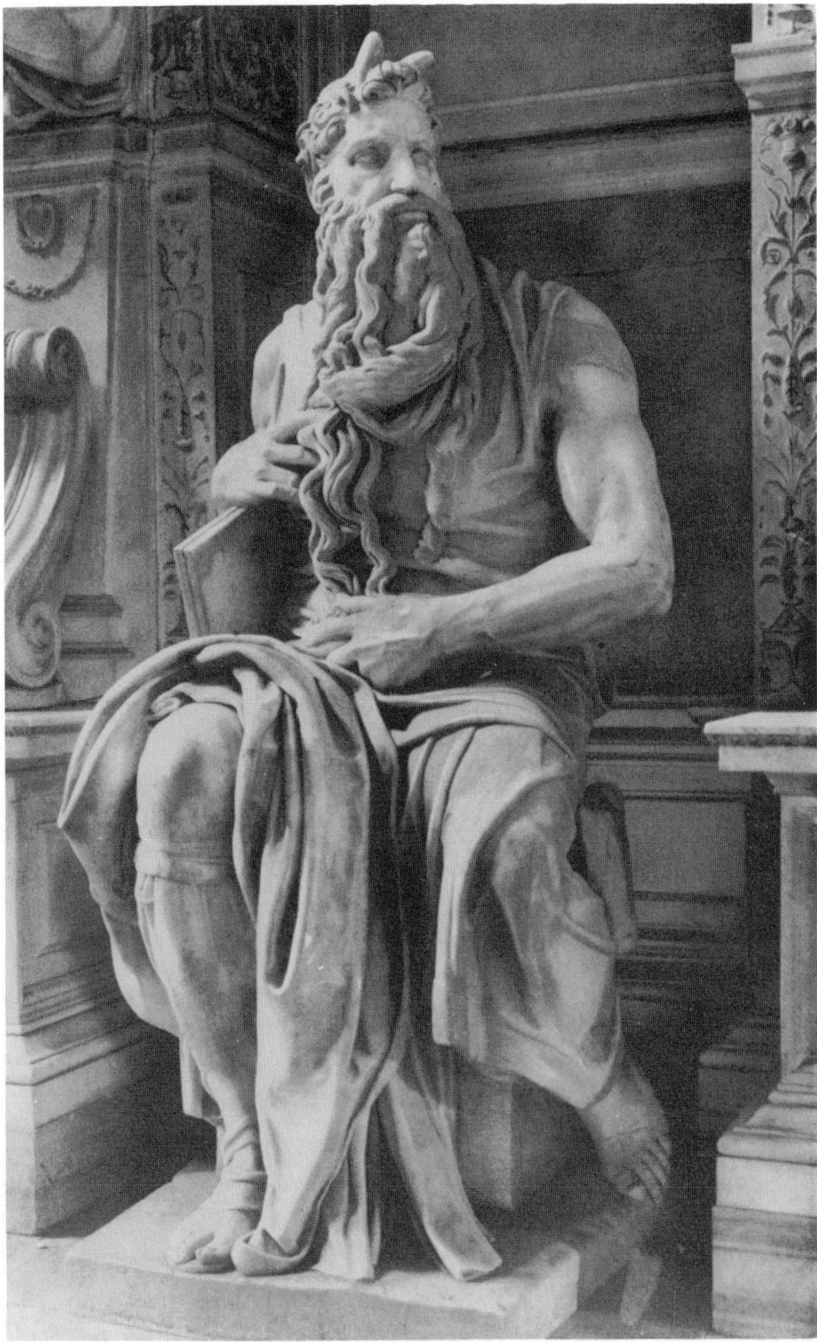

Figure 20. Michelangelo's statue of Moses. (Rome, San Pietro in Vincoli.)

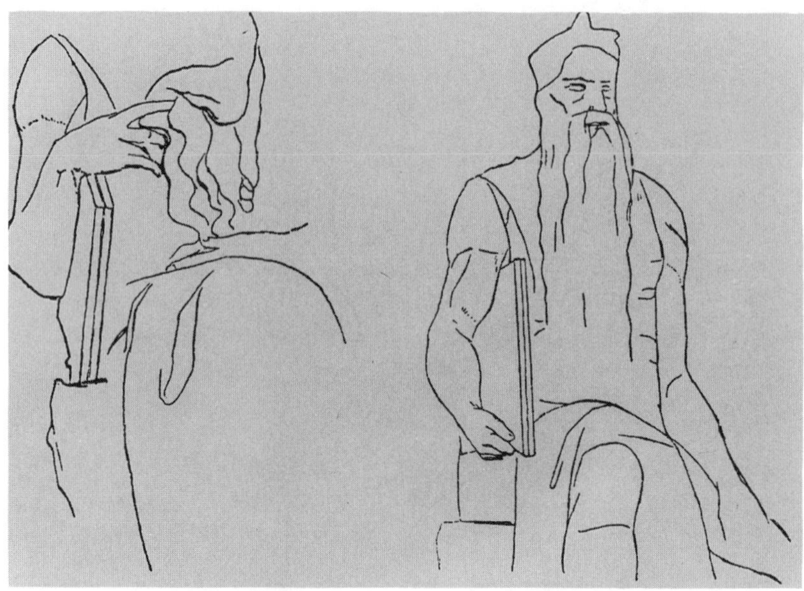

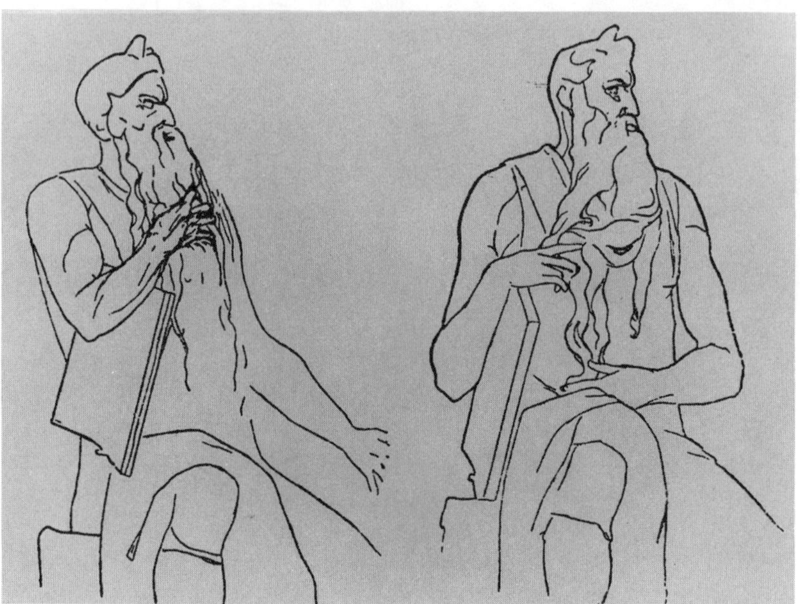

Figure 21. Freud's visualization of aspects of Michelangelo's *Moses*. Note the missing feet. (Freud, *Standard Edition,* 13:226–27.)

sion and main features of a picture, and by laying stress on the significance of minor details, of things like the drawing of the fingernails, of the lobe of an ear, of halos, and such unconsidered trifles" (*SE* 13:222). This is the stuff of psychoanalytic technique, according to Freud, which "is accustomed to divine secret and concealed things from despised or unnoticed features, from the rubbish-heap, as it were, of our observations" (*SE* 13:222). Here is the key to the sense of not being on "firm footing" in his reading. For Freud's reading stressed the "narcissism of minor differences" as integral to the epistemological basis of a "real science." Freud evoked the world of culture in his model for interpretation. Yet this world of culture mirrors the way the anti-Semite distinguished himself from the Jew, through the stress on the "narcissism of minor differences." And one of these "minor differences" in Freud's world is the meaning of the foot.

Freud's Autopsy of Gradiva's Foot

The depiction of the position of the feet of Michelangelo's *Moses* bears a striking resemblance to the position of the feet of a specific woman, who seduces a male (at least in his fantasy). That woman is the eponymous heroine of a novella by Wilhelm Jensen (1837–1911) titled *Gradiva* (1903). Introduced to the text by C. G. Jung in the summer of 1906, Freud published his interpretation in 1907.[108] It is the first complete study of a work of literature from Freud's pen (unlike his readings of *Hamlet* and *Oedipus Rex* in *The Interpretation of Dreams*). Given Freud's sense of himself as a "writer," a theme that haunts him from his early *Studies on Hysteria* to late in his life, there is much to be gained from seeing how he deals with a literary text, a text written within the tradition not of scientific language but of high culture.[109] As he noted in a conversation with Giovanni Papini as late as 1934: "I am a scientist by necessity, and not vocation. I am really by nature an artist. Ever since childhood, my secret hero has been Goethe. I would have liked to have become a poet, and my whole life long I've wanted to write novels." From the time he studied with Charcot (1885–86), he had "carried out the very same plan as Zola." "My oldest and strongest desire would be to write real novels, and I possess a mine of first-hand materials which would make the fortune of a hundred novelists. But I am afraid now it would be too late."[110] Zola's twenty-volume *Rougon-Macquart* novel cycle (1871–93) represented the degeneration of French society in the late nineteenth century through the case histories of specific families. The fantasy of writing novels after the model of Zola, tracing the family romance of the "degenerate" from generation to generation, is part of Freud's exculpation of the Jewish foot in his reading of Jensen's *Gradiva.*

Jensen's story seems to introduce us to a young archaeologist with a foot fetish.[111] The story, which Freud retells in some detail, revolves about the recognition, by the protagonist, a young German archaeologist named Norbert Hanold, of a reincarnated female figure in a piece of classical sculpture. The classical image, the *Gradiva,* was, according to Freud, a "sculpture [that] represented a fully grown girl stepping along, with her flowing dress a little pulled up so as to reveal her sandaled feet. One foot rested squarely on the ground; the other, lifted from the ground in the act of following after, touched it only with the tips of the toes, while the sole and heel rose almost perpendicularly. It was probably the unusual and peculiarly charming gait thus presented that attracted the sculptor's notice and that still, after so many centuries, riveted the eyes of its archaeological admirer" (*SE* 9:10). Jensen's own description begins: "Her head bent forward a little, she held slightly raised in her left hand, so that her sandaled feet became visible, her garment, which fell in exceedingly voluminous folds from her throat to her ankles. The left foot had advanced, and the right, about to follow, touched the ground only lightly with the tips of the toes, while the sole and heel were raised almost vertically. This movement produced a double impression of exceptional agility and of confident composure, and the flight-like poise, combined with a firm step, lent her peculiar grace" (fig. 22).[112] Freud rewrites the description so as to avoid the association with the voluntary exposure of the foot, the act of seduction that he captures in the image of the hysteric. Here the foot is a sign of beauty and grace. Freud has the figure given the name "'Gradiva'—'the girl who steps along'" (*SE* 9:11). Jensen has the protagonist call the sculpture "to himself Gradiva, 'the girl splendid in walking'" (Jensen, 148). The position of the feet, with the left foot resting on the ground and the right foot's toes barely touching the ground, is the mirror image of the position of the feet of Michelangelo's *Moses.*

Jensen's protagonist is convinced that "Gradiva's gait was not discoverable in reality; and this filled him with regret and vexation" (*SE* 9:12). It belongs to a work of art, a work that remains part of the unrediscoverable reality of the past; as Jensen notes, "It was a question of critical judgment as to whether the artist has reproduced Gradiva's

---

Figure 22. The plaster cast of the *Gradiva* from Sigmund Freud's study at 20 Maresfield Gardens, London. The original is in the Museum Chiaramonti in the Vatican. (Freud Museum, London.)

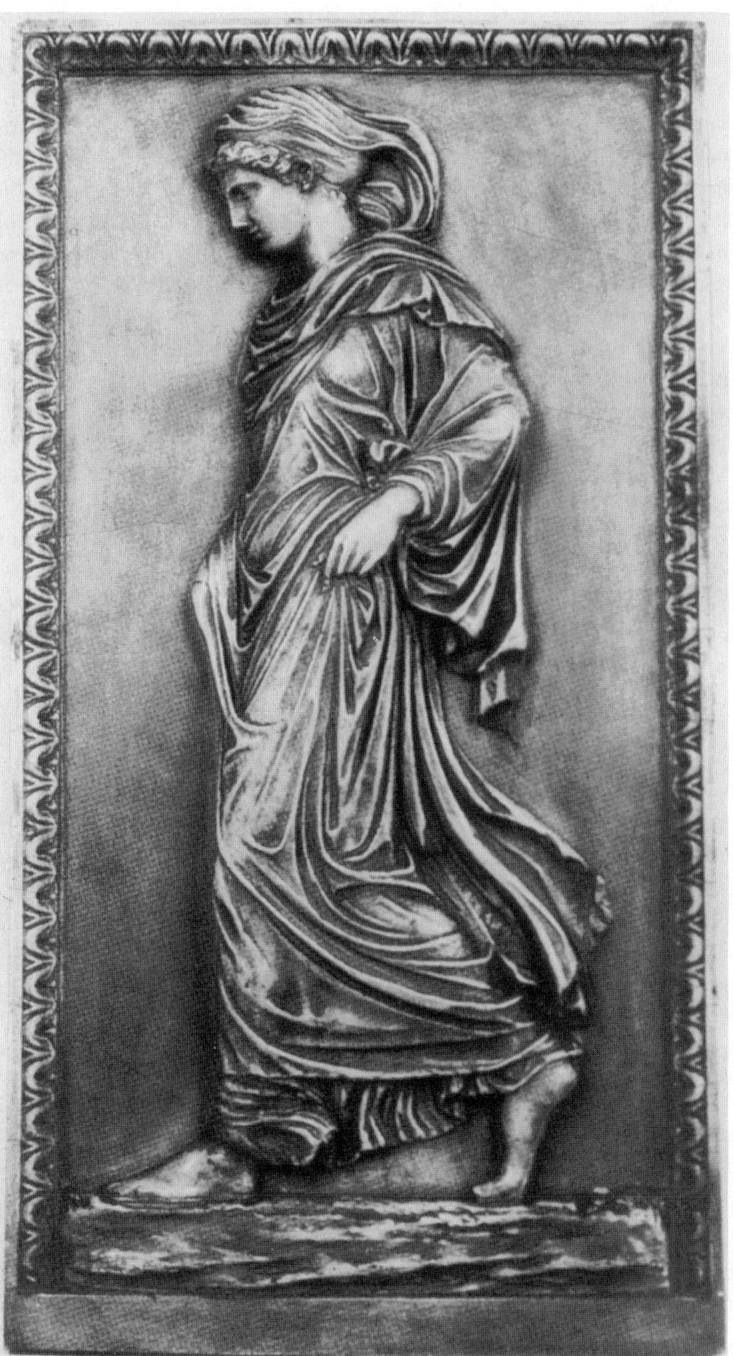

manner of walking from life. . . . The nearly vertical position of the right foot seemed exaggerated; in all experiments which he himself made, the movement left his rising foot always in a much less upright position" (Jensen, 151). Hanold spends his time observing the gait of many women, "some walked slowly, some fast, some ponderously, some buoyantly. Many let their soles merely glide over the ground; not many raised them more obliquely to a smarter position. Among all, however, not a single one presented to view Gradiva's manner of walking" (152–53).

One night he has a most realistic dream of the horrors of the explosion of Vesuvius in A.D. 79 in which he places the mirage of Gradiva, who "with buoyant composure and the calm unmindfulness of her surroundings peculiar to her . . . walked across the flagstones" (154). As a result of his dream he spontaneously decides upon waking to travel and eventually finds himself in Pompeii. There he spies Gradiva: "Her dress, which reached only to her ankles, she held lifted a little in her left hand, and he saw that in walking the sole of her slender foot, as it followed, rose for a moment vertically on the tips of her toes" (157). As quickly as she appeared, she vanished.

Instead of the idealized beauty of Gradiva, he suddenly finds himself among a swarm of young German tourists on their honeymoons. Their saccharine "billing and cooing" sends him into despair, making him see his own scientific discourse of archaeology as a "dead, philological language" (*SE* 9:16). "For the first time in his life he was compelled to observe his fellow human beings more closely with eye and ear. Although, from their speech, they were all his German countrymen, his racial identity with them awoke in him no feeling of pride, but rather the opposite one—that he had done reasonably well to bother as little as possible with the homo sapiens of Linnaean classification, especially in connection with the feminine half of this species" (Jensen, 161–62). Here is the crux of the story, for Hanold can see "for the first time . . . in his immediate vicinity . . . the mating impulse without his being able to understand what had been the mutual cause" (162). Racial selection is the basis for the selection of the marriage partner, and the marker for these parodied figures is their "North German tongue," which becomes for Hanold the discourse of the erotic (164). But this puzzles the young archaeologist, who confuses these lovers with the figures in his Pompeian dreamscape: "It struck him as remarkable that the two talked German, not Greek, to each other" (165). But what they are talking about is their own racial identity. He listens to them talk in Naples, having himself just visited the "sculptures and wall-paintings in the Museo Nazionale," where he would have seen the veiled erotic frescoes from Pompeii (166). The young German husband turns to his wife and says,

"I fear the sun there [in Pompeii] would be too hot for your delicate complexion, and I should never forgive myself that." To which she replies, "What if you should suddenly have a negress for a wife?" "No, my imagination fortunately does not reach that far" (167). Jensen's parody of the idea of correct races in their correct spaces, of the environmental definition of racial difference, allows us to see that it is in these comic characters and their unbridled eroticism that Hanold sees his own unfulfilled and unarticulated longing.

He goes on to Pompeii, where he suddenly sees the living Gradiva again walking on its streets. "Gradiva crossed the steppingstones with her calm buoyancy, and now, turning her back, walked along" (Jensen, 181). He is convinced that this is the reincarnation of the dead past, represented in the gait and foot of the beautiful young woman he sees. He "addressed her in Greek and then, when she did not reply, in Latin. Then with a smile on her lips: 'If you want to speak to me,' she said, 'you must do it in German'" (*SE* 9:18). For Hanold "it was not at all remarkable that she spoke German" but "that her voice . . . sounded as clear as her glance" (Jensen, 187–88). He is struck not by her language but by its beauty, a beauty that mirrors his aesthetic response to her gait.

But Freud stresses the reader's "humiliation." For, according to his reading, we have shared the protagonist's conviction that Gradiva was the relic of some lost past; she is now shown to us to be just as "real," that is, German, as the honeymooners whom the protagonist (and we) thought so ludicrous with their Germanic billing and cooing. Her language must be Greek, or at least Latin—but not German, the language neither of dead philology nor of sexuality. Here the "narcissism of minor differences" appears to provide the difference between the "reader" (Freud as the naïve reader, you and I) and the scientist (Freud as the commentator on the text). The reader has stressed those aspects that are trivial and has missed the central point, the sexual attraction of the protagonist to the *Gradiva*.

Freud makes much more of this twist than Jensen does. For Freud the question of language is a device employed to resolve the problem of recognition; for Jensen it is a sign of the absolute compatibility of the two characters, who literally speak the same language, are of the same race. For the identity of race and language is a standard claim of nineteenth-century anthropology, but not of ethnopsychology. The young woman's actual name is Zoë Bertgang. Her name is the German equivalent of Gradiva (someone "who steps along brilliantly" [*SE* 9:37]). And—she had been known to the protagonist when she was a child. Her father, Richard Bertgang, was a well-known professor of zoology whom Hanold had known in Germany. She eventually recognizes him, and there is a reconstitution of the sense of reality. For as Freud is at pains to point out, it is the residue of the past, with all of its affective dimension, that Hanold had projected into the form, the foot, and the gait of Gradiva. It is an act of unburying the past, as Freud himself noted in the margin of his copy (150), that is the "symbolic center" of the tale. The personal past of Norbert Hanold, his memory of Zoë Bertgang, structured his perception of the object, the bas-relief of Gradiva.

This recognition lends itself to the final resolution of the tale. The "happy end" of the future awaiting Hanold, who gestures to his new beloved to walk ahead of him: "A merry, comprehending, laughing expression lurked around his companion's mouth, and, raising her dress slightly with her left hand, Gradiva rediviva Zoë Bertgang, viewed by him with dreamily observing eyes, crossed with her calmly buoyant walk through the sunlight, over the steppingstones, to the other side of the street" (Jensen, 235). Suddenly he sees in the "real" woman the fantasy of Gradiva that he had created out of his memory of Zoë: the world is complete, the German has become a Greek who has become a German who has become a Greek. Freud commented in the margin of this passage: "Erotic! acceptance of fantasy-reconciliation." The erotic tension of this seeming resolution leaves the reader with the sense that it is in their fantasy that the relationship of the two is resolved. This fantasy is also that of the reader who sees in the two the ideal pair, walking off together into the sunlight.

Gradiva's foot is not a Jewish foot—quite the contrary. Indeed, if we read Jensen closely, the tale becomes one of a Germanic foot in all its glory: "'You recognized me again? In the dream? By what?' 'At the very first; by your manner of walking.' 'Had you noticed that? Have I a special manner of walking?' . . . 'Yes—don't you realize that? A more graceful one—at least among those now living—does not exist'" (Jensen, 196). If we free ourselves from seeing only through Freud's glass, it becomes evident that Wilhelm Jensen is a most interesting writer whose covert meaning in this tale may be elucidated. For it is a tale of appropriate marriage within the race, of permitted—indeed, encouraged—endogamous marriage; it is about the memory of the foot, the distant past, the appropriate object of desire. The natural mating of two like members of the same race reflects their cultural as well as their personal past. This is the theme of Jensen's tale, and it is one that Freud does not notice.

Wilhelm Jensen was a conservative, nationalist writer. Indeed, one of the mysteries about Freud's critical writing is the way he generally ignores contemporary Jewish writers and artists and concentrates on the European intellectual canon, which generally excludes Jews. It is not

Arthur Schnitzler and the complexity of his representations of memory and madness in his tales from the fin-de-siècle world of Vienna that capture Freud's critical attention (even though we know he read them and mentions them in passing in his essay on the uncanny),[113] but the work of Wilhelm Jensen, introduced to him by his Christian disciple C. G. Jung.

Who was Wilhelm Jensen? The illegitimate child of the mayor of Kiel and a servant, he was adopted by the daughter of the professor of botany at the University of Kiel. Trained as a physician in Wurzburg, Jena, and Breslau, he left his studies unfinished to turn to writing in 1860. He understood the psyche as represented in the dreams of Hanold as well as the very structure of his memories of the *Gradiva* as having been influenced by his medical studies.[114] He was heavily influenced by the late Romantic circle of writers in Munich, with its heavily nationalistic (and often explicitly racialist) bias. Jensen himself was not an anti-Semite, but he clearly accepted the reality of racial categories. An advocate of the works of the novelist Wilhelm Raabe, Jensen was the prototype of the northern German regionalist.[115] He was politically allied with Raabe in opposition of a pan-German political solution in 1866 and strongly supported the Prussian cause. This narrow, northern German view is reflected in his best-known work, especially his 1872 novella *Karin of Sweden,* which fixed his literary reputation. The dogmatic nature of his position is most evident in his anticlerical drama *The Struggle for the Reich,* a performance of which was disrupted in 1884 by a demonstration of Catholic students. Greatly influenced by the radical theologian David Friedrich Strauss, Jensen's views on race and nationhood were clearly reflected in his work.

If we read the *Gradiva* independently of Freud, it becomes the family romance of a race, the northern Germans, who find themselves in the classical world, which is itself German. Jensen employed a mimetic view of memory. Memory is suddenly real and representational in the sense that we know it from Francis Galton's photographs. The context of Jensen's story predetermines Freud's use of the reality, rather than the fantasy, of memory. Memory reduces the known to a set of codes—in this tale, the position of the foot, the gait of the young woman. In his explanation Freud drew on a clinical analogy and employed the model taken from Galton that he had used in *The Interpretation of Dreams,* but here he places it in a specifically diagnostic framework. For Galton's mode of representing human difference is a means of scientific representation. Freud tells the story of how he had lost a patient to exophthalmic goiter, the disease that more than any other was employed as a sign of the physiognomy of the insane during the nineteenth century.[116] (Graves' or Basedow's disease was thought to be neurological in origin in the nineteenth century.) One day years later a young girl entered his office, and he believed her to be his dead patient. "So after all it's true that the dead can come back to life," he thought (*SE* 9:71). It turned out that she was the sister of the dead woman and suffered from the same disease: "The victims of Graves' disease, as has often been observed, have a marked facial resemblance to one another, and in this case this typical likeness was reinforced by a family one" (*SE* 9:72). This disease is found most frequently in mature women and is caused by malfunction of the thyroid gland (fig. 23). Its signs are goiter, cardiac arrhythmia, increased apprehensiveness and fear, eyelid retraction, and a compulsive stare. For psychoanalysts the death of a patient (except through suicide) was a relatively unusual event. Its importance for Freud can be measured in the symbolic representation in the "specimen dream" (the "dream of Irma's injection"), which forms the centerpiece of *The Interpretation of Dreams,* of the death of a patient named Mathilde (*SE* 4:111–12). In his interpretation, Freud displaces the guilt about her death onto his friend and colleague Josef Breuer. Freud records this case of a patient's death (from Graves' disease) almost as a footnote, and yet its power, in terms of his own memory, is undiminished.

The face of the dead patient and the gait of the fictive Gradiva thus become observable, definable symptoms, like the impaired gait of the hysteric. But they evoke the past rather than the present. For the symptoms of Graves' disease point toward the fact that "hereditary disposition and psychical trauma play a large part in the development of the disease."[117] Here we have an individual past that duplicates the history of the family, a real past in which memory is mimetic. And if the most widely respected work on Graves' disease is examined, it is a specific group that is most at risk for this disease, because of its own self-destructive history. The anthropologist-physician Georg Buschan, in a prizewinning monograph published in 1894, commented that he was of the opinion that "the Jewish race was predisposed for Graves' disease . . . ; for in the case material Jewish family names or given names often appear. This is the result of the fact that the Jewish race is more highly predisposed to nervous illnesses."[118] And this is because of their more frequent intermarriage. Thus the face of the dead patient becomes that of the hidden nature of the Jew.

In Jensen's tale and in Freud's reading of that story, what triggers an evocation of the past is the memory of the foot and the gait of Zoë-Gradiva: "The childhood impression was stirred up, it became active, so that it began to produce effects, but did not come into consciousness" (*SE* 9:47). This image of the face and the gait that signifies the difference,

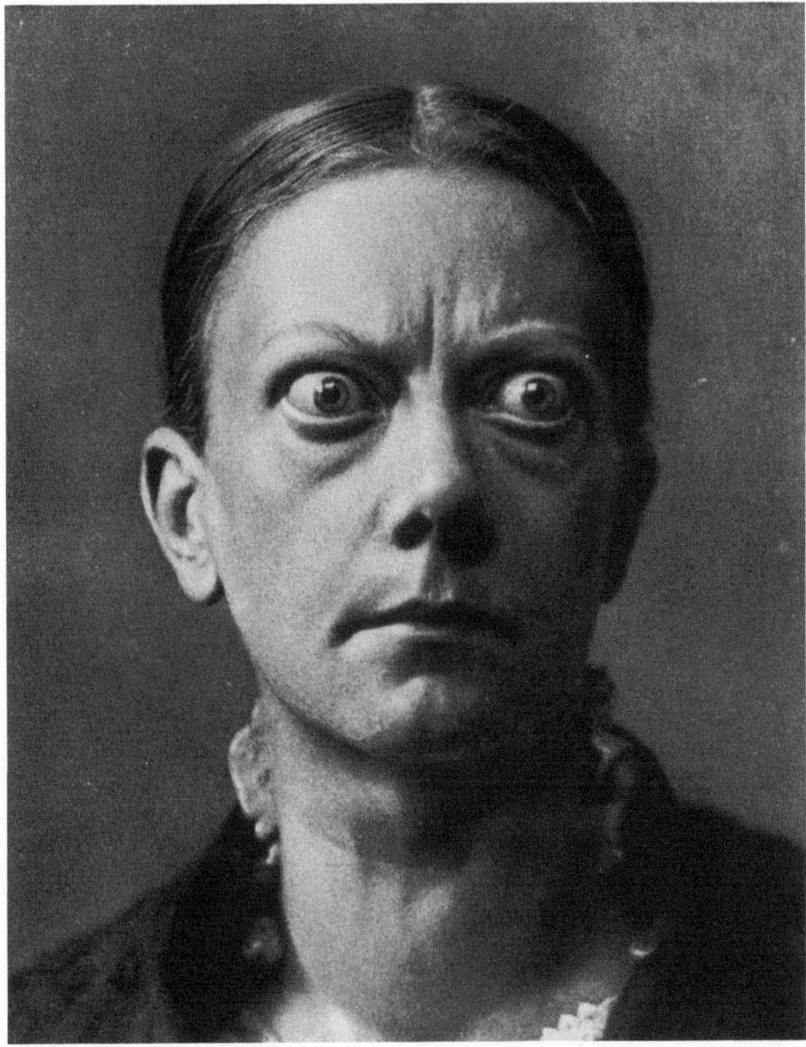

Figure 23. The physiognomy of a woman suffering from Basedow's disease. From Byrom Bramwell, *Atlas of Clinical Medicine* (Edinburgh: Constable, 1892–96). (National Library of Medicine, Bethesda, Md.)

the marked signs, are also the signs that Jensen builds into this tale. For what Hanold recognizes in the story is the racial attraction that he had for Zoë Bertgang. It was Hanold who translated the German name Bertgang into its Greek equivalent, creating the idealized portrait of the *Gradiva,* the German disguised as a Greek. Hidden within the Greek was the German; hidden within Freud's dead patient was the Jew. Each is "seen" through the signs that reveal their true nature to the observer, who is psychologically predisposed to be aware of the existence of such signs and their eventual meaning.

Hanold remembers the reality of the young woman he had known in Germany. There was an absolute relationship between this memory and her appropriateness as his sexual partner. Both are northern Germans, as signified by their Nordic names; both stem from the appropriate space. Indeed, the "humiliation" we are alleged to feel when Zoë Bertgang addresses Hanold in German is the embarrassment of being out of the correct space, of being in Pompeii. It is the embarrassment of the Westernized, acculturated Eastern Jew hearing the *Mauscheln* of the newly arrived *Ostjude* displaced onto the modern German tourist in Italy. But the hidden meaning is that the German she speaks (and that we are reading) is the cultural equivalent of Greek; it is the language of "truth" and "beauty," mirrored in the sight of Gradiva's foot.

It is certainly not a Jewish foot, deformed and marching to quite a different drummer, that Jensen represents in the tale. It is a healthy foot, and the attraction of Hanold to this foot is a healthy attraction. Unlike the fantasy of the hysteric who exposes her foot in order to seduce the male, or the psychoanalyst who has come through the process of transference to take the place of the male, the male gazing on the foot is healthy, is not a fetishist. His interest "in women's feet and their way of placing them . . . was bound to bring him a bad reputation both among scientists and among the women of the town he lived in, a reputation of being a foot-fetishist" (*SE* 9:46). But Freud frees the protagonist from the charge of being a degenerate, of having inherited his predisposition for foot fetishism:

> Furthermore, since our hero was a person capable of developing a delusion on the basis of such a strange preference, a strict psychiatrist would at once stamp him as a *dégénéré* and would investigate the heredity which has remorselessly driven him to this fate. But here the author does not follow the psychiatrist, and with good reason. He wishes to bring the hero closer to us so as to make "empathy" easier; the diagnosis of "*dégénéré,*" whether it is right or wrong, at once puts the young archaeologist at a distance from us, for we readers are the normal people and the standard of humanity. Nor is the author greatly concerned with the hereditary and constitutional

> preconditions of the state, but on the other hand he plunges deep into the personal mental make-up which can give rise to such a delusion. (*SE* 9:43)

The freeing of the protagonist from the charge of being degenerate plays off the charges against the Jew as a patient who shows the physical and psychological stigmata of degeneration. For it is the inbreeding of the Jew that leads to degeneracy, which impinges on even the physician's gaze. Freud constructs here a uniform "us" against the psychiatrists, placing himself among those unencumbered in seeing and therefore able to treat. Jewish inbreeding leads to degeneracy; Aryan inbreeding leads to health. The true physician in this case is not the Jewish psychoanalyst who frees the neurotic from her symptoms, but the racially identical lover. Hanold is cured by Zoë, who talks him out of his memories and his neurosis. She becomes his "physician" (*SE* 9:87).

Gradiva's body, the body of the physician, is that of an Aryan woman. It is her beautiful foot that reveals her power to cure. Her feet are represented in the identical position of the feet of the celebratory sculpture by the fin-de-siècle American Jewish sculptor and painter, Katharine M. Cohen, *The Israelite.* This was a life-size male figure clad in those loose "biblical" garments attributed to Temple Jewry, bearing a volume of the law. First exhibited at the Paris Salon in 1896 to great acclaim, this image was widely circulated as an engraving in fin-de-siècle European Jewish culture. The position is the position of movement, of action (fig. 24). For Freud, it was necessary to translate the image of the deformed Jewish male foot into the beautiful foot of the Aryan woman; the American Jewish female sculptor could represent it in the form of the beautiful body of the Jewish male. For Jensen and Freud, it is also a gait that incorporates the beautiful.

There is an odd postscript to the second edition of 1912, which seems to give us a great deal of miscellaneous material on Jensen and the *Gradiva.* Freud's postscript informs us where the sculpture is located as well as giving more information about Jensen, including the fact that his last novel "contains much material from the author's own childhood [and] describes the history of a man who 'sees a sister in the woman he loves.'"[119] This information, he notes, is to be found in a review of this most recent novel. Freud's invocation of the incest theme is very odd, in that Jensen had written to Freud on December 14, 1907, that "NO. I never had a sister, indeed, no blood relatives at all."[120] The review by Eva Gräfin Baudissin that Freud referred to in his postscript is very revealing. She describes the *difference* between the plot of the novel and Jensen's life, stressing that the incestuous moment in the novel does not have any parallel in Jensen's own life.[121] The novel, she comments, re-

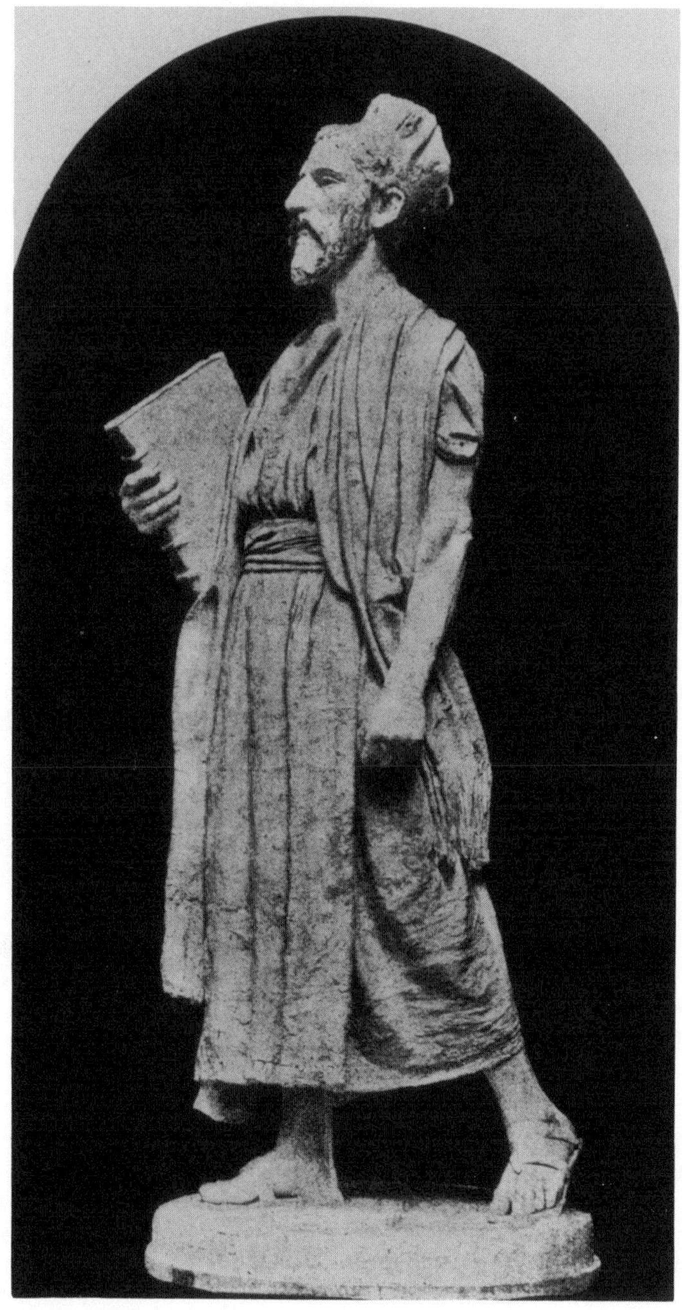

Figure 24. Katherine M. Cohen, *The Israelite*. This is a positive image of the Jewish male body. (Private collection, Ithaca, N.Y.)

flects a failed life, whereas Jensen's was apparently a successful one. What she does stress about the novel, which Freud evidently did not read, is that its hero, the surrogate for the author, is a "poor, homeless youth in which French, light blood mixed with German brooding." This racial theme is sounded in her reading of the book as the "suffering of a human being because he had never received what he had always sought: a German nation in the sense of an upright German man." The text is read, as the *Gradiva* can well be, as a reflection of the politicization of race in the fin-de-siècle novel.

The illegitimate Jensen is assumed in 1912 to have had some type of incestuous relationship with a sister who could not have existed. But Freud needed to see Jensen as one who was working out his own family romance in his tales, just as he had worked out his own identification with Hanold's mode of seeing in his reading of the text. The charge that the Jews are diseased because of their sexual practices, specifically their "inbreeding" or "incestuous" behavior, is one often lodged, as we shall see in chapter 4. In Freud's reading, Jensen becomes nothing more than an incestuous Jew. And his texts reveal this like a palimpsest: the limping, degenerate Jew as pervert becomes the northern German Protestant author as pervert. The signs of his sexual identity are inscribed in his text.

The motivating factor of Freud's evocation of the incest theme in his postscript to his reading of *Gradiva* may well lie in the conflicts that arose in 1910 and 1911 with that individual who introduced him to the text, C. G. Jung. It was Jung who suggested on reading Freud's interpretation of the text that in Jensen's work the central "*problem is one of brother-sister love*."[122] The implications for the very concept of brother-sister incest regarding the model of racial inbreeding would have been clear to Freud. Beginning in 1909 there was an increased stress on their relationship, which came to a head in 1912 over the question of incest and its meaning for the sexual etiology of neurosis. The postscript was written during Freud's conflict with Jung, and all that was positive in the initial reading of the tale is drawn into question by the association of the text, with its overt racial theme, and Jung's "anti-Semitic condescension."[123] It was Jung, the Aryan "crown prince," who had given Freud this text; in rereading his comments it became precisely that question—the question of the difference between Jews and Aryans—that appeared in the code words of incest and inbreeding. It was also because the point of conflict between Freud and Jung rested precisely in the arena of sexuality, with Freud advocating the centrality of sexuality as a universal experience and Jung beginning to deny this. The debates within the psychoanalytic circle about the meaning of incest and inbreeding reflect the strong ideological coloration of these debates by the racial biology and medicine of the time. Freud's own conflict with Jung is understood by Freud—and this is relatively explicitly stated in his correspondence with Jung—as an attempt to provide a universal, that is, not a Jewish, face for psychoanalysis. Freud's rhetoric of the time is revealing. He sees Jung as "Joshua" and himself as "Moses." It is, of course, the conversion of Jung into the Jew "Joshua [who] will take possession of the promised land of psychiatry" and Freud into the Egyptian "Moses" (given his later reading of this figure) that reverses the racial categories.[124] It is in the academic, medical discipline of psychiatry, not psychoanalysis, that Freud wishes to triumph, and there he sees his path blocked because he is a Jew. Freud's sense of Jung as the privileged individual collapses in 1913 with Jung's rejection of the central tenet of psychoanalysis, the sexual etiology of neurosis, and is sealed with the appointment of Ernest Jones as Jung's successor in the power structure.[125] Here the question of sexuality dominates even the importance of professional status.

William McGrath has related Freud's evocation of his identity with Moses, with all its images of the Jewish foot, to the dream Freud recounted a decade earlier of dissecting his own body.[126] In this dream Freud recounted how a representation of Ernst Brücke, professor of physiology at Vienna, gave him the task of dissecting his own pelvis and legs. The dream opened with the following scene in Brücke's physiological laboratory:

> Old Brücke must have set me some task; STRANGELY ENOUGH, it related to a dissection of the lower part of my own body, my pelvis and legs, which I saw before me as though in the dissecting-room, but without noticing their absence in myself and also without a trace of any gruesome feeling. Louise N. was standing beside me and doing the work with me. The pelvis had been eviscerated, and it was visible now in its superior, now in its inferior, aspect, the two being mixed together. Thick flesh-colored protuberances (which, in the dream itself, made me think of hemorrhoids) could be seen. Something which lay over it and was like crumpled silver-paper had also to be carefully fished out. (*SE* 5:452–53)

Freud goes on to describe a trip through the mountains where he finds himself among "Red Indians or Gypsies," still in possession of his legs.

Freud's interpretation of this dream centered on the dissection as the mental representation of his uncompleted self-analysis. He saw his self-doubt about this self-analysis as mirrored in the comments of Louise N., to whom he had offered a book, Rider Haggard's *She,* in lieu of his promised account of his own work.[127] The question of having the "legs to carry him" is, as we have seen in the use of the image of feet and gait in Freud's work, a reflection of the self-doubt implicit in the image of the Jewish feet. Here it is associated with the scientific enterprise, with the ability of Freud to undertake the duties of the research scientist. This ability hinges on Freud's control of the language of science, a language that is bound to a series of subtexts.

When Freud, following Brücke's dream direction, opened himself up, he found the sign of the Jew, the hemorrhoids associated in internal medicine with vascular diseases such as the intermittent claudication of Eastern Jews. There is a long connection between Jews and hemorrhoids. The Greco-Roman physician Galen already speaks of the digestive problems of the Jews in the second century.[128] A late fourteenth-century Hebrew translation of Bernard de Gordon's *Lilium Medicinae* (1305) contains the following passage: "The Jews suffer greatly from hemorrhoids for three reasons: first, because they are generally sedentary and therefore the excessive melancholy humors collect; secondly, because they are usually in fear and anxiety and therefore the melancholy blood becomes increased, besides (according to Hippocrates) fear and faint-heartedness, should they last a long time, produce the melancholy humor; and thirdly, it is the divine vengeance against them (as written in Psalms 78:66): and 'he smote his enemies in the hinder parts, he put them to a perpetual reproach.'"[129] The Hebrew translator adds to the final point: "What is written is a lie, and they who believe it lie." Hemorrhoids, like male menstruation (and indeed, all illnesses of the Jews), are a punishment for the Jews' denial of Christ. In 1777 Elcan Isaac Wolf had already commented on the relation between the Jews' sedentary way of life and the seemingly universal appearance of hemorrhoids.[130] This is a leitmotif in Jewish culture in Europe. One of the puzzles of the epidemiological literature on cancer is that Jews had such a low rate of rectal cancer given the very high occurrence of hemorrhoids among them.[131] But the image of hemorrhoids is associated in the medical literature with eastern European Jews, as Maurice Fishberg noted: "Among the Hasidim in Galicia and Poland a Jew without hemorrhoids is considered a curiosity. Physicians who have had experience among the Jews testify that it is rare to find a Jew who has passed the middle age without having his hemorrhoidal veins more or less enlarged. The Jews of eastern Europe attribute this condition to the habit of sitting during the greater part of the day on the hard benches of the *bet Ha-midrash* [school] while studying the Talmud."[132] Freud would have had this view of an Eastern Jewish predisposition reinforced by his reading of Ignaz Bernstein's collection of Jewish proverbs, to which he referred in a 1914 footnote to *The Interpretation of Dreams* (*SE* 4:132 n1). Among Eastern Jews, the inheritance of this illness becomes the stuff of folk wisdom: "A yiddishe yerishe is a gildene uder" (A Jew's inheritance is a golden vein, i.e., hemorrhoids) and "Vus yirushenen Yidn? Zurus un meriden!" (What do Jews inherit? Trouble and hemorrhoids!)[133] For the medical practitioner of the fin de siècle, "Hemorrhoids are an inherent part of the image of the Hassids of Galicia and Poland."[134] And indeed, Freud himself was a "chronic sufferer from an obscure abdominal complaint," and his adult life seemed fixated on his own "chronic constipation" with the resultant hemorrhoids.[135] Freud's body reveals itself to him as the body of a Jew. But even more so, it contains and defines the psyche of the Jew. For in W. Watkiss Lloyd's description of Michelangelo's *Moses,* which Freud read and annotated, the statue "conveys a feeling of the agitation expressed so frequently in the typical Hebraism, of bowels yearning for kindred in their tribulation or their perverseness."[136] This claim Freud questions with a large red question mark in the margin. For the "contemptuous indignation" of Moses may well be but a reflex of his "bowel" problem, a metaphor for the "common mental construction" of the Jew.[137]

And indeed, the "mental fright" with which Freud awakes at the close of the dream, like the "humiliation" of the reader of the *Gradiva,* is a reflex of his sense of the Jewish body. He concludes that the "mental fright" about the process is a "fresh allusion to the strange novel [Rider Haggard's *She*] in which a person's identity is retained through a series of generations for over two thousand years" (*SE* 5:455). This is precisely the rhetoric that Jewish scientists always evoke when they wish to place the origin of the disabilities of the Jew in the experience of the ghetto. It is the identity of the "eternal feminine" in the novel, but also the identity of the ghetto Jew with "feet of clay." While it is certainly correct that the image of the "eternal feminine, the immortality of our emotions," is present in Rider Haggard's novel, as Freud tells Louise N., it is also clear that this feminine aspect is a hidden aspect of the Jew, revealed in the dissection, a dissection that is hidden under "silver-paper." Freud provides this seemingly obscure reference for his reader in a note to the dream transcript: it is "the book by Stannius on the nervous system of fishes," which Freud remembers, in the account of another dream, was related to "the first scientific task which my teacher [Brücke] set me [which] was in fact concerned with the nervous system of a fish, Ammocoetes" (*SE* 5:413). This is of course not the only "scientific task" he performed in 1877. For the other one we must return to Trieste and the search, in Carl Claus's laboratory, for the elusive gonads of the male eel, the hidden sign of sexuality that distinguishes the male from the female. William McGrath is quite right to relate this dream to Freud's search for the Jew within, but Freud's Moses, like all Jews, is marked by "feet of clay."

Degeneration

The claim in Freud's analysis of Jensen's *Gradiva* that "we," his readers, would not have the same sympathy for the "degenerate" as we do for the neurotic builds on the discussion of the response to those whose innate difference is somatic. (The degenerate Jew would therefore be much less the object of sympathy than the neurotic anti-Semite, whose neurosis is a response to the nature of the Jew's body.) The "I" versus "you" structure of that argument stressed the desire for the general, not specifically Jewish, audience he wished to address in his *Gradiva* interpretation, but it also pointed up the difference between that audience, which would be out of sympathy with the degenerate, and the Jew, who was simply labeled degenerate because of the practice of sexual "inbreeding." Arnold Kutzinski, of the neurological clinic at the Berlin Charité, argued vociferously against this view in a popular Jewish journal in 1912.[138] He stressed the positive results of inbreeding, to counter the common wisdom that inbreeding led only to degenerate forms. Other views of the time removed the Jews from the category of the degenerate, since degeneracy was defined as the result of interracial breeding and the Jews were understood to be a "pure" race.[139] But for most at the fin de siècle, the degeneracy of the Jews came from sexual "perversions," such as inbreeding, and led to "perversions" such as the desire to intermarry.[140]

Early in his career Freud, like many of his contemporaries, even those not trained in science, saw the individual as well as the historical world in terms of the biological model of decay.[141] Such biologists were so convinced by the power of their explanatory model that they wrote philosophies of history as if the analogies to biology were literal.[142] Historians, especially conservative ones such as Houston Stewart Chamberlain, littered their works with the crudest parallels to biological development.[143] Within all these theories of history the problem of degeneracy held a major role in providing the explanation for the negative moments of history, just as it did in contemporary biology.

It is in Freud's earliest work on neurological diseases in childhood that the concept of degeneracy is first articulated. Freud, whose work on cerebral diplegia and multiple sclerosis put him in the forefront of thinkers on the neurological diseases of childhood, went to Paris in 1885–86 specifically to study the "secondary atrophies and degenerations that follow on affections of the brain in children" (*SE* 1:8). Although the term "degeneration" was used within the strict neurological sense given by Rudolf Virchow, that is, the endogenous decay of the cell, it is this early linkage between the concept of degeneration and childhood illness that colored Freud's thinking during this period. While he was in Paris, under the tutelage of Jean-Martin Charcot at the Salpêtrière, his interest moved from this original problem to the problem of hysteria. In his essay on neurosis (1894) Freud distinguished between degenerative neurosis, which had a primarily psychological etiology, and hysteria:

> In fact, hysterical illnesses even of troublesome severity are no rarity in children of between six and ten years. In boys and girls of intense hysterical disposition, the period before and after puberty brings about a first outbreak of the neurosis. In infantile hysteria the same symptoms are found as in adult neuroses. Stigmata, however, are as a rule rarer, and psychical changes, spasms, attacks and contractors are in the foreground. Hysterical children are very frequently precocious and highly gifted; in a number of cases, to be sure, the hysteria is merely a symptom of a deep-going degeneracy of the nervous system which is manifested in permanent moral perversion. As is well known, an early age, from fifteen onwards, is the period at which the hysterical neurosis most usually shows itself actively in females. (*SE* 1:52)

Most earlier work on childhood hysteria, as well as on the other endogenous illnesses cataloged by nineteenth-century medicine, had seen all childhood psychopathologies as proof of an inherent failing in the child.[144] Using the model of insanity *ex onania,* the weakness was seen within the child and was usually triggered by outside causes. Hermann Smidt, in his dissertation (1880) on childhood hysteria, argued for such a purely somatic origin of hysteria in children.[145] In Freud's earliest work a questioning of the somatic etiology of childhood psychopathologies was introduced. Yet in his extensive study of infant cerebral palsy (1897) Freud cited an extensive number of case studies to show the inheritance of the predisposition to specific neurological deficits in children, specifically those dealing with the impairment of gait.[146] The concept of "degeneracy" remained linked to childhood, to illness, and to childhood sexuality.

The French tradition ran parallel to his view. Charcot saw all neurosis including hysteria as "neuropathic," and Pierre Janet's view only refined this, seeing in the neurotic an inability to synthesize, which he called a "psychical stigmata," and evidence of the "degeneracy of hysterical individuals."[147] Freud maintained that the neurotic individual has some type of "pathological disposition," although such a disposition was in no way identical with individual or hereditary "degeneracy" (*SE* 3:48). Freud saw the roots of such pathologies existing prenatally, but he also equated the French formulation of this view, a view that had almost universal acceptance, with the concept of degeneration itself. Indeed, in all the later retrospective discussions of the history of psychoanalysis, Freud felt it necessary to draw the distinction between this earlier, more rigid manner of understanding the etiology of neurosis and his own views.[148] Quite often he will use the term *dégénération* rather than the equivalent German term (*Entartung*) to stress the French origin of this concept.

During this period, in his detailed correspondence with Wilhelm Fliess, the problem of sexual degeneracy as the model for psychopathology appeared as a major factor in their exchange. Freud attempted, in his draft outline "On the Etiology and Theory of the Major Neuroses," to distinguish between those psychopathologies that are the product of degeneracy and those that are the product of disposition (*SE* 1:187). Both categories placed the sources of the illness within the patient; the latter demanded an external stimulus before the illness manifested itself. Even with this modification, degeneracy remains the primary etiology. But Freud had postulated the role of trauma in the stages of some psychopathologies. In a letter to Fliess dated May 21, 1894, Freud still reduced the roots of all neurosis to four primary sexual etiologies, and degeneration remained central to all four categories.[149] Degeneracy remained the basis for the sexual etiology of neurosis. But degeneracy and disposition were too rigid for Freud, since they excluded the possibility of psychological influence. Freud simply equated degeneracy with inherent genetic error, and by August 1894 he began to move away from the concept of degeneracy as the root of sexual "enfeeblement" and toward the need for some type of psychological motivation for neurosis (90–95; see also *SE* 3:48). Yet in his paper on anxiety neurosis (1895), his first major attempt to undermine the concept of neurasthenia with its strong linkage to the role of degeneracy, Freud still gave credence to Paul Julius Möbius's category of "hereditarily degenerate individuals" as one of the etiologies for neurasthenia (*SE* 3:90, 1:106). In his paper on this question, "Heredity and the Neuroses" (1896), he still retained "syndromes constituting mental degeneracy" as a valid category but excluded obsessions from it (*SE* 3:146). This was a qualification of his rejection of degeneracy in the beginning of his paper "Obsessions and Phobias" (1894), which stressed the special place these neuroses had outside the category of degeneracy (*SE* 3:74). But there too Freud retained the idea that degeneration does exist and that certain psychopathologies must be attributed to it.

Freud worked on the concept of degeneracy, trying to recast it for his own needs. In January 1897 he wrote to Fliess completely restructuring the concept of degeneracy. His views evolved from somatic "disposition," the relation between inherent somatic factors and some type of psychological stimulus, to give the concept of degeneracy a greater psychological quality (*SE* 1:240–41). Degeneracy can be the inheritance of behavior patterns from one generation to another. The model for this is the view of the ethnopsychologists about the transmission of national characteristics. The existence of such earlier psychological structures played a major role in Freud's recasting the moment of degeneracy from prenatal influence to early childhood experience:

> An idea about resistance has enabled me to put straight all those cases of mine which had run into fairly severe difficulties, and to start them off again satisfactorily. Resistance, which finally brings work to a halt, is nothing other than the child's past character, his degenerate character, which (as a result of those experiences which one finds present consciously in what are called degenerate cases) has developed or might have developed, but which is overlaid here by the emergence of repression. I dig it out by my work, it struggles; and what was to begin with such an excellent, honest fellow, becomes low, untruthful or defiant, and a malingerer—til I tell him so and thus make it possible to overcome this character. In this way resistance has become something actual and tangible to me, and I wish, too, that, instead of the concept of repression, I already had what lies concealed behind it. (*SE* 1:266–67)

Character and not biology structures Freud's definition of degeneracy. Character is linked with the fantasy world of masturbation, following Kaan, and the concept of degeneracy has a specifically sexual context, as it does in late nineteenth-century discussions of neurasthenia.

In *Studies on Hysteria* (1895), written with Josef Breuer, Freud comes to terms with the pejorative implications of the term degeneration. His patients, even though hysterics, are in no way congenitally predisposed to hysteria. In the case of "Fräulein Elisabeth von R.," Freud first rejected the label of degenerate for the hysteric. This patient, the subject of Freud's first full-length analysis of hysteria, suffered "for more than two years from pains in her legs and . . . had difficulties in walking." Indeed, the very image of the complaint paralleled the clinical image of intermittent claudication: "She complained of great pain in walking and of being quickly overcome by fatigue both in walking and in standing, and that after a short time she had to rest, which lessened the pains but did not do away with them altogether." But Freud diagnosed this as a case of hysteria, eliminating all neuropathologies because of the way his patient spoke about the experience of illness. Her discourse marked her as a hysteric rather than as someone suffering from an organic illness (*SE* 2:104, 161, 135, 136–37). Freud's patient, whose real name was Ilona Weiss, was a Hungarian Jew. What Freud showed in his description was that the painful gait was in no way inherited but rather was the conversion into her hysterical symptoms of her association of her longing for her brother-in-law, who had accompanied her on a walk at a specific point in their relationship, with her father's impaired limb, which she used to bandage during his final illness. (Here the double meaning of "conversion" reappears—for her conversion signifies the shift from one mode of identity to another, from one set of associations to another. Freud, however, is very careful to avoid the religious term for conversion [*Bekehrung*] in this clinical context. He introduces the term *Konversion* in 1894 [*SE* 3:49]. However, the double meaning of "conversion" exists for this term but not for the more strictly theological one.) For Freud his successful treatment of his patient was proved when he spied her at a private ball "whirl[ing] past in a lively dance. . . . There is no excuse," Freud concluded, "for regarding [the features one meets with so frequently in hysterical people] as a consequence of degeneracy" (*SE* 2:160–61). Indeed, this case prefigured much of Freud's later discussion of the role the concept of degeneracy should play in the diagnosis of psychosexual pathologies.

In "Little Hans" (1909), Freud's argument created a rhetorician who condemns the child as hopelessly mired in the swamp of his own ancestry. "Little Hans," who grew up to become the noted opera director Herbert Graf, was (as we saw in chapter 2) Jewish, so that the repudiation of a generalized "degeneracy" repressed the hidden specter of a specific Jewish degeneration:

> But before going into the details of this agreement I must deal with two objections which will be raised against my making use of the present analysis for this purpose. The first objection is to the effect that Hans was not a normal child, but (as events—the illness itself, in fact—showed) had a predisposition to neurosis, and was a young "degenerate"; it would be illegitimate, therefore, to apply to other, normal children conclusions which might perhaps be true of him. I shall postpone consideration of this objection, since it only limits the value of the observation, and does not completely nullify it. . . . I think, therefore, that Hans's illness may perhaps have been no more serious than that of many other children who are not branded as "degenerates," but since he was brought up without being intimidated, and with as much consideration and as little coercion as possible,

> his anxiety dared to show itself more boldly. With him there was no place for such motives as a bad conscience or a fear of punishment, which with other children must no doubt contribute to making the anxiety less. (*SE* 10:100, 141)

By 1917 this voice, condemning all through the use of the term degeneracy, is the voice of "psychiatry" as opposed to the voice of the psychoanalyst:

> Psychiatry, it is true, denies that such things mean the intrusion into the mind of evil spirits from without; beyond this, however, it can only say with a shrug: "Degeneracy, hereditary disposition, constitutional inferiority!" Psychoanalysis sets out to explain these uncanny disorders; it engages in careful and laborious investigations, devises hypotheses and scientific constructions, until at length it can speak thus to the ego: —"Nothing has entered into you from without; a part of the activity of your own mind has been withdrawn from your knowledge and from the command of your will." (*SE* 17:142)

Degeneracy is the label for the Other, specifically the Other as the essence of pathology (*SE* 3:280). The sense of hopelessness and helplessness is what is captured by the label degenerate. Thus Freud rejected clinical psychiatry's label of the sexually deviant as the degenerate, again through the rhetoric of the prototypical "psychiatrist."

In his paper on a case of female homosexuality (1920), one of Freud's last uses of the term degenerate appears in this context (*SE* 18:149). The authority of medicine is the condemning voice that Freud mockingly quotes to illustrate its own limits:

> Perhaps you would like to know in advance, having in mind our earlier talks, what attitude contemporary psychiatry adopts towards the problems of obsessional neurosis. But it is a meagre chapter. Psychiatry gives names to the different obsessions but says nothing further about them. On the other hand it insists that those who suffer from these symptoms are "degenerates." This gives small satisfaction; in fact it is a judgement of value—a condemnation instead of an explanation. We are supposed to think that every possible sort of eccentricity may arise in degenerates. Well, it is true that we must regard those who develop such symptoms as somewhat different in their nature from other people. But we may ask: are they more "degenerate" than other neurotics—than hysterical patients, for instance, or those who fall ill of psychoses? Once again, the characterization is evidently too general. Indeed, we may doubt whether there is any justification for it at all, when we learn that such symptoms occur too in distinguished people of particularly high capacities, capacities important for the world at large. It is true that, thanks to their own discretion and to the untruthfulness of their biographers, we learn little that is intimate about the great men

> who are our models; but it may nevertheless happen that one of them, like Émile Zola, may be a fanatic for the truth, and we then learn from him of the many strange obsessional habits to which he was a life-long victim. Psychiatry has found a way out of speaking of "dégénérés supérieurs." Very nice. But we have found from psychoanalysis that it is possible to get permanently rid of these strange obsessional symptoms, just as of other complaints and just as in people who are not degenerate. I myself have succeeded repeatedly in this. (*SE* 16:260; see also 3:201 and 7:160)

The locus of this voice of authority is problematic. Is this merely the French medical tradition, with its general acceptance of Germany, against which Freud is arguing, or is this an internalized element of Freud's own system of belief that he is striving to overcome? If it is the latter—the internalized voice of the biologist in a struggle with the psychoanalyst—then other residual elements of this conflict should be found in Freud's work. The subject of Freud's comment, the "dégénérés supérieurs," is a category by which late nineteenth-century psychiatry defined the nature of creativity. It was also one of the explanations of Jewish creativity in cultural and scientific fields. In destroying the myth of the "dégénérés supérieurs," Freud was also protecting his own position as an innovative scientist from the accusation of being merely a clever but degenerate Jew. Ability, such as Zola's, which Freud admired and wished to emulate, is not one of the stigmata of degeneration.

Hidden within this rejection of the origin of psychopathology within the heredity of the individual is a fascination that links the role of heredity to sexual pathology, especially in the case of the Jews. The pejorative sense of "degeneration" that Freud saw in the use of this label distanced the essence of the Other. Freud observed medical science's need to differentiate between the normal and the degenerate as a means of drawing the line between the perfect and the perverse Other (*SE* 9:45). This observation, as I discussed in the analysis of Freud's essay on Jensen's *Gradiva* (1906), crystallized the problem that runs parallel to his own rejection of the medical/biological concept of the degenerate.

In *The Interpretation of Dreams* (1900) Freud had evolved a model of infantile sexuality as the basic developmental model of humanity. This view of chronological primitivism traced the movement of the infant from "egoist" to "moralist," a view compatible with earlier views of the acquisition of shame as the wellspring of morality: "For we may expect that, before the end of the period which we count as childhood, altruistic impulses and morality will awaken in the little egoist and (to use Meynert's terms) . . . a secondary ego will overlay and inhibit the primary one. It is true, no doubt, that morality does not set in simultaneously all along the line and that the length of non-moral childhood varies in different individuals. If this morality fails to develop, we like to talk of 'degeneracy,' though what in fact faces us is an inhibition in development" (*SE* 4:25). "Degeneracy" comes to have for Freud the sense of a faulty designation for the sexually pathological, inherent, immutable (*SE* 7:50).

With his *Three Essays on the Theory of Sexuality* (1905), the seemingly separate strands of childhood sexuality, the etiology of neurosis, perversity, and degeneracy merge, and the major shift prefigured in the passage above becomes evident, the shift from the model of sexuality to its historical analogy (*SE* 7:138–39). Although Freud attributed his shift in interest to Iwan Bloch's semipopular studies of sexuality in history, clearly Freud is to no little degree influenced by the contemporary debates concerning the nature of homosexuality and the role of hereditary predisposition in the development of the homosexual.[150] It is specifically in Freud's discussion of homosexuality that this is most evident. For homosexuality (at least in 1905) is not a "slipping back" into a more primitive or a more degenerate stage—it is being mired ("fixated") at an earlier stage in the developmental history of the individual. As Freud made abundantly clear in a long and convoluted footnote added in 1915, all human beings "are capable of making a homosexual object choice" at a certain point in their development (*SE* 7:145–47). The model for this "fixation at an earlier stage" can be found in the primary account of the history of sexuality written in the late nineteenth century, the opening chapter of Richard Krafft-Ebing's classic *Psychopathia Sexualis* (1886). There Krafft-Ebing writes the history of the human race as a history of the progress of human sexuality from the swamp of "primitive" sexuality to the most advanced form of modern Christian liberalism. Judaism and its sexual attitudes form an earlier stage. And it is at this stage that the Jews remain fixated.[151] Indeed, the construction of the idea of homosexuality, like that of the feminine, is redolent with qualities ascribed to the inherent nature of Jewish degeneration. Yet Freud's discussion of degeneracy in this passage is as a disease of civilization, parallel to the discussions of neurasthenia during the late nineteenth century. For Freud perversity is not necessarily degenerate (except in the ultimate sense that polymorphous perversity is inherent in all infants). Degeneracy is an illness of all individuals within Western civilization, not merely the Jews (*SE* 7:160). It is not merely the Jews who are fixated at an earlier stage of development. The Jewish body, as we have seen, was assumed to have suffered more than most from the effects of civilization because of its predisposition. For Freud this becomes not a Jewish problem but a human one. There are yet further contemporary overtones in this passage on degeneration and civilization.

Freud adopts a view of trauma in his view of sexual psychopathology that would seem much more at home in Ibsen's *A Doll's House,* in the figure of Dr. Rank, in the central figure in *Ghosts,* Oswald Alving, or in Michael Arlen's bestseller *The Green Hat.* It is the trauma of civilization, the illness that characterized it and condemns it, syphilis. For Freud civilization in its most degenerate sexuality passed the fear of syphilis, syphilophobia, from generation to generation (*SE* 7:236). The hidden decay of syphilis, its mythic relation to sexuality (assumed but not yet scientifically proved), its ability to destroy across generations, made it one of the late nineteenth-century paradigms for degenerative sexuality. It is also, in a special way, one of the means of explaining the dangers inherent in the Jewish body and how that danger is passed, like syphilis, from generation to generation. The theme became a topic of scientific consideration when, building on the work of Victor Augagneur, the concept of *hérédosyphilis,* which could be passed on from generation to generation, was introduced into the medical literature.[152] Prenatal syphilis became a form of congenital degeneration, passed not only from mother to child but across generations.

Freud had already made the fear of syphilis and its overt medical implications, the poisoning of the "bloodline," the subject of one of his illustrative anecdotes from his self-analysis of his "*Autodidasker*" dream in *The Interpretation of Dreams* (1900).[153] There all of the protagonists are Jews—the politicians Eduard Lasker and Ferdinand Lassalle, as well as Freud's brother Alexander. Freud mentioned that Lasker's death was caused by syphilis, while Lassalle "fell in a duel because of a woman." The precipitating event in the dream, according to Freud, was the presentation to his wife of a novel by the Austrian Jewish novelist Jakob Julius David about the decline and death of a writer. All the figures in this dream are men, all are Jews, and all are destroyed by the women in their lives. Freud transferred sexual pathology from the private, masturbatory sphere to the public, venereal one. Eduard Reich, as well as many other writers on public health during this period, projected at least some of his anxiety concerning sexuality and sexual pathology from masturbation to syphilis, moving from a degenerate endogenous model to a degenerate exogenous one.[154] In masturbation the evil lies in the degeneracy of the individual; in syphilis, in the degeneracy of the Other, the prostitute. Sexuality can become contaminated through an external source rather than in the light of any inherent failure of the individual. Late nineteenth-century discussions of the prostitute, like discussions of the Jew, centered on whether she was inherently degenerate (the view of Lombroso) or whether she merely had a disposition for prostitution, which was triggered by her economic circumstances (the view of Parent-Duchatelet).[155]

Freud favored the former view, since his comprehension of sexuality stressed its inherent nature. Libido theory, with its view of the inherent polymorphous perversity of the infant, is not far removed from the view that perversity is the disposition of all human beings, including the prostitute (*SE* 7:192). Likewise, the view that the Jew had a special disposition to diseases associated with sexuality is universalized through a similar process. This is an extrapolation from the view that a special subclass of degenerates carries the stigmata of perverse sexuality rather than its rejection.

But for Freud sexuality is not "degenerate." In reversing the paradigm of degeneracy, sexuality becomes, in Freud's thinking, the antithesis of degeneracy. Sexual selectivity, inbreeding, has been understood as the source of degeneracy among the Jews. For Freud it becomes a positive force, preserving the "common mental construction" of the Jews. Freud undermined the view that sexuality, especially in terms of the Jews, leads to decay. He observed the descent of a ciliate infusorian as reproducing to the 3,059th generation with "no signs of . . . degeneration."[156] Freud continued with an analogy in *Beyond the Pleasure Principle* (1920), seeing in this absence of decay the vitalism inherent in sexuality:

> Let us, however, return to the self-preservative sexual instincts. The experiments upon protista have already shown us that conjugation—that is, the coalescence of two individuals which separate soon afterwards without any subsequent cell-division occurring—has a strengthening and rejuvenating effect upon both of them. In later generations they show no signs of degenerating and seem able to put up a longer resistance to the injurious effects of their own metabolism. This single observation may, I think, be taken as typical of the effect produced by sexual union as well. (*SE* 18:55; see also 1:187)

Thus Freud's earliest and his last use of the concept of degeneracy employed Rudolf Virchow's sense of inner decay of the cell. Freud, however, reversed his perception of the pathological nature of sexuality and its importance within the degenerative model.

Freud needed to draw on historical data to delineate more clearly his views concerning perversion from generation theory. The cyclical occurrence of perversion only within highly developed cultures still implied degeneration. In 1917, in the *Introductory Lectures,* he reformulated his reading of Bloch from 1905, seeing perversion as a universal presence, limited neither in its historical manifestation nor in its geographical locus (*SE* 16:307; see also 16:320, 18:243, 23:152). Degeneration is no longer a category through which to diagnose the etiology of mental illness. Freud had already stressed this in his dismissal of the false rhetoric of psychiatry, which used the concept of the degenerate to defame the Other. In the striking opening paragraph of his "Thoughts for the Times on War and Death" (1915), Freud had attributed his labeling of the Other as degenerate to the "anthropologists":

> In the confusion of wartime in which we are caught up, relying as we must on one-sided information, standing too close to the great changes that have already taken place or are beginning to, and without a glimmering of the future that is being shaped, we ourselves are at a loss as to the significance of the impressions which press in upon us and as to the value of the judgements which we form. We cannot but feel that no event has ever destroyed so much that is precious in the common possessions of humanity, confused so many of the clearest intelligences, or so thoroughly debased what is highest. Science herself has lost her passionless impartiality; her deeply embittered servants seek for weapons from her with which to contribute towards the struggle with the enemy. Anthropologists feel driven to declare him inferior and degenerate, psychiatrists issue a diagnosis of his disease of mind or spirit. Probably, however, our sense of these immediate evils is disproportionately strong, and we are not entitled to compare them with the evils of other times which we have not experienced. (*SE* 14:275)

This is the view Freud repeats a decade later in his birthday letter to Ernest Jones in 1929:

> The first piece of work that it fell to psychoanalysis to perform was the discovery of the instincts that are common to all men living today—and not only to those living today but to those of ancient and of prehistoric times. It called for no great effort, therefore, for psychoanalysis to ignore the differences that arise among the inhabitants of the earth owing to the multiplicity of races, languages, and countries. (*SE* 21:249)

Science has moved from its neutral stance; it has become the means of defaming the enemy. But this had always been the tradition of racial biology during the preceding decades, some of it practiced by Jews. Science had never been beyond nationalism. One wonders, did Freud also have in mind work such as that by his friend and colleague Leopold Löwenfeld on the "psychopathia gallica"?[157] Or his later comments in 1921 on the strongly anti-German tone of the study of mass psychology by Wilfred Trotter (who would become his physician in his English exile) (*SE* 18:118)? Trotter wrote of the "maniacal tone" of the German debates about the superiority of the German race as "the representatives of God's thought on Earth. . . . Now we understand why other peoples pursue us with their hatred. . . . So the Jews were hated in antiquity because they were the representatives of God on earth."[158] (Trotter is quoting Werner Sombart.) "We [meaning the British physician] seem forced to assume some actual lunatic condition in the German people." The Germans were simply insane, claiming, like the paranoid, to be in direct contact with the deity. In virtually all of his readings of this material Freud has effaced the racial tradition that existed in the debates about the enemy during this period. It is indeed to the French anthropological tradition of modern psychiatry with its pseudoscienticism that the term degeneracy is most indebted. In dismissing this label as false rhetoric, Freud is able to move the category of degenerate from its sexual context and place it where it belongs, in the realm of political rhetoric. But, as with his attempt to do this in his 1896 essay on heredity, he is unable to articulate the special position in which he is placed as a Jewish scientist. For to articulate this would be to call into question the basic neutral stance of the science from which he derives his status. Degeneracy for Freud is no mere biological category but one that implies the specific comprehension of the historical process in which he is himself implicated. The charge of degeneracy, specifically the degeneracy of the Jew, was to be found in one other major arena of late nineteenth-century and early twentieth-century medicine. It was to be found within the forensic literature concerning Jewish sociopathy—the criminality of the Jew. Just as Freud transmuted the charges of the innate difference of the Jewish psyche and the Jewish body into the rhetoric of psychoanalytic difference, so too he undertook to displace his anxiety about Jewish criminal identity, which we discussed in chapter 1, onto quite different medicalized categories.

4

SEDUCTION, PARRICIDE, AND CRIME

Jews and Criminal Sexual Activity

By the end of the nineteenth century, the Jewish criminal had become a case for the medical scientist. The association between Jews and crime is an older tradition that is embedded in the image as well as the reality of German Jewry. It has canonical form in Friedrich Schiller's *The Robbers,* a drama that was, in general, a favorite of acculturated German-speaking Jews because of its revolutionary message cast in the acceptable language of high culture. It was a play from which the youthful pupil Sigmund Freud memorized a long passage as a typical school exercise.[1] It is also a text that, in its representation of the heritability of circumcision among the Jews, reflects the relation between the mind of the Jew and his indelibly marked body.[2] For, at least according to his own deceitful account, Schiller's character, Moritz Spiegelberg, was born circumcised. But if the mark of circumcision scored the body of Schiller's prototypical Jewish criminal, his lying, criminal soul also reflected his Jewishness. He alone of all the bandits in Schiller's play was presented as a pathological criminal. One can plausibly argue that Schiller's image reflects the existence of bands of Jewish highwaymen, which was well documented at the close of the eighteenth century and the beginning of the nineteenth. But it is equally important to note that those criminals in central Europe who were not Jews were tied to the overdetermined image of the Jews through the use of a criminal lingua franca based on Yiddish.[3] But these were highwaymen and bandits, counterfeiters and confidence men whose social status was no different than that of marginal figures from other socially stigmatized groups. All shared the marginality of the Jew. The inclusion of a truly Jewish criminal among Karl Moor's band of brigands was a means of separating such natural criminals from those forced into a life of crime through circumstances. Karl Moor's own forced and illegitimate exile from the middle class into a world of crime is contrasted with the situation of the true criminal, the Jew. Jews were presumed criminal by their nature, much like the lower classes.

By the conclusion of the nineteenth century the idea of the Jew as criminal had become part of the psychiatric literature on forensic pathology. By the fin de siècle the image of the Jewish robber was a staple of the literature that attempted to understand antisocial activities as a pathology of the human mind. Jews look different, according to Cesare Lombroso's primary German disciple, Hans Kurella, and they speak differently—they *mauscheln*. That difference is the difference also found in criminals, who bear the "typical stigmata of their heritage."[4] Nowhere is this clearer than in the fin-de-siècle monograph on Schiller's *The Robbers* by the famous criminologist Erich Wulffen.[5] Although the central focus of Wulffen's text is the criminal nature of both (!) brothers, he pays attention to the special language of Spiegelberg. Spiegelberg is a "libertine" who has an "inherited criminal character" that can be read in the very form of his skull (44, 65). Central to Wulffen's discussion is the representation of Spiegelberg's claim to be a Jew. The Jewish criminal, like all other criminals, had become part of the world of medicine, for the signs of degeneration marked the Jewish criminal.

The criminal is as necessarily visible as the Jew, and the signs of criminality and of Jewishness merge. Thus the criminal, like the Jew, has a specific, measurable gait. Citing work by Albert Gilles de la Tourette,[6] Cesare Lombroso presented a table measuring the difference between the normal gait, the gait of the criminal, and the gait of the epileptic.[7] The criminal's stride is longer (because of his robust body form); he moves ever more away from the center and more toward the right. It is the asymmetrical, the misshapen, the ugly that mark both the Jew and the criminal. The beautiful can never be truly criminal. According to Cesare Lombroso, "physical beauty is equivalent to a noble spirit" (2:3).

Lombroso's view on the fixed physical form of the criminal reappeared within the debates about "constitution" that have a major role in the continuation of this tradition after the beginning of the twentieth century.[8] This reaction to the Darwinian view of the mutability of form is best captured in the debates about the attempt, in the 1920s, to apply the body-type thesis of Ernst Kretschmer to racial biology.[9] This debate repeated a series of claims concerning the relationship between race and constitution during the late nineteenth century. Kretschmer's three body types (asthenic, athletic, pyknic) were associated with specific forms of mental illness. Given the general assessment that there was a close correlation between race and mental illness, it was not long before this leap was made. Ludwig Stern-Piper, in a lecture at the 1922 Southwest German Psychiatric Conference, took the three body types outlined by Kretschmer and claimed that "they are basic racial types."[10] He took the obvious association of disease with body type and gave it the no less evident racial association. Kretschmer answered in the next issue, distancing his views from those of Stern-Piper.[11] He saw the existence of all three body types in all races; indeed, he saw a certain contradiction between the very concept of "racial" types and body types. Stern-Piper returned to the argument stressing the inherent racial makeup of each individual and the link among body type, illness, and race.[12] This debate became joined when clinicians such as the Munich physician Moses Julius Gutmann attempted to work out which mental illness dominated among Jews. Given the dominance among Jews, Gutmann noted, of the asthenic body type, with a long, lanky body, one would imagine that there would be a predominance of schizophrenics, but his work seemed to indicate that manic-depressive psychosis was the dominant form of mental illness.[13] The way the Jew looks, like the way the criminal looks, was scientific evidence of the Jew's sociopathic condition.

This debate echoed the assumption of nineteenth-century forensic psychiatry that the criminal was marked by the stigmata of degeneration. For Cesare Lombroso the criminal was an atavistic form, a throwback to earlier and uglier stages of human development: "The germs of moral insanity and criminality are found normally in mankind in the first stages of existence in the same way as forms, considered monstrous when exhibited by adults, frequently exist in the fetus."[14] The appearance of the criminal, according to the physiognomy of criminology, is similar to that of the Jew: he has very mobile facial characteristics but a "cold, frozen gaze."[15] The criminal also evinces a prominent and marked nose. Dark hair is six times more frequent among criminals than blond hair.[16] If criminality is not written on the face, it is imprinted on the brain. For the Viennese Jewish anatomist Moritz Benedikt, it is a reflex of the biology of the brain and is marked in the brain's structure. It is a hidden factor, unlike Lombroso's stigmata, which are written upon the body. Like Lombroso, Benedikt sees the criminal as a different race or degenerate variant,[17] but in the work of the Italian Jewish forensic psychiatrist the role of race is dramatically understated though still present. Of the 220 male criminals Lombroso photographed, including 23 Americans, 1 Englishman, 2 Frenchmen, 18 Italians, 164 Germans, 8 Jews, and 4 Russians, none showed the typology of race except "for the 8 Jews, who show a Semitic type."[18] Lombroso, as is true of the discussions of the nature of Jewish criminality, accepts that Jews are more criminal in specific economically defined areas. But "the percentage of crimes among Jews is always lower than that of the surrounding population; although there is a prevalence of certain specific forms of offences, often hereditary, such as fraud, forgery, libel, and chief of all, traffic in prostitution, murder is extremely rare."[19] Race plays a factor, according to Lombroso, but he also remarked that Jews are usually less evident among criminals (though they are very visible among the insane), even though there are Jewish criminal families. He attributed the substantially higher rate of insanity to "intellectual overactivity."[20] This view that sees the criminality of the Jew as a reflex of disposition was widely followed. Max Sichel, who noted that endogenous marriages were becoming more infrequent among Jews at the fin de siècle, also noted that this seemed to have no effect on the rate of insanity, since it was a disposition of the innate nature of the Jew, not the result of degenerative inbreeding.[21] Carl Heinrich Stratz, in a pamphlet read by Sigmund Freud, argued quite the opposite. For him all the "degenerate stigmata" associated with the "Jewish type," especially the form and structure of the face (including the "protruding eyes with their powerful upper lid"), were signs of the "inbred type": "Excessive inbreeding transforms itself into indecency, . . . for not only do the advantages [associated with inbreeding] increase over time but so do the disadvantages, until the increase of the latter finally makes individual life impossible."[22] The degenerate is also the criminal, and the criminal's nature is written on his body by his inheritance. (For this Aryan scientist, the only cure for the Jewish [degenerate] type was crossbreeding.) The movement from the sexuality of the Jew as the cause of the Jew's criminality to the sexual nature of the Jew's criminality is an easy one.

In the fin-de-siècle medical literature there is a clear association of the Jew with sexual crimes, with criminal perversions. This is an ancient topos that harks back to Tacitus's description of the Jews as the "projectissima ad libidinem gens"—the most sensual of peoples. By the close of the nineteenth century it had become part of the new forensic literature in Germany that described the nature of the Jews as it was stated in one of the standard forensic studies of the time: "Further, it must be noted that the sexuality of the Semitic race is in general powerful, yes, often greatly exaggerated."[23] Or as John S. Billings, the leading American student of Jewish illness and the head of the Surgeon General's Library in Washington, noted, when Jewish males are integrated into Western culture they "are probably more addicted to . . . sexual excesses than their ancestors were."[24] The "sexual" male is "dark" (Biérent), or has a "dark complexion" (Bouchereau), or has "brown skin" and a "long nose" (Mantegazza).[25] Jewish physicians of the period understood the implications of this charge. The Viennese Jewish physician Hanns Sachs, who was involved in the earliest development of psychoanalysis, commented in his memoirs on this version of the "timeworn prejudice that the Jewish . . . mind was abnormally preoccupied with matters of a sexual nature."[26] Some Jewish scientists of the fin de siècle, such as the Munich neurologist Leopold Löwenfeld, were forced to confront this charge and were unable to dismiss it. Löwenfeld argued, in a study of sexual constitution published in 1911, that the role of racial predisposition in structuring the sexual drives could be confused by the mediating role that climate, nutrition, or culture can play.[27] But he and his Jewish contemporaries such as Iwan Bloch had no doubt that racial identity did play some role in structuring sexual constitution. Freud's Jewish lodge brother and one of the original members of the Viennese Psychoanalytic Society, Eduard Hitschmann, believed that "neuroses, psychoses, suicides, etc. play a more important role among the Jews, . . . they have many more sexual experiences than others and—a fact that must be particularly emphasized—take them much more seriously."[28] The Jews' mental state, specifically the psychopathologies associated with them, is closely linked to their intense sexuality.

In terms of the medical world of the fin de siècle the criminality of the Jews was also a major factor in understanding their sexuality. The discussion about the nature of Jews and their relation to the world of antisocial activity became a central theme in the medical literature of the late nineteenth century. The statistical evidence of forensic psychiatry argued for a greater rate of criminality, in some specific spheres, among the Jews. Such activity was read as being not only sociopathic but also psychopathic; it was a sign of the degeneracy of the Jews because of their endogamous marriages and the resultant inbreeding.[29] The etiology for the Jew's hysteria, for example, like the hysteria of the woman, was to be sought in "sexual excess,"[30] specifically in the inbreeding within this endogenous group: "Being very neurotic, consanguineous marriages among Jews cannot but be detrimental to the progeny."[31] This view was even advocated by Rudolf Virchow, whose liberal views on the ability of Jewish acculturation were paralleled by his sense of the dangers of Jewish consanguinity.[32] Virchow pointed out the much greater occurrence of inherited diseases among the Jews. Such dangerous marriages were labeled as a criminal activity, even when such "inbreeding" was not consanguineous. In historical terms, writers such as Houston Stewart Chamberlain could comment on the origin of the Jews and its "refreshingly artless expression in the genealogies of the Bible, according to which some of these races owe their origin to incest, while others are descended from harlots."[33] This was answered, at least in the data gathered by Jewish social scientists and their medical allies, in the claim that either the totality of the image presented was incorrect and correct statistical data could be amassed or that a higher incidence could be found but only for certain crimes (usually economic ones) or among specific subsets (such as Eastern Jews).[34] These were linked in the view that the "destructive impact of certain professions (such as that of the stock market speculator) on the nerves predisposed individuals to commit sexual crimes."[35] What is most striking is the counterargument; the Jewish "immunity" for sexual crimes, such as incest, was stressed by other groups.[36] Such immunity was often read as a form of latent criminality, a hidden disposition that was simply not triggered because of the sexual barriers erected by Jewish religious practices. This literature must be set against the ubiquitous charge of Jewish criminal sexuality that haunted European culture of the fin de siècle.

The face of the Jew and that of the sexual criminal had merged in the course of the fin de siècle in the figure of "Jack the Ripper" as an eastern European Jew.[37] The "real" parallel to the fantasy about the Jewish Jack the Ripper as a sexual monster was played out in the courts of London in the accusation of murder lodged against the eastern European Jew Israel Lipski in 1887, the year before the Ripper murders.[38] Lipski was hanged that year for having murdered a pregnant woman by pouring nitric acid down her throat. Her exposed body was discovered with Lipski hiding beneath the bed. His case was widely debated, since it was charged that he had been accused because he was an eastern European Jew. The assumption was that Jews had a more intensely violent sexual nature. This was not seen as an individual aberration. The charge was made in 1894 in the anti-Semitic newspapers in Germany that Jack was an eastern European Jew functioning as part of the "international Jewish conspiracy."[39] This image of the Jewish Jack the Ripper rested on a long association of the Eastern Jew in the West with the image of the mutilated, diseased, different appearance of the genitalia. It is especially in the image of the Eastern Jew as criminal (as described in Western literature) that this view seems to be fixed. The overall medical view is that Jews in the East demonstrate a higher incidence of criminal insanity than do Western Jews. Whereas Eastern Jews argue that they actually evince a lower rate of criminality,[40] the overall assumption among Western forensic scientists, both Jews and non-Jews, is that the Eastern Jew is dangerous. The Jewish psychiatrist Rafael Becker, reporting from a Jewish mental hospital near Warsaw, noted that 13 percent of the mental patients examined for their legal competency were Jews.[41] In Vienna the legal attempt to identify those who were not German "by race or language" during the early 1930s led to an ongoing representation of the Eastern Jews in Austria as the source of all criminality, including sexual crimes.[42] The theme of the criminality of the Eastern Jew continued into the Nazi period. Joachim Duckart documented the history of a "criminal community" of Eastern Jews back into the eighteenth century.[43] Though it has been argued that Jews, especially Eastern Jews, presented an overwhelming majority of those individuals involved in sexual commerce in Europe and South America from the 1880s through the beginning of the 1930s, the image of the Jew as sexual criminal in the medical and forensic debates of the fin de siècle rested on the special, sexualized nature of the Jew.[44] The debate about race taints all other views of the social reality of the period.

Within the major psychoanalytic work dealing with criminality, a study written by the Berlin psychoanalyst Franz Alexander and the jurist Hugo Staub in 1929, there is absolutely no mention of a Jewish predisposition for any type of crime.[45] Indeed, race has completely vanished as a category of analysis. Only "idiots, paretics, schizophrenics, and epileptics" are considered under the label of those criminals showing a "biological etiology" for crime. All other crimes are committed either by neurotics, whose unresolved Oedipus complex provides the psychological basis for their acts, or by "normal" criminals, whose acts are examples of the weakness of character deformed by a negative social context. Alexander and Staub evoke all the rhetoric about the Jewish criminal—on all sides of the issue—but in completely removing the category of race from their analysis, they make criminality universal rather than racial. Sexuality becomes the hallmark of the neurotic criminal with his unresolved Oedipus complex; inheritance is the sign of the "born criminal" suffering from mental deficiency or impairment; and the social milieu marks the "normal" criminal. The authors do not create a nosology of crime. They do not place any group in a special relation to any of these categories. In doing so they avoid all the debates about the special status of the Jews in relation to the world of sexuality and crime.

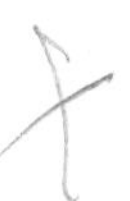

The Jew remains the representation of the male as outsider, the act of circumcision marking the Jewish male as sexually apart, as anatomically different. For fin-de-siècle medicine, madness was marked not only on the face but also on the genitalia. In the case of the signs of mental degeneration, "precisely the anomalies of the genitalia are of extreme importance and are rarely found alone."[46] The prostitute was the embodiment of the degenerate and diseased female genitalia in the nineteenth century.[47] From the standpoint of the normative perspective of the European middle class, it is natural that the Jew and the prostitute, Jack and his victims, must be in conflict and that the one "opens up" the other, since both are seen as "dangers" to the economy, fiscal and sexual, of the state.[48] This notion of the association of the Jew and the prostitute is also present in the image of "spending" semen (in an illicit manner), which dominates the literature on masturbation in the eighteenth and early nineteenth centuries. For the Jew and the prostitute are seen as negating factors, outsiders whose sexual images represent all the dangers felt to be inherent in human sexuality.

The desire to explore this world of Jewish sexual identity became a theme in the early psychoanalytic literature. Otto Rank wrote an essay, "The Essence of Judaism," in December 1905.[49] His argument tied together a number of the threads from the medical and forensic literature of the fin de siècle and reversed their implications. Society, Rank argues, moves toward ever greater sexual repression until it "reaches the neurotic stage of antisexuality, a disturbance of consciousness." This disease state is one not yet reached by the Jews, since they have preserved themselves at a more "primitive," "relatively favorable stage of the repression process" through their closer ties to nature. Echoing Otto Weininger's parallel, Rank notes the now-positive, primitive sexuality of the Jews: "Like woman, they have remained 'unchanged.'" The "essence of Judaism is its stress on primitive sexuality." And this is like the wellsprings of artistic creativity, for artists, individually, arise from a repression of sexuality. Jewish sexuality, unlike that of the artist, provided the impetus for the selection of "specifically Jewish professions, which are simple, sensible attempts at preventing nervous illness." As a result Jews "became physicians. For the Jews thoroughly understand the radical cure of neurosis better than any other people. . . . They brought matters to such a point that they could help others, since they have sought to preserve themselves from illness." Here we have the entire repertoire of charges: Jews engage in perverse, atavistic sexual practices; they are sexually like women; they have a special relationship to mental illness and its cure. All of these charges are those leveled at the Jew as sexually diseased, and all of them are reversed by this Viennese Jewish literary critic and psychoanalyst. In 1912 Rank published his extraordinarily influential study of incest as a motif in culture.[50] Here too the universalization of the charges of sexual criminality is turned into a comment on the polymorphous nature of human sexuality.

In contrast to the popular image of the Jew as a sexual criminal, much of the medical literature about Jewish criminality during the late nineteenth and early twentieth centuries assumes that the Jew is by nature a "white-collar" criminal, a criminal who commits economic crimes. This is also an underlying assumption of the literature concerning Jewish sexual criminality, but it is made much more explicit in the literature analyzing the Jewish white-collar criminal. In 1906 Willy Helpach sees the increase of economic criminals as an "occupational disease" of the Jews. Rather than an "occupational psychosis," it is an "occupational error" passed on from generation to generation, "as it is learned at the father's knee. It expresses itself in the inability to feel oneself into specific directions. It is not easy to express this feeling, a feeling that even unprejudiced observers have against the Jews as having something foreign in their souls."[51] It is part of the common mental construction of the Jew. But more central to the medicalization of the image of the Jew is the range of other crimes about which there is a substantial debate in the fin de siècle, the crimes that relate to sexuality: incest, sexual abuse of minors, rape—all the crimes that filled the rich anti-Semitic literature circulated on the streets. How is Jewish sexual selectivity, supposed to be a form of inbreeding rather than endogamous marriage, understood in the forensic literature of the period, when it is converted into a reading of the Jewish predisposition for criminal sexual activity such as incest and inbreeding?

The medical literature of the early twentieth century documents the greater rate of "inbreeding" and the resultant degenerative diseases among Jews.[52] In both Germany and Austria "inbreeding" is a criminal act. It is assumed to be a cause for moral as well as physical degeneration; thus it not only is a crime but is the source of crime. It is the disease of the city.[53] As Richard Krafft-Ebing noted: "Large cities are hotbeds in which neuroses and low morality are bred, *vide* the history of Babylon, Nineveh, Rome and the mysteries of modern metropolitan life. . . . The episodes of moral decay always coincide with the progression of effeminacy, lewdness and luxuriance of the nations. These phenomena can only be ascribed to the higher and more stringent demands which circumstances make upon the nervous system. Exaggerated tension of the nervous system stimulates sensuality, leads the individual as well as the masses to excesses, and undermines the very foundations of society, and the morality and purity of family life."[54] The decadence of civilization, of the city, is inexorably linked with the sexual exclusivity of the Jew. In *Mein Kampf* Hitler notes this link, thinking back on his fin-de-siècle experience in Vienna: "No, the fact that our big city population is growing more and more prostituted in its love life cannot just be denied out of existence; it simply is so. The most visible results of this mass contamination can, on the one hand, be found in the insane asylums, and on the other, unfortunately, in our children. They in particular are the sad product of the irresistibly spreading contamination of our sexual life; the vices of the parents are revealed in the sicknesses of the children."[55] And Hitler states the doctrine of racial purity: "For since this question primarily regards the offspring, it is one of those concerning which it is said with such terrible justice that the sins of the fathers are avenged down to the tenth generation. But this applies only to the profanation of the blood and the race. *Blood sin and desecration of the race are the original sin in this world and the end of a humanity which surrenders to it*" (249; emphasis in the original). Incest and racial pollution through crossbreeding are parallel sins for Hitler and for the time.

Nowhere is this linkage made more evident than in Thomas Mann's parodic novella *The Blood of the Walsungen* (1905). This tale of brother-sister incest ends, at least in the first version, with an emphasis on the sexual exclusivity of the Jews. The brother has just consummated his relationship with his sister, and she ponders the fate of her German fiancé. This is, according to Auguste Forel in the standard sexual handbook of the day, "a psycho-pathological form of incest associated with morbid appetites in the families of degenerates."[56] It is also, according to J. G. Frazer, one of the most widespread taboos among "primitive" peoples, since it is the most common of such activities.[57] He concludes the tale in its unpublished first edition with two Yiddishisms, a sign of the damaged and at the same time sexualized discourse of the siblings. Mann's father-in-law, Alfred Pringsheim, so objected to the inclusion of Yiddishisms to represent the hidden *Mauscheln* of the Jews—"We robbed [*beganeft*] the non-Jew [*goy*]"—as a sign of the siblings' ethnic identity that Mann suppressed the planned publication of the story.[58] The novella, which Mann reedited in 1921 to eliminate the Yiddishisms, echoed the sense of the corruption of both "modern life," as typified by the Wagner cult, and the Jews. The Jews, through their lack of redemption, are morally weak, and this manifests itself in the most primitive manner, through incest. This theme is one found throughout the literature of the period.[59] Indeed, Adolf Hitler, never the most original of thinkers, simply summarized "Jewish religious doctrine" as "prescriptions for keeping the blood of Jewry pure."[60] The view that within the Jews' sexuality is hidden the wellspring of their own degeneration haunts the overtly sexual imagery of anti-Semitic writings from the end of the nineteenth century. The Jew, the most visible Other in late nineteenth-century Europe, is also the bearer of the sign of the most devastating sexual stigma, the act of incest. In the one novel on this topic by a German Jewish writer, Kurt Münzer's novel *The Path to Zion* (1907), brother-sister incest among Jews is paralleled to the seduction of Christian women by Jewish men. The language Münzer places in the mouth of the Jewish figures is overly emotional and reveals their own incestuous predisposition.[61] Münzer's representation of Jewish sexuality accepts all the stereotypes of Jewish incest of the time and casts them, quite seriously, into the rhetoric of the Wagnerian myth that Mann parodies. And this in a novel dedicated to "my sister Adele"!

The Statistical Arguments about Incest

The debate about Jewish sexual crimes provides a further reading of the idea of the hidden nature of the Jews. Latent criminality becomes a component of their "common mental construction." In 1881 there appeared an anonymous anti-Semitic pamphlet titled *The Jews' Role in Crime,* which began by asking its audience to inquire not "Où est la femme?" in searching for the origin of crime, but "Where is the Jew?"[62] The Jew became the substitute for the woman as the source of criminality in society. The author cited the following statistics from the 1871 Prussian census. In 1871 Jews made up only 1.3 percent of the population. Thus there were 16,636,990 Protestants, 8,625,840 Catholics, and 339,700 Jews (or "one Jew for every seventy-four Germans"). But they were accused of crimes against morality 20 percent more often than Catholics or Protestants (Catholics, 372; Protestants, 703; Jews, 18). And this argument was made by the author across every arena of criminality. The argument is explicit that Jews are by their very nature criminals and that all areas of criminality, including sexual crimes such as incest, rape, and sexual abuse of minors, find them overrepresented.

This pamphlet called forth an immediate and intensive rebuttal on the part of Jewish social scientists. S. Löwenfeld attempted to answer it, labeling it a "statistical cry against the Jews."[63] Löwenfeld's argument was that though Jews may be accused of certain crimes more frequently than other groups, their conviction rate was actually lower than for either the Catholic or the Protestant population; indeed, they represented less than half the number of convictions to be expected from their representation in the population. He stressed this in specific areas, such as sexual crimes. In 1885 Ludwig Fuld, a lawyer in Mainz, published yet another tabulation of the "relation between religion and criminality." Relying on the 1881 Prussian criminal census, his tabulation of sexual crimes noted that the sexual abuse of minors and statutory rape were the most often punished moral crimes among Jewish men but were also widespread among non-Jews. Incest, on the other hand, was so rarely to be found that he sees its absence among Jewish men as a relic of the biblical injunction that punishes this crime with death. He sees the lower rate of conviction of Jews for the crime of incest as an atavism that can be traced back to the ethnopsychology of the Jews.[64] At the same time, the French Jewish community, in reviewing the crime statistics in France during 1885, argued that these statistics were "an honor to the Jews," since they revealed a much lower incidence in all areas including incest.[65]

The debate about Jewish criminality, with its subtext about the higher or lower incidence of sexual crimes among Jews, was serious enough that when the Committee to Defend against Anti-Semitic Attacks began its publication series in 1896, its first statistical study was directed against the literature on Jewish criminality.[66] The statistics on sexual crimes reported in this study are revealing. Covering the period from 1882 to 1892, the statisticians found that instead of the forty-four cases of incest projected for the Jewish population based on its representation in the population, only seven convictions were found; in the case of "unnatural inbreeding" [*Inzucht*], twenty cases were found as against the fifty predicted, and there were twenty-one cases of "crimes against morals," which was the number projected.

In 1905 Arthur Ruppin, the founder of Jewish social statistics in Germany, reported similar statistics from the period 1899 to 1902.[67] Ruppin's rationale for the substantially lower rates of sexual crimes is the "greater education of the Jews" (9). Ruppin's work is reflected in his basic study of the sociology of the Jews published in 1904.[68] This view is seconded by Bruno Blau in a pamphlet in 1906, which, however, admits to a higher incidence of certain crimes (such as slander) because of the "temperament" of the Jews.[69] Here the contrast between evaluations based on nature or nurture can be judged. Ruppin saw the educational level of the Jews as a reflex of the older religious tradition now secularized. This is precisely the aspect of the Jewish mind that is most often evoked when the discussion is of the negative impact of the stresses of civilization on the Jews, given their predisposition for mental illness. Blau's comment on the temperament of the Jews looked at a characterological argument for criminal activity. Character, however, was formed by social stress, by the ghetto experience, according to many commentators. What was clearly an argument based on experience reveals itself to be analogous to one based on inheritance and vice versa. This can be most clearly seen in the comments of Erich Wulffen, one of the leading criminologists of the early twentieth century, in his 1910 handbook on sexual crimes: "The Jew is marked by his intellectual gifts, which in general serve as a preventative against the commission of crime. His ability to think logically and his cleverness provide an antidote to his passion and his sexual excitedness. In other [than sexual] crimes, especially fraud and perjury, these characters are a predisposing criminal factor."[70]

The view that race was a primary factor in criminality became the focus of debate after the beginning of the twentieth century. In the second volume of the primary German periodical on criminology founded by the most eminent criminologist of his day, Gustav Aschaffenburg, there is a long essay on the topic of race and criminality by the physician

Richard Weinberg from Dorpat/Tartu (Estonia).[71] Weinberg argued that criminality is inherently a reflex of race, that it is an inherited proclivity of a group. In looking at the Jews, Weinberg notes the "general tendency of the Jews for mental illness," and he sees this as a sign of their racial degeneration (727). This degeneration has a clearly psychological aspect. It is the result of the mixing of races, a sign of the alteration of the character of the second generation of mixed racial types (729). Madness and criminality result from racial mixing, and both are forms of psychological degeneration as represented by physical signs. This is the view of the ideological originator of modern biological anti-Semitism, Count Gobineau, who saw degeneracy of a people as the direct result of the decline of racial homogeneity.[72]

The madness of the Jews, their predisposition to disease, was a result of their inbreeding, much as the noble families of Europe had decayed (and lost power) and the population of the Swiss villages had degenerated. This view is stated quite directly in the standard textbook of psychiatry of the fin de siècle, that of Emil Kraepelin.[73] Simon Scherbel, a Polish Jew and the son of a rabbi, presented his dissertation to the medical faculty of the Berlin University in 1883 on the topic of consanguineous marriages. He is confronted with an absolute contradiction. How can the "laws of Moses, which are for the most part still valid for Protestants," advocate the marriage of their "daughters within the tribe"?[74] For it is evident that these laws have "a negative result." Jews have higher incidences of deaf-mutism and mental illness.[75] Scherbel responds that Jews have the necessary disposition for such illnesses, because of their economic or professional status or because of some factor yet unknown, which is triggered more frequently than in their non-Jewish counterparts. The laws that forbid consanguineous marriages are an attempt to avoid "incest and immorality" in families (43–44, 9). The entire debate on consanguineous marriage, from a religious as well as a medical point of view in the 1920s, was summarized in the *Jewish Lexicon*.[76] The essay by Felix Theilhaber stressed that the result of such marriages is an increased rate of mental illness among the offspring.

In 1909 further statistics are brought to argue a decrease in the conviction rate for Jews accused of sexually related crimes.[77] In Aschaffenburg's journal, the chief of the Dutch Bureau of Legal Statistics published an essay that asked quite directly: "Is it racial criminality, or is it a criminality that is a product of social circumstances?"[78] He presented the Dutch figures for the period from 1896 to 1906 and argued that "in spite of the various circumstances in which Jews live, they show the same pattern of criminality" (197). And this is especially true in the tendency to commit sexually related crimes. They may show fewer cases of incest and sexual criminality, but they are much more involved in the publication of pornography. For de Roos, their criminality is the result of the "combination of the natural disposition and their social and economic circumstances" (205). Thus in 1911 Rudolf Wassermann was forced to confront the question of the "racial" cause of Jewish criminality directly. Spurred on by de Roos's essay, Wassermann stated his position most clearly: Jewish criminality mirrors the criminality of the society in which the Jews find themselves and is a purely social reflex rather than the result of inheritance.[79] And indeed this is the general view within the German-speaking Jewish scientific community.[80] Franz von Liszt attempted to further Wassermann's views, stressing that the criminality of any group, including the Jews, sprang from the specific social location.[81] What is different in Liszt's approach is that he assumed that the choice of profession was a reflex of the "common mental construction" of the Jews.

It is striking that none of the studies suggested the evident control for testing such assumptions: the rate of criminality and the types of crimes committed by Jewish converts and their offspring. The assumption would be that conversion, given the contemporary discussion of its intent, would at least change the social localization of the converts and would permit them to engage in other professions, some of which were de facto barred to Jews. The rate of the commission of sexual crimes would also be reflected (positively or negatively) in the change of the structure of the family and of the social context of the Jew. The taboo about seeking to examine converts can be attributed to the anxiety on all sides about the implications of boundary crossing.

It is important to clarify what these various "sexual" crimes were. Incest in the German legal and forensic discourse of the fin de siècle is *Blutschande,* the violation of the blood.[82] The origin of this concept is that there is a real "pollution" of the blood by the sexual contact between relatives.[83] Its origin is the concept of the *sanguis contumelia* of Roman law.[84] Incest is understood as being "unnatural" because it comes from an "unnatural" desire and may lead to "unnatural," that is, unhealthy, offspring. Incest is a question of law, though there is a substantial debate among forensic scientists about its universal applicability or historical foundation. But it is also seen as a loss of control: "That the mentally ill tend to commit incest is easily explained, for the mentally ill there is complete loss of control as well as the law of the shortest way."[85] Incest thus marks the atavistic nature of the mentally ill. In the course of the nineteenth century this concept moves from signifying incestuous behavior to meaning the violation of the purity of the race.[86] It is no longer the violation of the taboos created within the narrower definition of the social unity (such as the family); rather, it becomes a definition of the boundaries of the wider unity, such as the race. Commit *Blutschande* and you violate the newly biologically defined taboos inherent in the purity of the racial stock. This act pathologizes the very concept of race by defining what will and does cause racial degeneration, for the very concept of *Blutschande* implies the degeneration of the race into illness and moral corruption.

It is little wonder the very debate about "incest" was fraught with racialist undertones. For Magnus Hirschfeld, the great German Jewish sexologist, it was a moral, not a legal, question. The term he and other researchers of the period preferred was *Unzucht* (indecency) rather than *Blutschande* (incest). *Inzest* (incest) was forbidden sexual contact between related individuals, but not necessarily related by consanguinity. This view was also stressed by Hermann Rohleder, who distinguished between incestuous relationships, which were forbidden by law, and "inbreeding," which he interpreted as any sexual contact within the wider blood relationship.[87] Thus German and Austrian law at the fin de siècle punished sexual contact between in-laws.[88] The Christian preoccupation with the Jewish custom of the levirate marriage, a man's obligation to marry the widow of his brother, comes into clear conflict with these European traditions.[89] Within the German understanding of the Jew's sexuality, this aspect of Jewish ritual practice had been a central focus. The "reader" appended to one of the very first grammars of Yiddish written in German, which was to be used to train missionaries to the Jews in the seventeenth century, consisted of two texts: one on leprosy and one on the levirate.[90] The link between the diseased nature of the Jews and the Jews' marital practice was long established. It is unimportant that by Talmudic times such marriages were seen as objectionable; indeed, Abba Saul viewed them as equivalent to incest. This obligation could be avoided through the institution of the ceremony of *chalitsah*.[91] Even though the levirate was not a common ritual practice in nineteenth-century Europe, it remained a subject of endless fascination. In his history of marriage, one of Freud's major sources, Edvard Westermarck, evoked the practice among the Jews in his discussion of the levirate. He cited the obligation "of a man to marry the widow of his brother if he died childless, and the firstborn should succeed in the brother's name 'that his name should be not put out of Israel.'"[92] This type of marriage was one of the keys to the European debate about incest in the nineteenth century.[93] It is the incestuous implications of the levirate that underlie the charge of brother-sister incest often lodged against the Jews. For a sexual relationship between a brother-in-law and his sister-in-law was considered in German and Austrian law to be the legal equivalent of brother-sister incest. C. G. Jung's charge that Freud had sexual relations with his sister-in-law Minna Bernays, whom he called his "sister," is an evocation of this calumny.[94]

For German Jewish scientists such as Hirschfeld, "Incest is the most frequent crime of solitary farms and narrow proletarian domiciles,"[95] not of the middle-class dwellings of Berlin or Viennese Jewry. It is in these venues, marked by endemic goiter and insanity, that the signs of the degenerate are permitted to be found. Another German Jewish sexologist and psychiatrist, Max Marcuse, noted that "all human beings stem from inbreeding, for the original sexual relationships were incestuous. . . . In people, the marriages of consanguineous parents often evidence severe illnesses and deformities. The dangers of inbreeding can be illustrated by the degeneration and disappearance of many noble families, the racial pathology of the Jews, and the endemic constitutional inferiority of people living in mountain villages, in which the inhabitants tend to mix only with themselves."[96] The acceptance of the view that inbreeding (and certainly incest) results in the decline of the group was commonplace and was often applied to the Jews as an explanation, as we have seen, for a number of pathological conditions. The "cure" for the disease of Jewishness would be exogenous rather than endogenous marriage. The cure would be to marry outside the group. In 1904 Heinrich Singer had argued against such positions. For him it is an error to imagine that Jews suffer from the physiological results of inbreeding. "Mixed marriages," he writes, "as the sole cure and preventative of the collapse of the race are not necessary."[97] Such a cure can be accomplished by Jews' moving into professions that are healthier and by youths' undertaking a "hygienic, body-building education."

The analogy between the historical sexual inbreeding (*Inzucht*) of the Jews and the geographically bounded inbreeding of those "in the mountains" was also made by the biologist Albert Reibmayr in 1897. Although Reibmayr discussed both the positive and the negative aspects of inbreeding of the species for the "culture" of the group, he finally came to understand inbreeding as obstructing progress. For him there is a regression to inbreeding that occurs later in a group's history, as in his microhistory of the Jews. Exogamy marked a higher level of development, and endogamy marked the beginning of the degeneracy of the group.[98]

Within the early psychoanalytic literature the debate about "blood" and *Blutschande* played a very minor role. However, it did appear in one marginal but revealing essay by Hermann Runge, an Aryan analysand of Georg Groddeck.[99] Published in Groddeck's house journal, it discusses the general consternation patients reflect when they come to a physician. Patients in Germany immediately attempt to localize the source of their own disease. "I believe it is in the blood," such patients tell their physicians. Much like the French preoccupation with livers and the American with hearts as the inevitable source of disease, Runge asserted, for Germans at the beginning of the twentieth century the potential source of all pathology was the blood. In a sensitive and complex manner, Runge linked this fascination with a German preoccupation with blood, as in the pact with the devil in Heine's ballet scenario of *Faust.* But most important, Runge relates this anxiety to the fear of incest, of *Blutschande.* The incest taboo for Runge reflects anxiety not only about the integrity of the body but about that of the community. The cultural context of this anxiety, which Runge links to a reading of the meaning of the Aryan body, reflects on the scientific awareness on the part of Aryan and Jewish physicians of the internalization of the apprehension about social identity and sexual contact as it lies "in the blood"—a description of a racial as well as a social pathogen.

The confusion surrounding the very concept of incest surfaced in the forensic literature of the fin de siècle. In 1907 Rudolf Wassermann published his basic introduction to the question of Jewish criminality.[100] Wassermann accepted the question as appropriate for statistical evaluation, even though there had been a debate in the criminological literature about the effectiveness and appropriateness of using "religion" as a criterion for the tabulation of such statistics. Wassermann, using the criminal census figures in Germany from 1899 to 1902, tabulated a slightly lower (about 10 percent) rate of sexual crimes on the part of Jews. But he also noted that during 1895 there had been a 10 percent higher rate of these crimes among Jews. In general Jews committed more crimes against public morality than did Christians, but Christians showed a much higher incidence of incest (4–5, 39–41, 46–47).

For Wassermann, and for many other commentators of the period, the Jews' lower rate of sexual crimes was closely tied to lower alcohol consumption. This motif, also linked to the lower incidence of syphilis among Jews, presented a social practice linked to the inheritance of sobriety. Hugo Hoppe, the author of the standard study of Jews and alcohol, saw the Jews as less likely to commit such crimes because they drank less.[101] Jewish abstinence provided the key to the lower rate of incest. Incest was a crime, as Hirschfeld had noted, committed when one was completely out of rational control. The insane provided him a perfect model, and alcoholism or at least drunkenness provided precisely the same context. Alcoholism remained the major "social" context of sexual abuse, although it was seen as an inherited trait that passed other, more devastating inherited traits on to the children of alcoholics. Zola described his *Nana* as the "story of a girl descended from four or five generations of drunkards, her blood tainted by an accumulated inheritance of poverty and drink, which in her case had taken the form of a nervous derangement of the sexual instinct."[102] If alcoholism leads to sexual degeneration and perversity, then the absence of such sociopathic acts among the Jews must be the direct result of their abstinence.

The debates about Jews and alcohol reflect the overall debates about predisposition as opposed to socialization. Wassermann noted that the more visible Jews are in society, the more they are placed in a position where alcohol consumption is desirable.[103] Thus the latent criminality of the Jews can be triggered and they can commit sexual crimes. In 1909 Wassermann added to his argument about the social context of the Jews' criminality, seeing the changes of the patterns of Jewish criminality as a reflex of the changes in social status of the Jews.[104] He calculated that 59 percent of all sexual crimes were committed under the influence of alcohol. Alcohol consumption among Jews remained relatively low into the 1920s.[105] Incest figures for Jews during the period from 1899 to 1916, although higher than in the previous decade, also remained remarkably below those for all other groups.

Mixed Marriages: No Answer to Incest

Now, if Jews were criminals and criminally insane (or at least morally insane) because of their "inbreeding," then the clear alternative would be to marry beyond the boundaries of the group. The assumption is that Jews show their racial pride in their refusal to marry outside their group.[106] This endogamy is based on the historical claim of the Jews to be the "chosen people," a theological view that is medicalized and pathologized within European culture by the fin de siècle. There is the claim by non-Jewish scientists, such as the Munich physician Curt Michaelis, that the sexual selection of the Jews lies at the bottom of the racial hatred the whole world feels against them. It is the disdain the Jews show to the rest of humanity that is at the core of anti-Semitism.[107] For Jewish physicians such as Alfred Nossig, the claim to be "chosen" is seen as a purely psychological response to the oppression of the Jews. It is part of their striving for preservation and fulfillment (Michaelis, 1–4). It is also seen, even by Jewish scientists (and especially by those espousing proto-Zionist or Zionist views), as being a reflex of the necessary racial selectivity of the Jews.[108] The biological results are in every case a reflex of this "inbreeding."[109] Certain positive qualities arise, such as the greater immunity to diseases such as syphilis, but there can be negative results. The claim on both the Jewish and the non-Jewish sides is that Jews always undertake breeding with a sense of direction: "For

Jews today always approach marriage with cold calculation."[110] When a Jew chooses to marry outside his group, this is also presumed to be purposeful. The assumption at the fin de siècle is that the Jew (always the male Jew) "breeds up" to "improve [his] blood through the admixture of 'Aryan' blood of a Christian girl" (177). It strengthens the race: "The Aryan woman, regardless of whether she is German, French, English, or Russian, comes from races that possess extraordinary warlike, state-creating abilities, and are in addition filled with the burning desire for the independence and the greatness of their nation. If we could breed into the entire Jewish youth these qualities in the sense of Zionism, then the entire Jewish question would be solved."[111] Indeed, there is the view that consanguineous marriages may well be advantageous in producing more males and mixed marriages disadvantageous in producing more females. Edvard Westermarck, one of the pioneers in the sociology of marriage, noted that "Jews, many of whom marry cousins," have "a remarkable excess of male births," whereas "mixed marriages produce only girls."[112] This view provided a rationale for mixed marriages that would strengthen the "race" and escape the dangers of degeneration through inbreeding.

The biological arguments about mixed marriages are equally complex. They presented a conflation of the biological and social rationales for the implications of race in its most intense form. Carl Claus distinguished various possibilities for the races in the present. Central to his interest is the viability of "mixed" races. Some of the crosses that create the artificial "races" are fertile, others are not. He argued for the essential mutability of species and races. But in doing so he cited a contemporary authority that "artificially bred races behave similarly to real species; they have an analogous range of forms and an analogous stability; they too show reduced fertility when producing bastards; and the bastards, like those of the species, have strange forms that can arise in no other way." It is "the closeness of kinship and not some unknown plan of creation [that] forms the invisible bond that links the organisms in different stages of similarity."[113] Claus's biology of relationships and his categorization of the race were typical for the time. It is biology that determines all relationships. He stressed the differences among human beings as biological and illustrated this difference with the claim that interbreeding would lead to infertile monsters. Although Claus's examples do not deal with human interbreeding, his voice represented the majority during the late nineteenth century.

August Weismann, who showed the fallacy of the belief in acquired characteristics, outlined three models for the crossing of species in a chapter titled "Plant-Crossings [*Pflanzenbastarde*] as an Example of Racial Character" in his seminal study of reproduction in 1892. For Weismann the offspring of a "crossing" could have three forms: first, the qualities of both parents might appear in the offspring; second, the qualities of one parent or the other might dominate; third, the qualities of first one parent and then the other might dominate in the offspring.[114] Hidden within this pattern, as Weismann noted, was always the possibility of a regression to an earlier type (392–402). In an earlier study, Weismann noted that crossing can, but need not, have the effect of rejuvenating a species. This positive result has been understood as an atavistic return to the earlier power of the pure race. Weismann rejected any such reading, stressing only the formal observation of the changes in the offspring.[115] Weismann, unlike Galton and many other biologists, is very careful to take his examples from the plant world. But the application to the world of racial biology is very clear. And indeed, the vocabulary of "crossing," such as the use of the term "bastard" for the product of the crossing, is present within the racial biology of the day. The implication of the "reversion to type" precluded any real sense that one could shed the previous generation's racial identity through intermarriage.

An analogous discussion of the meaning of "crossing" within ethnolinguistics is found in the views evolved by Wilhelm Wundt. Wundt was fascinated by the implications of "language mixing and mixed languages" and saw these as biological, even though he was extremely careful not to postulate them as racial or essential.[116] For Wundt the usual model of the "mixing of language" is that of the "lower" races accepting the language of the "higher" races, since the "higher race is usually more dominant than the lower race in its impact on the language" of the offspring of a mixed culture. As a result, the "appropriated language is relatively little altered, while the mother tongue . . . degenerates through the acceptance of the new language." The result is a "jargon." His example is the thieves' language in Germany, which reveals aspects of its Hebrew origin. Wundt did not posit an absolute relationship between "race" and "language." Rather, as an ethnopsychologist, he saw the linguistic environment as formative. The German-speaking child, for example, has a different "racial physiognomy" than the English-speaking one, but if the environment shifts, the child (unlike the adult) can also shift relatively easily (1:294, 395, 609). The mixing of languages and the creation of a degenerate "jargon" is caused by adults and mirrors the debate about the negative impact of racial mixing. Adults of a lower race will "revert to type," revealing the degeneracy of their race through their mixed language. Mixing can result in lower forms of language, although Wundt, like Weismann, is extremely careful to avoid any overt political references. Missing (even from his discussion of thieves' cant), for example, is any discussion of the Jews and their "mixed language," Yiddish. The meaning of "mixing" within the most up-to-date science of the fin de siècle, even in that science that self-consciously opposed models of biological determinism, evoked these models in a direct manner.

The power of the ethnopsychological debates about the implication of race mixing can be been seen in a text well known and generally well received by Freud (*SE* 18:83–85, 96–97). William McDougall's *The Group Mind* (1920) was the "state of the art" of the debate about group psychology when Freud wrote his "Group Psychology and the Analysis of the Ego" (1921). McDougall's book rests on the argument of the "innate mental constitution" of the "various branches of mankind."[117] Of all of the races, the "Semitic stock . . . is one, which widely scattered, seems to present certain constant peculiarities." These are the "result of a long continued process of selection, comparable with the natural selection by which, according to Darwin, animal species are evolved." And they are little changed by outside pressure: "In order to realize fully the influence of race, we must consider peoples whose culture and much else that enters into their social environment has been impressed upon them from without. We then see how little the social environment can accomplish in the moulding of a people, when it is not congenial to and in harmony with the racial tendencies." Thus, "the crossing of races," according to McDougall, results in only two possible social models, both "in harmony with old established popular beliefs, and with what we know of the crossing of animal breeds." The first is the result of the mixing of "inferior" races with superior races. The result is twofold: "a general lack of vigor, which expresses itself in lack of power of resistance to many diseases and in relative infertility" and "a lack of harmony of qualities, both mental and physical." These are precisely the qualities ascribed to the offspring of Jews and Aryans in the literature of the period: they are diseased and malformed, both psychologically and physically. For McDougall this risk "more than justifies" the British colonial "objection to intermarriage with those other races which Englishmen have upheld wherever they have settled" (111, 113, 117, 242–43, 244). For Jewish scientists reading such material in central Europe, this debate had been part of their social reality since the beginning of civil emancipation at the opening of the nineteenth century.

The Napoleonic Sanhedrin, convened in 1807, recognized marriage between "Israelites and Christians when concluded in accordance with the civil code."[118] The reformer Samuel Holdheim argued in 1843 that the prohibition against intermarriage did not include followers of monotheistic religions. In 1844 Ludwig Philippson proposed to the rabbinical conference at Brunswick that marriage between Jews and the adherents of any of the monotheistic faiths was "not prohibited" as long as the children were raised as Jews. This view was accepted widely in reformed circles (and was supported by neo-Orthodox scholars such as Samuel Raphael Hirsch). Opposition to the permission for intermarriage grew (coming from, among others, Ludwig Philippson) as the practice became more and more common. By 1898 there were 100 mixed marriages of Jews in Vienna and 847 purely Jewish marriages.[119]

An alternative explanation of the attraction of the Jew to the non-Jew is one of class. Through the 1880s the popular image of the mixed marriage was one in which non-Jewish men (often poorer members of the nobility) married wealthy Jewish women.[120] By the fin de siècle the image had changed remarkably. Jewish men were marrying non-Jewish women and were marrying women of a class below themselves. Karl Abraham, in a paper published in 1914, translated this desire of Jewish men to marry Aryan women as a form of "neurotic exogamy" by which the desire to have an incestuous relationship within the immediate family is reversed and projected into the rejection of those within the greater group as potential objects of sexual interest.[121] The first example Abraham notes, however, is the absolute antithesis of the image of the Jewish male's attraction to the Aryan woman. His initial clinical case is that of a "blond northern German male" who is attracted only to "dark-haired, brunette women of a different race" (228). Indeed, he is so repelled by members of his own group that he is not even attracted to those who speak his own dialect! Only then does Abraham provide a series of cases of Jewish males who are disgusted by Jewish women, since they see in the Jewish woman the forbidden relationship with mother or sister. This is accompanied by exaggerated love or hate. For Abraham such a neurosis can manifest itself as Jewish self-hatred, and a form of that self-hatred is the Jewish male's attraction to the Aryan. Mixed marriage is therefore a form of neurosis—a "flight from incest or from the family" that depends exclusively on the racial identity of the (female) object of desire. Gender here becomes subsumed under race as a category of identification—the attractive sexual partner is by definition someone of the other race. The desire to marry outside the group becomes for Abraham a pathological sign, as surely as an anxiety about open spaces or heights.

Mixed marriages between Jewish males and Aryan females would (according to traditional Jewish law) make the offspring totally non-Jewish. But such images of the criminal male forced to marry outside the group as a defense against incestuous attraction also echoed the anti-Semitic image of the Jew as the seducer of the defenseless non-Jewish female. Here the pathological image of the mixed marriage was understood as a compensatory act that at least avoided incest. And this image was also tied by Jewish psychoanalysts to the act of circumcision. Otto Fenichel commented:

> The drastic reminder of the sanguinary puberty rites of the primitives has been replaced by less drastic measures during the course of history. The Jewish circumcision, although practiced on the infant, is still comparatively drastic. It has remained a really sanguinary operation on the genitals. The knowledge of this fact on the part of the uncircumcised has undoubtedly increased the feeling of uncanniness which the Jew gives them. It has helped to lend a more precise form to the indefinite fear that a retaliation on the part of these curious people is imminent; this retaliation assumes a sexual form. The Jews will do something to the little girls of other races in the same way that they do something sanguinary-sexual to the little boys of their own race.[122]

Here the image of the hypersexual Jew seducing Christian young women is infiltrated with metaphors taken from the charges of both "blood libel" and "blood defilement." All are read as responses to the body of the male Jew.

The image of the hypersexual male Jew, parallel to the image of the hypersexual black in German culture of the period, led Jews to understand that their sexual practices could be the source of political tension. In 1918 a Catholic priest tied this to the Jews' unbridled sexuality as mirrored in the form of their bodies. He commented how a young male Christian was seduced from a life of purity by "three young Jews who every evening undress completely in his presence, make fun of the uncircumcised, tell him to listen to what is going on in the conjugal bedroom and persuade him to bring a girl of his acquaintance." The priest goes on to comment that the Jews bring to the "peasant girl the erotic element (in spite of the brutality and coarseness with which they treat her) which is . . . so different from the severe Christian view upon the body and sexual functions. . . . The sexual relation with a Jew is in the eyes of the Church a particularly aggravating circumstance in view of the familial connection established by the coitus, the danger of the child being educated in the Jewish religion, and the 'mixing' of Christian and Jewish blood."[123] This became the central theme of one of the best-selling anti-Semitic novels of the early twentieth century, Artur Dinter's *Sin against the Blood* (1918). This text provided a narrative description of the Galician Jew Burghamer and his seduction of blond Aryan women in order to corrupt the Aryan race. Dinter's text also supplied a long, pseudoscientific appendix to document the "reality" of his claim.[124] This charge is turned on its head in one of the most extraordinary novels of the early 1920s, *The City without Jews* (1922) by the Viennese Jewish writer

Hugo Bettauer. Bettauer acknowledged that one of the wellsprings of anti-Semitism is this sexual competition. Here the Jewish male is seen as "noble, and if he marries a Christian girl, he is overly generous to her. They don't drink. . . . It is possible that the anti-Semitism in the male population of Vienna had become so strong, so fanatic, because the young men with their swastikas couldn't deal with the fact that their Jewish competition stole the prettiest girls!"[125] Such mésalliances haunted the nightmares of Christian Vienna, appearing even in the dreams of Freud's non-Jewish patients (*SE* 6:67). In these dreams they were even made responsible for the errors of the Austrian postal system (*SE* 6:223). And Freud was sufficiently attuned to this theme that he saw it as a natural part of the associative process in therapy.

Such forbidden relationships were common enough that they became the stuff of clinical anecdotes. The sexologist Albert Moll saw in the hypocrisy of many of the moralists of his time a mask for their sexual interest across either race or gender. He notes that many homosexuals, while leading a gay life-style, pursue a very moral relationship with women. He follows this with the anecdote of one of the leaders of the "Christian" party in the Parliament, who spoke out for "throne and altar, for Christianity and morality." One day his Jewish mistress is in the audience and asks him, "How can you lie so?" He answers, "It's our job."[126] The lying nature of the Jew and the Jew's corrupting sexuality are reversed here. The sign of the inherent corruption of the politician is that he lies and that he has a Jewish mistress. These are the classic signs of Jewish male identity projected onto the negative image of the non-Jew. Male Jews lie, and one sign of their lying nature is their ability to seduce non-Jewish women. The traditional view of both medical science (which was in line with most Jewish and Christian religious opinion of the time) stressed that "it would require an almost impossible amount of large toleration for a Christian maiden . . . to regard union with a Jew as anything other than unnatural."[127] The unnaturalness of such relationships is that they couple individuals who are (according to both scientific and religious sentiment) inherently incompatible.

The opposing view to the claim that mixed marriages could lead to an improvement of the Jewish race is also to be found. Such marriages are dangerous because they are basically diseased, if not infertile. This view was present into the 1890s and beyond. In 1894 the philo-Semitic publishing house of J. Schabelitz in Zurich published a pamphlet under the title "The Decline of Israel," by a "physiologist."[128] For this scientist as author, the Jews as a religious community no longer exist at the fin de siècle; the race itself is in danger of vanishing, for "the purpose of religion is the preservation of the race." Even mixed marriage will not retard this process, for "individual marriages between Jews and Christians have little purpose physiologically and are of importance only when they lead to the addition of new blood under new circumstances. At present this is not imaginable, since the general, national practices are now to be found among the Jews and influence their progeny exactly as they influence those of the Christian population." It is not prejudice that will lead to the disappearance of the Jews (whether this is good or bad is never made quite clear), but rather the nation with which "they mix and that permits their characteristics to become lost" (11, 15, 16).

The widely circulated fin-de-siècle view that the Jews were in danger of vanishing was best known through the work of Felix Theilhaber in 1911.[129] Theilhaber's work on the "decline of the Jews" (its title prefigured Oswald Spengler's *Decline of the West* of 1918) presented the demographic case for the disappearance of the Western Jew in greatest detail. He accepted most of the negative evidence, including the greater incidence of disease and insanity, as signs of the degeneration of the Jews. Indeed, he relied heavily on the medical authorities for the evaluation of the clinical status of the Jews as the object of special study, without ever calling their findings into question. Medicine has a much greater authority for him than do other arenas of proof, such as social statistics. Central to his argument is the decline in the Jewish birthrate because of late marriages, the emancipation of Jewish women, and mixed marriages.

According to Theilhaber, mixed marriages have an especially low rate of reproduction. Indeed, he notes, were it not for the "primitive sexuality of the *Ostjuden,*" the figures concerning the birthrate of the Jews in Germany would be even worse (93). Theilhaber's view of the eventual disappearance of western European Jewry was anticipated by Arthur Ruppin in 1904.[130] Ruppin warned that there was "danger of gradual extinction" of the western European Jews while the birthrate of eastern European Jews continued to rise.[131] The view that the Eastern Jews' behavior was the antithesis of Western Jewish (i.e., acculturated Western) sexual practices arose in an intense debate during the meeting of the Viennese Psychoanalytic Society on May 24, 1911, about Werner Sombart's study of the Jews and capitalism.[132] Wilhelm Stekel countered Ernst Federn's view that only through Christianization did the Jews become ascetic by noting that for the Eastern Jews, with their early marriages, asceticism was in the form of monogamy. In the discussion of Sombart's contention that Jews sublimate their sexuality into economic channels, Freud commented that Judaism as a religion had a central role in eliminating "perverse" sexuality, in that it "channeled all libidinous drives into reproduction." Thus the sexual practices of the Eastern Jews became the sign of the social control of the libido by culture.

Felix Theilhaber's argument was that the Jews were a dying race. Max Marcuse argued that it was the cultural value of the Jews, not their existence as a race, that was worth trying to save. It was a "unique case in eugenics" that could teach everyone about the dangers inherent in ignoring "the general German population politics, which is based on evolving a psychologically and psychically strong and culturally vital racial core and which ignores all racial and religious identity."[133] Mixed marriage was a further form of assimilation.

The central view of the time, a view that is dominant in the debates in the nineteenth century about interracial marriages between blacks and whites, is that "it is almost as if nature did not want such marriages [of Jews and non-Jews]. Nature revenges herself by branding mixed marriages with the mark of infertility."[134] Marcuse's views attempt to answer this general sentiment of the time—that mixed marriages produce weak or few offspring.[135] Indeed, for Marcuse the very act of marrying outside the group is a sign of pathology. It reflects a "sexual antipathy against 'members of the same race.'"[136] His exception is the Eastern Jew, whom he sees "for internal as well as external reasons" as immune to the possibility of mixed marriages. Indeed, Marcuse sees the difference between the Eastern and the Western Jews as being as great in "their blood and their character" as the difference between groups such as the French and the Germans (702, 730). These families, like the family of Sigmund Freud, have a much higher rate of reproduction than even the norm for the society they live in. Marcuse's rationale for the higher rate of mixed marriages is the urban location of Jews, their late marriage, and the economic and social level of the partners. These people have the greatest chance of meeting and marrying outside the group.

But the belief in the indelibility of the Jewish race, of the drop of ink that stains even when it is diluted, was much too powerful to be dismissed even by Jewish scientists of the period. The Jena zoologist Gustav Jaeger quotes the early nineteenth-century convert to Christianity Eduard Gans to the effect that "we Jews do not lose our stench even to the tenth crossbreeding."[137] The Viennese physician Leo Sofer argued that "in the second or third generation following a mixed marriage, a dissolution takes place. No longer are offspring with a definite mixed character produced, but the source dissolves, so that a percentage of the offspring again are of the pure, original racial stock."[138] Or, as Werner Sombart noted, "What clearly results is that the Jewish physiognomy often comes through in children of a mixed marriage, so that even after generations the addition of Jewish blood becomes evident, certainly to the anger and sorrow of the parents who wished to 'assimilate.'"[139] This is Francis

Galton's view of "reversion towards the typical center of their race" when unlike individuals mate and reproduce.[140]

These children of Jews and non-Jews, these *Mischlinge,* are Jews, but Jews in heightened form who bear all the stigmata of degeneration that exist in incestuous or inbred families. Like the sign of congenital circumcision, the mark of the decay of the Jew is present even (or especially) in the *Mischling:* "The children of such marriages [between Jews and non-Jews] . . . even though they are so very beautiful and so very talented, seem to lack a psychological balance that is provided by pure racial stock. We find all too often intellectually or morally unbalanced individuals, who decay ethically or end in suicide or madness."[141] There is no place one can hide; there is no means of becoming invisible. One's Jewishness appears even more clearly when one marries out of the faith, for it appears on the face and in the character of one's offspring. In these individuals the negative qualities are associated with those very qualities that seemed to motivate marriage outside the "race." The intellectual quality of the male is paralleled by the sexual attractiveness of the female.[142] This labeling of beauty as a sign of degeneration is of course an ironic reversal of the standard awareness of the role of beauty in the process of sexual selection as presented in the late nineteenth century. This is the alternative to Lombroso's argument, which sees beauty as the very proof of the moral individual. Darwin, as well as his opponents such as the sociologist Edvard Westermarck, sees in the physical beauty of the female (as opposed to the strength of the male) the markers of positive sexual selection.[143] This attempt to reverse a hundred-year-old tradition of aesthetic relativism by making beauty a biological mechanism leads Darwin and other thinkers to postulate standards of absolute beauty. It reflects the age-old debate about the "beautiful" as opposed to the "ugly" races.

The *Mischlinge* are the end product of the process of Jewish degeneration, which produces children who reveal the hidden racial difference of the Jews, their "blackness."[144] In addition to their moral, psychological, and physiological failings, all inscribed so that they can be read by the physician, the *Mischlinge* also are proverbially creative. This is a negative quality of the Jew that has its roots in the nineteenth-century discussion about the relation between genius and madness. And for the Jews this creativity lies in their use of the German language.[145]

The *Mischlinge* are so diseased because of their ancestry that their Jewishness will out. Wilhelm Stekel, the Viennese Jewish psychoanalyst, provided an extraordinary case study of a foot fetish that paralleled Freud's own evocation of the meaning of the Jewish foot in his work.[146]

Stekel can distinguish between Freud's account of the protagonist of Jensen's *Gradiva* and the account of the "orthopedic fetish" of Stekel's homosexual patient, a twenty-seven-year-old Viennese physician named Otto with a Russian mother, a German father, and a grandmother who was Jewish. His prime fetish is binding his feet and legs to encumber them and give him sexual satisfaction. Stekel began his account with the comment that his patient "was very sensitive about his ancestry because he wanted to be a 'real German'" (1:47). Stekel detailed the relationship of the fetish to the ambiguity of the patient's position as a *Mischling*. He recounted the following dream:

> I am at lunch and two corps students from Riga whom I know sit opposite me. One of them is red-faced and I don't like him. He asks me: "Are you a Catholic or a Christian?" I: "I'm a Christian." He: "Is it possible that you are not a Christian?" I: "Yes, I'm a Jew." He: "And you dare to sit in here?" The other one who was a little more sympathetic also said that I would have to leave. (1:253)

The authority of the student is but a mask for the anxiety the patient feels about his status in regard to the authority symbolized by the fraternity (corps) system. And this is in turn read by Stekel as a manifestation of the anxiety he feels about his own body. For his body is different—not from that of the corps students but from that of his father: "My father is circumcised. At an early age I found out that the foreskin of my penis is something valueless. I would pull it back, but it always slipped forward again" (1:261). The contrast of his uncircumcised body with the circumcised penis of his father is read by Stekel in terms of the Oedipus complex, for the authority of the father is in the size and form of his penis. This is coupled by Stekel with the interpretation that Otto had actually had intercourse with his sister when he was a child. Here neurosis is tied to a series of realities—all associated with the Jew in fin-de-siècle Vienna and all universalized by the Jewish psychoanalyst as part of the Oedipus complex. The status anxiety of being revealed as a Jew because of one's race identity is represented in all those qualities that are associated with the Jew: the hobbled legs, the deformed penis, the charge of brother-sister incestuous activity. All these symbolic references come from the vocabulary of race associated with the Jew in turn-of-the-century Vienna.

The hidden secret of the Jews is thus their sexuality, mirrored in the male Jew's body and in the Jews' avoidance of sexual contact outside the race. Is this the "knowledge of Jewish intimate ways that one spoke of only among ourselves" that angers Freud?[147] It is a secret knowledge shown by George Eliot in *Daniel Deronda* (1876), which Freud mentions to Martha Bernays. For George Eliot's novel, with all its philo-Semitic rhetoric, is a tale of how Deronda is fated to marry Mirah, a Jewess, and thus avoid the taint of race mixing. The secret sexual attraction the Jews show in the novel, the special gift Deronda shows in learning Hebrew, all reflect on the secrets attributed to the race.[148]

Freud's own complex reaction to the question of mixed marriage appears in his relationship with his own children, who (if they married at all) married Jews. In the memoirs of his analysis with Freud in 1935, the American Jewish psychiatrist Joseph Wortis recounted his quizzing Freud about the meaning of assimilation, which Wortis endorsed. Freud stressed the risk of mixed marriages, for "the chances for success seem greater in a Jewish marriage: family life is closer and warmer, and devotion much more common. My married children have all married Jews, though it may be that they would have married Christians if they had found the right one."[149] The stress on the positive "common mental construction" of the Jews as reflected in the structure and nature of the family is found in the works of Freud's scientific contemporaries such as Havelock Ellis, who stressed that the "superiority of Jewish over Christian children . . . and their lower infant mortality, seem to be entirely due to the fact that Jewesses are better mothers."[150] And yet the question of marriage beyond the group remained open.

Freud, Incest, and Blood

Now that we have framed the movement from the trauma theory to the seduction theory within the debates about conversion and baptism, it is clear that the universalization of incest and parricide in Freudian theory follows the contours of the arguments about the criminality and sexual proclivities of the Jews. The image of an original crime in the phylogenetic sense is part of Freud's anthropological argument, which frames his sense of history. Much as in Richard Krafft-Ebing's cultural-historical introduction to his study of human sexual pathology, sexuality is seen as a universal force that, however, has a specific history. It is a teleological history that places Jews at the stage above "primitive man" and on a lower level of sexual sophistication than Christians. The Jews (like the Egyptians, the Greeks, and the Teutons) showed "a high appreciation of virginity, chastity, modesty, and sexual fidelity," while "Christianity raised the union of the sexes to a sublime position by making woman socially the equal of man and by elevating the bond of love to a moral and religious institution."[151] This is the historical parallel to his argument about the individual's evolution from an incestuous love of the parent and its attendant conflicts. It is important to note that in contrast to psychiatric writers such as Krafft-Ebing, the early psychoanalytic writings on the history of parricide, specifically A. J. Storfer's monograph on this topic, do not discuss the Jews in any form.[152] They focus on the "primitive" peoples described in classic ethnological studies or within the Greco-Roman classical world.

In his earliest writing, Freud saw the incest taboo as the sacrifice that "human beings . . . [make] for the benefit of the larger community." They "sacrifice a portion of their sexual liberty and their liberty to indulge in perversions. The horror of incest (something impious) is based on the fact that, as a result of communal sexual life (even in childhood), the members of a family remain together permanently and become incapable of joining with strangers. Thus incest is anti-social—civilization consists in this progressive renunciation."[153] This view resonates with the theme sounded later in "'Civilized' Sexual Morality and Modern Nervous Illness" (1908) as well as in *Totem and Taboo* (1912–13): civilization is a force that represses the atavistic polymorphous sexual nature of the original human being. But it is also clear that this is precisely the argument used against Jewish sexual selectivity by physicians such as Paolo Mantegazza in the late nineteenth century. The rationale for understanding the incest taboo as a force that moves the individual out into the world, forming social and sexual relationships with other peoples, is the same as that opposing Jewish sexual selectivity. Freud's ambivalence here is evident. Is it good to give up the ingroup and "become capable of joining with strangers"? Society says it is, and society structures the individual's response.

The fantasies of parricide and incest framed by the Oedipus complex become one male Jew's answer to the charge of incest or inbreeding lodged against the Jews.[154] It is Freud's attempt to present as a universal phenomenon the very core of the argument about the origin of Jewish disease, the problem all Jews face: if they "inbreed," as Freud did, they are diseased and criminal and predispose their children to disease; if they marry outside the group, they are diseased and degenerate.[155] It is not only that Freud avoided the proposed and truly consanguineous marriage with the daughter of his older half brother Emmanuel, whom he visited in Manchester upon finishing the gymnasium. Freud's own marriage would have been understood as endogamous in terms of the racial biology of his time since he married "within the race," and that would have been sufficient to place him and his children at risk.

Freud's formulation of the Oedipus complex, with its evocation of murder and incest, and his historical extension of this model in *Totem and Taboo* to the roots of human experience also rearticulates the specific complex of charges concerning criminal sexual activity brought against the Jews at the fin de siècle. Using a variation on the image of the atavistic criminal introduced by Lombroso, Freud projected the charges of sexual license made against the Jews into primeval history, seeing the original crime, the murder of the father by his sons, as the psychological root of human nature.[156] The Oedipus complex is but the repetition in the individual's fantasy of the phylogenetic experience in the primal horde. It is the result of the "common mental construction" of all human beings, but it is also marked by the institution of the incest taboo. Every infant, Jewish or not, desires the opposite-sex parent. What the social repression of such polymorphous perversity demands is the universal suppression of this desire. This is precisely what is demanded of the Jews—that they cease the practice of endogenous marriage. But the Jews refuse to do this. Like circumcision, it has become part of their "common mental construction." Thus the Jews are dangerous members of society, not only as violators of the economic laws that control the excesses of the marketplace, but also in sexual terms.

Other Jewish scientists of the fin de siècle simply dismiss or modify Freud's argument. Magnus Hirschfeld and Max Marcuse both saw the incest taboo as a fairly recent phenomenon of Western (read Judeo-Christian) culture, unrelated to the psychosocial development of the infant. Indeed, Marcuse denied the concept of infantile sexuality. They see the incest taboo as a cultural phenomenon of the West. They attempted to separate the debate about incest from the Lombrosian model of atavism by arguing that the incest taboo was a social phenomenon totally unrelated to any biological or ethnopsychological imperative. Marcuse dismissed the question of a biological rationale for the incest taboo as early as 1915.[157]

For Freud it is not a cultural phenomenon but rather a historical and developmental one. These views evolved during the period from the mid-1890s to 1910 and are best represented in Freud's study of "some points of agreement between the mental lives of savages and neurotics"—the subtitle of *Totem and Taboo* (1912–13). Freud's study is an anthropological excursion into the inner world of the past, a world that will be given its necessarily "Jewish" face in *Moses and Monotheism.* But it is in *Totem and Taboo* that the evocation of the "mind of primitive man," to use the title of Franz Boas's answer to such fin-de-siècle readings of the phylogenetic image of the "savage," is best outlined and presented.

Freud carefully structured his argument concerning "inbreeding" in this text. He argued in *Totem and Taboo* against the purely biological views of Edvard Westermarck, the founder of the sociology of the family, as well as those of Havelock Ellis, both of whom see in the incest taboo "a horror of intercourse between near kin," as Westermarck put it (*SE*

13:122). According to Havelock Ellis, children raised together are simply too familiar with one another: "All of the sensory stimuli of vision, hearing and touch have been dulled by use, trained to the calm level of affection, and deprived of their potency" (*SE* 13:122). While such familiarity would lead to the rejection of individuals one was raised with, Ellis stressed the factor of race—endogamous marriage—as a means of preserving the quality of the individuals in the group. He argued for the primacy of race as a criterion for selecting a marriage partner: "The indiscriminate thrusting of men and women into marriage, without regard to the supreme question of their fitness to be the parents of a fine race . . . could only lead towards racial degeneracy and moral disorder."[158] Freud contrasted this view with the insight that such familiarity within families is in no way the equivalent "of the biological fact that inbreeding is detrimental to the species. A biological instinct of the kind suggested would scarcely have gone so far astray in its psychological expression that, instead of applying to blood-relatives (intercourse with whom might be injurious to reproduction), it affected persons who were totally innocuous in this respect, merely because they shared a common home" (*SE* 13:123). The arguments about incest seemed to transcend the debates about inbreeding and consanguinity. And yet Freud's sources, such as John Lubbock, cited the case of the Jews in terms that evoked charges of incest. Thus Lubbock noted that "Abraham married his half-sister, Nahor married his brother's daughter, and Amram his father's sister; this was permitted because they were regarded as relations. Tamar also evidently might have married Amnon, though they were children of David."[159] Lubbock's example is meant to show the power of matrilineal descent; his rhetoric illustrates the incestuous nature of Jewish historical practice.

For Freud the incest taboo arises precisely because of the incestuous longing of every child for the opposite-sex parent. It is the unconscious attraction of Oedipus to his mother. It cannot have anything to do with an understanding of the dangers of inbreeding: "Not only must the prohibition against incest be older than any domestication of animals which might have enabled men to observe the effects of inbreeding upon racial characters, but even today the detrimental results of inbreeding are not established with certainty and cannot easily be demonstrated in man" (*SE* 13:124). Here Freud echoed a basic view of the biology of his time: We cannot know anything in detail about the effects of inbreeding, and, if we cannot, how do we imagine that the "savage" could? This is a fascinating denial of many of the assumptions of the period on the part of non-Jewish as well as Jewish physicians and forensic scientists, who argued quite clearly that inbreeding and its more egregious form, incest, led to specific physiological and psychological deficits in the children of such marriages. The very attraction of marrying within the "blood" could be seen as a neurotic symptom revealing the psychopathology of the consanguineous partners themselves.

Freud cites as his authorities Émile Durkheim and Charles Darwin, both of whom relativized the question of incest. As a Jew, Durkheim, like Freud, needed to universalize the basic assumption that Jewish inbreeding produces a certain set of physiological and psychological errors in development.[160] Durkheim accepted the higher incidence of mental illness ascribed to the Jews in the statistical literature of the fin de siècle but also stressed their lower suicide rate.[161] (This was against the overall sense that the suicide rate among *assimilated* Jews was extremely high.)[162] His explanation for both rested on the external, environmental context for this definition of Jewish risk. Durkheim equated the incest taboo with exogamy and saw it as analogous to other ritual taboos associated with blood. The question of "blood" lies at the heart of Durkheim's discussion. When he examined the nature of Jewish endogamous marriage, he accepted the greater risk of the Jews for disease (especially mental illness such as neurasthenia), but he also saw their greater resistance to the destructive social pressures on them as the result of consanguineous marriage.

The incest taboo and its racial analogy are incorporated in Freud's own discussion of the "horror of blood," which he views as a universal trait, pathologizing the menstrual experience of women. This he linked to the fantasy of the meaning of "mixing one's blood": "In one case, in which education had succeeded in postponing sexual knowledge especially late, a fourteen-year-old girl, who had already begun to menstruate, arrived from the books she had read at the idea that being married consisted in a 'mixing of blood'; and since her own sister had not yet started her periods, the lustful girl made an assault on a female visitor who had confessed that she was just then menstruating, so as to force her to take part in this 'blood mixing'" (*SE* 9:222–23). The fantasy of the young girl, reading books about the mixing of blood (as in much of the fin-de-siècle literature on Jewish sexuality), is that she can mix her blood with that of another female and produce offspring. This is the case when immature minds, such as those of children, understand the metaphors of incest and inbreeding literally.

Charles Darwin, who wrote on the immutability of the appearance of the Jews as well as the potential for the inheritance of circumcision, had a special place in Freud's sense of the status of science in his time. Darwin's argument concerning inbreeding is on the surface scientific and distanced. In his study *The Variation of Animals and Plants under Domesti-*

cation (1868), he commented on the "evil effects of close interbreeding." This is where he saw the origin of the incest taboo.[163] He silently drew on his personal experience, for he, like his older sister, had married consanguineously.[164] Darwin, like Freud, dismissed the view that the incest taboo is instinctual. He cited, in the *Descent of Man*, the view that "men during primeval times may have been more excited by strange females than by those with whom they habitually lived."[165] He doubted that "consanguineous marriages, such as they are permitted in civilized nations, . . . which would not be considered as close interbreeding in the case of our domesticated animals, cause any injury."[166] His proof for this is provided by his own son's statistical work, work that, one assumes, he could not have undertaken had there been a "blood taint" owing to his parentage. George Darwin's statistical work, which was widely circulated in Germany, argued against an increased rate of mental illness among certain families because of the marriage of cousins. But he pointed out the increased rate of certain diseases, including mental illness, among the British aristocracy. He also localized the increase of mental illness in urban areas.[167] The Jewish response to George Darwin's work was complicated. Joseph Jacobs evoked Darwin's essay to dismiss the contention that "the neurotic tendency of Jews is due to these consanguineous marriages. . . . [T]his view is no longer credited among medical men, who regard consanguinity in marriage as aggravating any diathetic tendency in a family, but not as causing the tendency per se."[168] Mental illness was a prime feature of the Jewish family, but according to Jacobs it was not the result of inbreeding. Marcus Adler commented that Darwin's work showed the lack of a causal relationship between inbreeding and increased rates of mental illness, stressing that Jews "live in densely populated districts." But he commented that the increase of Jewish mental illness was also the result of the "common mental construction" of the Jews, who were "more addicted to head work than to manual labour, and to many of them being of a rather nervous temperament."[169]

The incest taboo is not seen by Freud as the result of the "impair[ment] of racial characteristics" (*SE* 15:210). Indeed, "a human being's first choice of an object is regularly an incestuous one, aimed, in the case of the male, at his mother or sister, and it calls for the severest prohibitions to deter this persistent infantile tendency from realization" (*SE* 16:335). Here we have the echo of the special status of the incestuous Jews and the power of their religion to force them not to commit incest. This is the explanation that sees the latent criminality of the Jews become the latent "universal criminality" of all human beings, to use Wilhelm Stekel's phrase.[170] Sarah Kofman has noted that Freud conceptualized "the enigma of woman along the lines of the great criminal rather than the hysteric."[171] If this is accurate, then the original model for the "great criminal" may well have been the incestuous Jew.

Freud saw the ultimate answer for the meaning of incest and inbreeding in the anthropological approach of J. G. Frazer. Frazer wrote in his *Totemism and Exogamy* (1910) that "the ultimate origin of exogamy, and with it of the law of incest—since exogamy was devised to prevent incest—remains a problem nearly as dark as ever." Freud subscribes to "Frazer's resigned conclusion. We are ignorant of the horror of incest and cannot even tell in what direction to look for it. None of the solutions of the enigma that have been proposed seems satisfactory" (*SE* 13:125). It is the unknowable, the unspeakable center of existence. Incest, which links male Jews and all women as the seducers and corrupters not only of individuals but of entire races, is also at this very core of the unknowable. The Jewish mind and the sexuality of women are all mired in this swamp of unknowability.

The debate about "inbreeding" and the question of the offspring of such marriages arise within psychoanalytic theory in 1908. Karl Abraham gave a very controversial talk before the conservative Berlin Society for Psychiatry and Nervous Disorders on November 9, 1908.[172] For Abraham, drawing on Freud's incest theory, the question was not only what happens to those who intermarry but whether intermarriage itself can be seen as a form of neurosis. Abraham evoked the structure of the argument that Freud later hints at in the postscript of his reading of *Gradiva,* that in highly neurotic families the forbidden love for the sibling can be projected onto the permitted love of the close relative. Indeed, such individuals may not have the capacity to extend their libido toward strangers. Abraham stressed that such attraction can be the result of psychopathologies as well as giving rise to them in offspring. Given this image of the neurotic family as creating the environment where the sexual selection among the offspring tends to be incestuous or at least symbolically so, not a word is mentioned about the Jews as the prime example of marriage with close relatives. It is only within the sheltering pages of *Imago,* in his 1914 paper on "neurotic exogamy" discussed above, that Abraham can return to this topic and reveal the invisible subtext on Jews and intermarriage that framed this question in the minds of his listeners.

The response of his audience at the beginning of the discussion was more or less as Abraham had expected. There was an immediate attack by Abraham's cousin Hermann Oppenheim on the idea of infantile sexuality that was the underlying assumption of the paper. Abraham had taken the precaution of citing Oppenheim and Theodor Ziehen, professor of psychiatry at Berlin, at length about the neurosis of children. These discussions were intense but retained a "scientific" tone, according to Abraham, until "a very pushy member, B., whose conversion to Christianity has proved only partially successful, assumed a moralizing tone more suited to a public platform. I had evoked among others [the Swiss writer] Konrad Ferdinand Meyer . . . as an example for love for the mother. This is unheard of. German ideals were now at stake. Sexuality was now even attributed to German fairy tales, etc. . . . The whole Association should express their disapproval of this new trend."[173] This intense response is an evocation not merely of Freud as the Jewish psychoanalyst and of psychoanalysis as the new Jewish sexualized science, but of the underlying anxiety Jewish scientists felt about their own vulnerability. Psychoanalysis is a sexualized science because its practitioners are Jews and Jews are overly sexualized. Indeed, Hanns Sachs observed that among the most vituperative critics of psychoanalysis were Jews who needed to "prove their full assimilation of Teutonism by 'outheroding Herod.'"[174] All Jews were at risk. Conversion would not protect one from the inexorable genetic laws that inbreeding was assumed to follow.

Freud's own response to the question of the sexuality of the Jews came in a debate at the Viennese Psychoanalytic Society on January 3, 1907, following the presentation of a paper by Alfred Meisl on the basic drives of "hunger and love." Meisl evidently discussed the question of the Jews and sexual selection in his paper. Wilhelm Stekel responded by simply dismissing Meisl's discussion, since "modern biologists have completely discarded the concept of race."[175] Freud carefully positioned himself vis-à-vis Meisl's paper, balancing its strengths and its weaknesses. He clearly saw "Meisl's explanation of the racial characteristics of Jews to be incorrect. Natural selection [in the choice of sex object] plays a minor role in humans" (*Protokolle,* 1:83; trans., 1:88). Freud dismissed the question of Jewish sexual selection as a biological reality in shaping human beings. Meisl evidently took the critique of Stekel and Freud to heart. Even though his paper was (according to him) in press, its published version contains not a single reference to Jewish sexual selectivity.[176]

If Freud's rejection of the concept of the degenerate was keyed to his perception of the misuse of racial arguments during World War I, it was only at the very end of his life that he was able to give inbreeding a positive connotation. In the 1930s Freud used the image of inbreeding in discussing the movement of history and the theories of Karl Marx: "I really believe that it was gunpowder and fire-arms that abolished chivalry and aristocratic rule, and that the Russian despotism was already doomed before it lost the War, because no amount of inbreeding among the ruling families of Europe could have produced a race of Tsars capable of withstanding the explosive force of dynamite" (*SE* 22:177). Inbreeding is a positive factor producing ever stronger individuals, rather than a negative factor producing ineffectual degenerates (and often associated with the decline of the nobility in Europe). And by the time Freud wrote *Moses and Monotheism* in the late 1930s the image of incest and inbreeding had been given a purely positive valence: "It was taken as a matter of course that a Pharaoh should take his sister as his first and principal wife; and the later successors of the Pharaohs, the Greek Ptolemies, did not hesitate to follow that model. We are compelled, rather, to a realization that incest—in this instance between a brother and sister—was a privilege withheld from common mortals and reserved to kings as representatives of the gods, just as similarly, no objection was taken to incestuous relations of this kind in the world of Greek and Germanic legend" (*SE* 23:121–22). The Greek and German legends are the reflection of the cultural residue of the pan-European theme of incest so detailed in its documentation in the work of Otto Rank. It was Rank who documented the universal appearance of brother-sister incest. But for Jews at the fin de siècle this was not a vague, universal charge. The fascination with the levirate and the association of this practice with brother-sister incest made the Jews the prime example of incestuous behavior at the turn of the century. Thomas Mann's literary parody of the Jewish involvement in the Wagner cult—the siblings' incest mirrors the actions of Siegmund and Sieglinde in Wagner's *Die Walküre*—reflect the translation of culturally significant literary traditions, such as those of Greece, northern Europe, and Egypt into the tawdy, tasteless reality of upper-class German Jews. Wagner only represented Aryan incest on the stage; Mann's Jewish protagonists enact it in their bedroom.

The special nature of Jewish sibling relations, especially between Jewish brothers and sisters, was a standard aspect of the early twentieth-century image of the Jew. Aryan brothers and sisters, as adults, were understood to have a "cousinly" relationship, whereas that between Jewish brothers and sisters developed into one mirroring the paternal or maternal relationship between mother and male child or father and female child.[177] This sense of the innate difference of the development of bonds within Aryan and Jewish families stressed the interchangeability of parental and sibling relationships in Jewish families. Thus the move from the incest of brothers and sisters to that of parent and child is already inscribed in the way German popular culture understood the different implications of Jewish sibling relationships.

Thus it is brother-sister incest, not mother-son or daughter-father incest, that is the literary representation of Jewish, corrosive hypersexuality. Freud displaced this onto the traditions of the Egyptians and the myths of the Teutonic tribes. He provided a universal context for a very specific theme, that of Jewish incestuous practice and its results. But what he does in moving this theme into the universal, into the fantasy of the Oedipus story, is to translate brother-sister incest into mother-son incest. Of all the charges against the Jews in the popular and forensic literature of the fin de siècle, this particular one is missing. Not brother-sister incest, with its Jewish overtones, is reflected in human development, but rather the relationship between the mother and her son. When the myth of Jewish incest is transmuted into the Oedipus theme, what is added is the act of parricide, the murder of the father which is linked to the incestuous act.

Freud's movement of sexuality from a quality solely associated with the genitalia, indelibly marked on the Jewish male, reworks the very question of the sexual into an issue of "psyche" rather than "soma." But the secret aspect of the Oedipus complex is not the desire to possess the mother; it is the desire to destroy the father. Parricide becomes a sign of degeneracy of the Jew. For parricides, at least in the forensic literature of the period, are *always* degenerates.[178] The parricide is a criminal whose will has degenerated, who is impulsive, and whose character shows a "limitless egoism."[179] He is a mimic, often copying the criminal actions of other parricides. And he is the offspring of diseased parents: "who is guilty, the parents who gave them life."[180] The parents are guilty of their children's degeneracy, the sign of which is the act of parricide. Like the Jews, the parricide shows the overt signs of degeneration. The heightened sensibilities of the Jews lead to their mental collapse, to their becoming like parricides, and they enact this by their own suicide.[181] The increased rate of suicide among Jews is linked to the "decline of the Jews." The murder of the parent, like the murder of the self, is an act of psychological decay.

It has been long evident that Freud's construction of the Oedipus complex deals exclusively with "male" sexuality. Indeed, Freud's construction of the "Electra" complex is so riddled with inconsistencies that it shows the asymmetry of his representation of male and female experiences. The asymmetry can also point up the difference between the sexuality of the Jew and that of the Aryan, as represented in the culture of the fin de siècle. Freud's view stressed similarity and a difference between a masculine and a feminine experience of sexual attraction. The female child begins by having a masculine active libido, by believing she is a male, and by being attracted to the mother (as is the male child). When she discovers that she is anatomically different from the male, that she is castrated, she turns to the father as the primary focus of her libidinal energy. The developmental movement of the female is analogous to that of the male Jew, who sees himself as a male within society until the society, reacting in horror to his circumcised state, points out his lack of masculinity.[182] This is done by denying him social equivalence with other males—in the cultural understanding of his body and in the assumption of his place within the social fabric. He then comes, as Freud pointed out in his discussion of Otto Weininger, to disparage himself and to identify his failures with those weaknesses the culture associates with the feminine. This becomes a neurosis similar to the "masculinity complex" of the masochistic women in Freud's essay "A Child Is Being Beaten" (1919), who continue to long for a penis and deny their own anatomy. It is clear that the very definition of the "masculinity" of the Jew was in doubt within the debates about racial biology during the fin de siècle. It is the sexuality of the Jew that is mirrored and distorted within the Oedipus complex. The fantasy, not the biological reality, of incest is represented here. The sexual crimes of the Jews, which mark them as diseased, are no longer qualities of their "common mental construction"; they are part of the mind-set of all human beings.

Freud found the social and cultural location for sexual crimes documented in a work that he read with intense interest in 1931. Georg Fuchs was a literary critic in Munich who was imprisoned for a political offense in the late 1920s. In prison he wrote a memoir that provided some insight into the nature of prison conditions and the "types" found in German prisons in the Weimar Republic.[183] This was one of several such firsthand accounts of "lowlife" in the Weimar Republic, which appealed to intellectuals as "authentic" representations of social oppression. Fuchs presents a wide range of figures, including a twelve-page profile of an individual convicted of incest. The profile fits all of the discussion of the "natural" forces that are suppressed by civilized behavior. Johannes Gürtler was an illegitimate child who became a brewer and then a peasant farmer. A Protestant, he married into a Catholic family in a small Catholic village, had three daughters, and in time had sexual intercourse with his oldest child. Fuchs's response was that Gürtler was doing what everyone else in that "primitive" community had done, but that he was prosecuted for the crime because of the enmity of the local priest. Indeed, Fuchs's report of the discussion of Gürtler's wife with the priest in the confessional stressed that her husband was not a real Christian: "A Jew is almost better than he!" (232). Gürtler was convicted and had served five years of a seven-year sentence (which Fuchs felt was unfair) when Fuchs met him in prison. Freud read this volume closely. He would have found his views of the vitality of "primitive" peoples substantiated. He would have seen the suppression of such incestuous traditions by organized religion. And he would also have been able to extract a case study on the dangers of intermarriage—for the persecution of Gürtler, even by his wife, is attributed by Fuchs solely to the hostility of the Catholic church to marriages outside the faith. Freud would not have seen the suppression of incest understood by the "liberal" Fuchs as a positive force in society. Freud's response to this volume and to Fuchs's letter to him (and to many other leading cultural figures of the day, including Jakob Wassermann) was that Freud felt himself to be "*persona ingrata,* if not *ingratissima,* with the German people—and moreover with the learned and the unlearned alike."[184] It is as a Jew that Freud responds to this "noble, wise, and good" book: in the discourse of Fuchs's study there appear all the qualities ascribed to the Jew, but placed within other, equally egregious stereotypical representations.

For Freud, the murder of the parent, the striking out against the figure of authority, is embedded in the distant past, in the world of the ancestors of all human beings. It is not overtly a "Jewish" problem until *Moses and Monotheism* (1938). And yet the debate about parricide, about the Jew as murderer, had already been evoked and evoked one of the most striking tendencies of the late nineteenth century to recall and reinstitute older charges against the Jews. For that period was the age of the evocation of the blood libel: that Jews killed Christian children and used their blood in making the unleavened bread they ate during Passover. It served as a cure for the diseases of the Jews, especially those associated with their own bleeding, such as the menstruation of males. This reversal of the charge of parricide is clear. We find not children killing parents, but adults killing children, and all these crimes are tied to the mysteries of blood.

The history of the charge that the Jews, either historically or in the present, sacrificed to the god Moloch has an uninterrupted tradition at least back to the Enlightenment.[185] Thus Voltaire argued that "Jewish Law expressly ordered the immolation of men dedicated to the Lord. . . . Human blood sacrifices were thus clearly established. No historical detail is better attested. A Nation can only be judged by its own archives."[186] In the early nineteenth century this view was repeated by Georg Friedrich Daumer, though he placed the Jews' blood rituals in the present rather than in the distant, biblical past. Daumer brought this charge up to date by evoking the 1840 accusation that the Jewish community in Damascus murdered a friar to obtain blood for their rituals. The theme of the murder of the Christian, especially the Christian child, by the Jew never vanishes in nineteenth-century thought.

Freud lived at a moment when the charge of blood libel could be read regularly in the newspapers of Vienna.[187] In 1882 the charge appeared in Hungary; in 1899 in Czechoslovakia; in 1891 on Corfu; in 1911 in

Kiev.[188] The Hungarian case Freud would have found documented in one of his anthropological sources, Americus Featherman's *Social History of the Races of Mankind* (1891).[189] Featherman provided a stinging attack on the narrow-minded bigotry that lay behind such accusations. In Corfu the charge led to riots that decimated the Jewish community; in the Austro-Hungarian empire, to sensationalist trials that were the talk of everyone in Vienna.[190] Indeed, it was difficult to pick up an issue of the Viennese *New Free Press* without reading about the lodging of the blood accusation somewhere in Europe. At least fifteen cases appeared between 1881 and 1900.[191] For example, on November 26, 1899, there is a long article about the attempt to hide the body of a dead infant in a Jewish bar in Podgorze near Crakow. Karl Kraus, a Viennese Jewish satirist, commented on the poor taste of respectable Christian citizens of Vienna, who assured their Jewish neighbors that they were sure they were incapable of committing ritual murder![192]

The court cases that often resulted from these charges were widely covered and intensively debated throughout the German-speaking world. It was T. G. Masaryk, the founder of the Czech republic, who published one of the most widely cited attacks on the very idea of the blood libel during the trial of Leopold Hilsner in 1899, which resulted from the murder of Agnes Hrůza in Polna (Bohemia).[193] The charges against Hilsner had great currency in Vienna, even reaching the floor of the parliament in Vienna.[194] It was also seriously debated in the Prussian Chamber of Deputies[195] and was discussed in the medical literature of the period.[196] There were also widely read pamphleteers and newspaper writers who espoused quite the opposite view. Notable among them was the Prague theologian August Rohling, who had the ear of the Austrian minister of education beginning in 1883.[197] The Jews' murder of Christian children became an element of the forensic rhetoric of the time.

Freud himself commented on the mental state of the chief witness against Joseph Scharf, who was accused of having murdered Esther Solymosi at Tisza-Eszlar in Hungary during 1882.[198] He also presented an extraordinary account of this case in his 1888 translation of French Jewish physician Hippolyte Bernheim's study of suggestion.[199] Bernheim described the background of the Tisza-Eszlar case in great detail. He recounted how a fourteen-year-old Christian girl in the village vanished and how thirteen "unlucky" local Jews were arrested and accused of her murder by the public prosecutor, who "was a great enemy of Israel" and had a "blind hatred" of the Jews. The public prosecutor seized the thirteen-year-old son of the caretaker at the synagogue and held him for three months, isolated from his family. The child then proceeded to give detailed testimony as to how he observed the murder of the girl by three

Jews through a keyhole in the synagogue door, and he continued to claim this even under cross-examination: "I saw it!" Eventually the accused were freed, "justice prevailed, and all friends of Hungary and the civilized world could breathe freely."

Bernheim wanted to understand why the child would have given such monstrous testimony. He dismissed the idea that he was simply blackmailed into lying because of threats to himself and his family. Rather, he assumed that the child came to believe he had actually seen the events described to him by the public prosecutor. Bernheim sets the scene: The "small, weak child, raised in the direst poverty, is brought before this august person, who incorporates all justice and power." This "poor, isolated being is overwhelmed by him" and listens as he describes the Jews as "a damned race, who see it as their pious undertaking to spill Christian blood, in order to dampen the dough for the unleavened Easter bread." The power of the rhetoric of this figure has an "impact on the weak character" of the child, and this "extreme suggestion permeates his hypnotized brain." He comes to believe that he actually saw the events described to him by the public prosecutor.

Bernheim proposed that the child's testimony was a "retrospective hallucination, such as one can generate in a deep trance." This model carries within it all the aspects of Freud's later, major debt to Bernheim—the replacement of the world of trauma with the world of fantasy. The testimony of the child, like that of Freud's neurotics, was evidently false, but why was it false? Not because he was consciously lying but because he had come to believe the reality of an event he had imagined rather than experienced. The reason for this was the suggestibility of the child (the product of his environment) and the presence of this larger than life figure of power and authority (the father surrogate). When Freud returned to the model Bernheim had presented, it too was without any act of overt hypnotism. The power of the neurotic's fantasy life was that it shaped the very sense of the neurotic's body. The child, who came to believe he had seen a murder committed by his coreligionists, was the original neurotic. The only thing he could do was forget what he had seen.

The Jews responded to these charges of ritual murder by forgetting, and what they eventually forgot was the meaning of their bodies and of their racial identity. In *The Psychopathology of Everyday Life* (1901) Freud recounts what, according to him, comes to be an often-cited and much debated bit of psychoanalytic lore—his analysis of the inability of his traveling companion to remember the correct wording of a quotation from Virgil. Through a web of associations Freud moved the young man from the repressed word (*aliquis*) to the murder of Simon of Trent by the Jews: "'I am thinking of the accusation of ritual blood-sacrifice which is brought against the Jews again just now, and of Kleinpaul's book in which he regards all of these supposed victims as incarnations, one might say, new editions of the Saviour'" (*SE* 6:10). Rudolf Kleinpaul's book on human sacrifice was, however, one of the Christian defenses of the Jews.[200] (Kleinpaul's further work was well known to Freud [*SE* 5:351, 8:94, 129, 13:58–59].) Like the noted Berlin Lutheran Orientalist Hermann Strack's more famous (and more extensive) attack on the legend of the blood accusation, it presented a rebuttal of this libel within a liberal Christian context.[201] Kleinpaul not only discussed the parallels between the blood accusation and the celebration of the Christian Mass but, more carefully, examined the replacement of the supposed human sacrifice to the "old Semitic god Moloch" with the ritual of circumcision.[202] In 1897 Freud had speculated on a similar pattern concerning a "primeval sexual cult . . . in the Semitic East" and its practice of ritual circumcision.[203] This aspect of Kleinpaul's text is never mentioned by Freud's traveling companion, but it formed a central part of the debates about the meaning of circumcision in the medical as well as the popular literature of the period.

The circumcised penis is the symbolic displacement of the earlier barbaric ritual murder practiced by the Jews in the Near East. To translate this into psychoanalytic terms, following Theodor Reik, circumcision was a form of symbolic castration, which was intended to prevent incest.[204] This unspoken and unsought association provided the missing link in Freud's own train of associations, for the blood accusation was associated by Freud's traveling companion, under Freud's not very subtle tutelage, with the assumed pregnancy and proposed abortion of the young man's Italian (Christian) companion. Mixed marriages are dangerous; they end in children who need to be destroyed. The association Freud made culminated in the "sacrifice of St. Simon [of Trent] as a child." It is the death of the child, here the Christian child, with its Italian mother, as the substitute for the Jewish child, the potential sacrifice to the god Moloch, which takes place.

Fritz Wittels provided a conflation of circumcision, castration, and the libel about ritual murder in his 1924 unauthorized biography of Freud. He summarized Freud's account of the association of circumcision and castration as follows: "The unconscious confounds circumcision with castration, and therefore believes the Jews to be cruel. Those who castrate their children are capable of committing any atrocity, and are therefore capable of committing ritual murder. The unconscious thus despises the Jews because they have been castrated, and at the same time dreads them because they castrate their own children."[205] The movement from castration to ritual murder (as the crime the Jews are charged with) is Wittels's own attempt to destroy the link that had been made between the Jew's body and the Jew's actions. It placed the question of the meaning of circumcision and the reading of the Jew's putative actions on the same plane and thus impugned the anti-Semitic reading of both.

Jews of the fin de siècle reflected the powerful tensions associated with the meaning of the "blood libel" and its reflection of their present state (in terms of either body or mind). Freud would have found the rationale for the blood libel spelled out in the scholarly literature he cited. And it related to the diseased nature of the Jew's body. W. Robertson Smith noted that "in legal sacrifices of the Hebrews blood was never eaten, but . . . sprinkled on the worshippers, which . . . has the same meaning." In general, this tradition vanished except as it was "retained in certain special cases" such as "the purification of the leper."[206] Blood sacrifice and the diseased Jew are expressly linked in this practice. The association of the Jews and blood sacrifice was a constant theme in the scholarly literature of the fin de siècle, either as a means of reconstructing the "primitive" history of the Jews or as a means of distancing present-day Jewry from these practices. But lurking behind this discussion was the model Herbert Spencer had applied to the "primitive Hebrews," the view that there was "a forgetting of that which was familiar at an earlier mental stage." For Spencer it is evident that while certain concepts may "seem ridiculous" to "advanced peoples," they most certainly "had forefathers who held these primitive conceptions."[207] Hidden within the "common mental construction" of the Jew may well have been the history of "blood sacrifice."

The debates about the blood libel were also part of the debate about the origin of circumcision, the tradition that marked the Jew's body as different. For the ancient practices of the Jews, the human sacrifices that were supposed to mark their rituals, had become symbolically reduced to the act of circumcising their young males instead of killing them.[208] Freud's rhetoric concerning the Oedipus complex places all these concerns into a broader, universal context: not Jews, but all individuals wish to kill their parents (not the parents to kill their children); the degenerate parricide becomes the mark of the human psyche in its most "primeval" or "atavistic" form, a form that needs to be harnessed and controlled by the civilizing impulses of the superego.

It is in one of the most overtly Jewish of Freud's dreams presented in *The Interpretation of Dreams,* his dream of the "Myops," that all these themes are linked with the Oedipus complex and with the hidden language of the Jews. In this dream, which is, as we have noted, connected to a number of Jewish themes (from Theodor Herzl, the founder of modern Zionism, to the syphilitic and limping Jew), there is a scene in which "a female figure—an attendant or nun—brought two boys out and handed them over to their father, who was not myself. The elder of the two boys was clearly my eldest son; I did not see the other one's face. The woman who brought out the boy asked him to kiss her goodbye. She was noticeable for having a red nose. The boy refused to kiss her, but, holding out his hand in farewell, said 'Auf Geseres' to her, and then 'Auf Ungeseres' to the two of us (or to one of us)" (*SE* 5:442). Freud's interpretation evoked Theodor Herzl, the "Jewish problem," and the "concern about the future of one's children." And he explained to his readers the two "unknown" terms he used in the dream: *Geseres* is "a genuine Hebrew word . . . and is best translated by 'imposed suffering' or 'doom'"; *Ungeseres* is "a private neologism of my own." He provides the meaning of this neologism in its association with "'leavened-unleavened' bread," which the Jews "in memory [of the Exodus] eat . . . at Easter." The word *Geseres* itself came about through the association of the "Myops" of the title, with its cyclopedic root, and the narrator of the dream, Professor M., whose son has developed an eye disease. As his infected eye healed, his healthy eye became infected: "The boy's mother, terrified, at once sent for the doctor to the remote spot in the country where they were staying. The doctor, however, now went over to the other side. 'Why are you making such a "Geseres"?' he shouted at the mother, 'if one side has got well, so will the other.'"

Freud reads this dream in light of his Jewish identity and the relationship to his own sons and to his own father. The key to Freud's partial reading is his philology: for him *Geseres* is a Hebrew word.[209] As the doctor's own exclamation indicates, it is in fact a Yiddish word, for given the form in which Freud presents it, with its *-es* ending, it cannot be Hebrew. The doctor speaks in *Mauscheln,* evoking the specter of the Eastern Jewish parvenu in the dream and reinforcing the sense of marginality the dream itself represented. This marginality is the link between the Eastern Jews (with their *Mauscheln*) and the unleavened bread, the "source" of the charge of blood libel. For it is on "Easter," not Passover, according to Freud, that the Jews make unleavened bread. It is, of course, Easter that commemorates the Resurrection of Christ, who was, according to the language of the church during Freud's day, murdered by the perfidious Jews. It is the charge not only of parricide but of deicide, the killing of the son of God, that is lodged against the

Jews. And it is by the blood of Christ that this perfidy can be cleansed. Both parricide and deicide are marked on the Jew's body through his ritual circumcision.

The child sacrificed by his father by remaining a Jew is reflected here as well as the father sacrificed by the child. (Is it the father here sensing the competition of the child or sensing his own inability to articulate his anxiety about his son's risk?) Freud evoked the powerlessness his own father narrated when he told him how he stepped out of the path of an anti-Semite who had knocked his hat in the gutter of a Freiburg street (*SE* 4:197). Within the dream of the "Myops" are many of the themes of incest, of crime, of sacrifice that are present in the Jews, including the question of their criminality. This criminality, the charge of parricide and deicide, all become associated with the biological definition of the Jew. The Jews' immutability means also that they will never be safe within the anti-Semitic world of European culture, no matter what their gifts or abilities.

Freud struggled with the argument about the special relation of Jews to the world of crime to the very end of his life. In a 1938 essay published in Arthur Koestler's émigré periodical, *The Future,* Freud quoted an unnamed (and according to him, only half-remembered) source on the Aryan responses to anti-Semitism.[210] Whether or not this source actually existed, Freud's quotation of this extremely long passage rejected the argument that the Jews "have many disagreeable qualities" and that "their race, compared with our own, is obviously an inferior one." Rather, Freud's source (and Freud himself) stressed that Jews, as a race, have "somewhat other characteristics and somewhat other faults." And that in "some ways they are our superiors." Among those ways are the fact that "they do not need so much alcohol as we do in order to make life tolerable; crimes of brutality, murder, robbery and sexual violence are great rarities among them; . . . their family life is more intimate. . . . Nor can we call them in any sense inferior" (*SE* 23:291–92). By 1938 the charge of Jewish criminality (or the immunity of Jews from specific forms of criminality) becomes, even for Freud, a touchstone of the debate about the Jewish predisposition to specific tendencies and must finally be rebutted.

Placing Freud's response to the claims of the biology of race about the special nature of the Jewish body and mind in the context of the medical literature of his time may imply that the construction of images of difference within medicine ceased with the Shoah. What is most striking is that—even within psychoanalysis—the claims about the meaning of the Jew's body did not cease with the 1940s. Claims about the special nature of the Jew's body helped position certain psychoanalysts before 1938 and, most strikingly, following the Shoah.[211] It is this repetition of the claims concerning the special nature of the Jew within the medicine of Freud's time—each variation with its own special motivation and special focus—that can conclude this study of medicine and identity at the fin de siècle. For the book begins at the close of the nineteenth century and concludes at the close of the twentieth—with some of the same images of the Jewish body continuing to exist with the specialized world of psychoanalytic discourse.

CONCLUSION
THE LIFE OF A MYTH

Sigmund Freud struggled his entire life to overcome the prejudices of his age. His conscious opposition to racism in his writing and thought was to no small degree shaped by the meaning of being Jewish in the culture he was born into. He belonged to that group targeted as different and dangerous. As an acculturated Jew in the European Diaspora, he could not help responding, in complex and often contradictory ways, to the image of the Jew found in his world. But it was not only within the general culture that such images of the Jew existed. The metaphors about Jewish difference and danger were made concrete in the medical discourse about Jewish pathology and predisposition for disease. Freud, as a medical scientist, was exposed to and understood the complexity of the implication of biological determinism within the medical science of his time, since it was a discourse about himself.

The fin-de-siècle epistemological problem that resulted from the powerful presence of racial ideology within a positivistic philosophy of science confronted Jewish physicians with a potential inability to be "real" scientists. How could the neutral gaze of the "real" scientist and the corrupt gaze of the Jew be identical? How could the observing healer and the observed patient be one? This double bind helped structure the rhetoric of the scholarly work for scientist-physicians such as Freud. Freud strove to resolve the conflict between being the physician who heals and being the patient who is the object of treatment, a conflict fueled by the neutrality demanded of the scientist-physician, by transmuting precisely those qualities that marked him as different into aspects of the system and rhetoric of psychoanalysis. Yet traces of this problem remained within the new science of psychoanalysis.

Nowhere is the epistemological debate about the status of the Jewish scientist more strikingly transmuted into the rhetoric of psychoanalysis than in the question of countertransference, the impact that the unconscious feelings (often negative) of the analyst have on the analytic process. The debate about countertransference, which swirled about Freud during his own lifetime but which he only marginally recognized, reflected on this general problem of the therapist's neutrality while excluding any reference to racial identity.[1] In 1910 he demanded that the analyst recognize countertransference as a problem to be "mastered," for "every psychoanalyst only gets as far as his own complexes and inner resistances allow" (*SE* 9:144–45). Neutrality is a state the therapist must at least attempt to approach. Even toward the end of his life, Freud's anxiety about Sándor Ferenczi's clouding of the boundary between analyst and analysand pointed toward the continued importance of this distinction for him.[2] In "Analysis Terminable and Interminable" (1937), he rejected Ferenczi's "mutual analysis" in the light of the stated and necessary difference between analyst and analysand (*SE* 23:221–22). His example, though clouded by the anonymity he placed on the account, is his own analysis of Ferenczi. Freud discusses Ferenczi's "antagonistic attitude to the analyst" but cannot see his own reciprocal hostile attitude toward the analysand. Ferenczi's discovery, in his analysis of R. N., that within the analytic situation there were powerfully repressed emotional responses on the part of the analyst had called the neutrality of the analyst into question. This view of an uncertain boundary between analyst and patient was difficult for Freud to accept, since it made his role as neutral listener behind the couch ambiguous. Such a qualification would have evoked the epistemological conflict present in the definition of the Jewish medical scientist. As late as 1937, Freud needed a boundary between the observer and the observed as a valid and validating line of demarcation.

Freud's self-definition as a scientist accepted the indispensable distinction between patient and physician because the world of science in which he functioned made this distinction a primary one. And there was no arena where this was more clearly exposed than in the debates about the biology of race and its pathological significance. This is not to assume that the conflicted question of the relation of the Jewish physician to the rhetoric of race is the sole social determinant of the discourse of Freud's work. On the contrary—the internalization of questions of national identity, class, family structure, and gender certainly provided further conflicted moments in his sense of self, as they did for others of his generation. In addition, of course, one can evoke a wide range of personal qualifications—such as his relationship with his own parents as well as their internalized representation—that also helped structure the way he came to understand the world. Freud elected to be a physician. Yet this choice heightened the meaning of his Jewish identity, for he could never remove himself from the anti-Semitism that clouded his professional choice throughout his entire adult life. Anti-Semitism haunted the medical profession, from the brilliant and innovative surgeon Theodor Billroth's condemnation of Jewish medical students in the 1870s to the very halls of the medical faculty of the University of Vienna in the 1930s, which "were filled with Nazi announcements and with their inflammatory propaganda. There were frequent student riots at the university—especially at the medical school—in which Jewish students were beaten up and sometimes seriously injured."[3] But even more than the anti-Semitism of the social setting, the very fabric of medicine assumed the Jews' innate, pathological difference.

The demands of medical science for the neutrality of its practitioners and the inability of the Jew to fulfill these demands provide a fragmentary frame for understanding Freud's identity. Freud's search for identity is reflected in his creation of psychoanalysis as a new science. This is true even in the debates in the late 1920s about lay (nonmedical) analysts. Freud sees them escaping the limits of medical indoctrination but still able to be true scientists undertaking the "unprejudiced reception of the analytic material" (*SE* 20:220). Such powerful residual moments of scientific positivism, even in the light of a redefinition of the relation of the analyst to traditional medicine (and as his nonphysician daughter, Anna, began to enter the analytic community as his evident successor), are shaped by the initial conflict concerning the neutrality of the observer present within the rhetoric of race in the science of his times.

Though such an intense presupposition helps shape the rhetoric of psychoanalysis, it is vital to remember that the origin of a theory does not vitiate its ultimate validity. Psychoanalytic explanatory models are indeed the very ones that provide the structure to analyze the unconscious conflicts and their resolution that appear within the very discourse of psychoanalysis. Therefore, to dismiss the conflict with the rhetoric of scientific racism as not germane to psychoanalysis—that is, as not existing in the literal sphere of psychoanalytic theory as a topic—ignores the powerful and often compelling implications of psychoanalytic theory for the examination of the process of superego formation. Certainly an awareness of the process of externalization and its ramification is necessary to sense the power ascribed to the rhetoric of difference.

Joseph Sandler, the former Freud Memorial Professor of Psychoanalysis at the University of London, has pointed out the complicated pattern of externalization of those conflicts existing within the self into the world.[4] Such a model can lead to a more careful discrimination of the implications of countertransference.[5] As Heinz Hartmann noted as early as 1939, all discussion of the processes of internalization, the way individuals become gradually aware of their dependency on the world about them, must rely on the view that such behavior reflects the direct stimulation of the external environment.[6] The "dialogue with the introject" to which Sandler refers may indeed be a projection onto the external world of the internal, bipolar image of the self, of the self understood as the projection of the introjected ideal object and bad object. But its coloration, the language in which this externalization is housed, is taken from one's life experience. Little wonder that Freud's externalization in the formulation of his own theories of such an internalized conflict is clothed in the rhetoric of the science that shaped it and from which it wished to distance itself—the language of biological determinism.

Freud's necessary reshaping of the rhetoric of the biology of race is keyed to the centrality of this material for the very science within which (and against which) he felt he had to position himself. Rafael Moses evokes an analogous problem of externalization in another highly structured, power-laden institution—the army.[7] The army is a "rigidly structured organization which does not allow for much direct expression of negative feelings." Here the feelings of aggression generated by the powerlessness of the soldiers are projected onto the sergeant major. Such a social situation, according to Moses, replicates the projective mechanisms to be found full blown within the internal world of the psychotic. As Melanie Klein observed: "In psychotic disorder this identification of an object with the hated parts of the self contributes to the intensity of the hatred directed against other people."[8] But Moses argues that such a projection onto an Other of those aspects of the self internalized as "bad" can take place within "normal" social structures, such as the army. Political oppression, Freud noted in a letter to Jung on January 22, 1911, creates a climate in which the oppressed become fascinated by the mechanisms of psychological distancing.[9] No greater moment of distancing can be found than in Freud's own relation to the medicalization of race during his time, and no more powerful rhetoric for the "bad" object can be found than the language of anti-Semitism rampant in European culture during the nineteenth and early twentieth centuries. And the world of medical science appears as highly structured and power oriented as any other social institution in the culture of the time. Indeed, the growing prestige of the science of medicine in this age of the final secularization of theology into science made the claims of this institution on power seem appropriate to its contemporaries.

Moses' view of the role externalization plays within the political process in the army rings true in the light of an examination of Freud's scientific world. The social structure of medicine and its attendant power provides a compensation for the frightening autonomy gained with the awareness of the individual's separation from the world of the caregiver. It also provides a language as well as a means for locating the "bad" object outside the self. "I," the physician, know and can control the "diseased" and "dangerous" patient, who represents all the anxiety about loss of control over the self that is inherent in all our fears about separation, decay, and death. But what if there is an overarching category that inexorably and immutably makes the physician an extension of the patient, that bridges the imagined and needed chasm between the constructed sense of one's own power and the powerless now understood to be present in the Other? What if one must be simultaneously physician and patient? And what if not only the world of medicine but the general culture sees individuals as "bad" or "dangerous" or "diseased"? At this moment the internalized sense of the bad object is externalized into the world not as a paranoid fantasy but as an appropriate distancing of a negative discourse about the self. And yet it cannot even be truly externalized as long as the social structure of medicine provides the primary context for the individual's sense of identity.

This was not solely a "Jewish problem" (to use the formulation of the time) in medicine. One can turn to other groups in other historical contexts (such as African American physicians in the United States during and following Reconstruction, or women physicians in Europe and the United States during the late nineteenth and early twentieth centuries) who confront much the same global problem—they wish to assume a professional identification as physicians and share the status (and power) of that role.[10] Yet they find the very discourse of medicine presents the group they are assigned to as damaged and at risk. But each individual and group resolves the question differently according to the resources available to them in the particular time and place.

An analogy can be seen in precisely the involvement of African Americans in the debates about the pernicious impact of segregation in the United States during the course of the mid-twentieth century. William E. Cross, Jr., has clearly shown the complexity of this argument.[11] Many African American psychologists needed to accept a totalizing view of African American impairment and the resultant self-hatred because of the claims of the liberal academic social science of the time, which saw unacceptable social contexts as necessarily leading to psychopathology. The models existing in those academic institutions African Americans were permitted to enter provided virtually only such totalizing models (taken, not coincidentally, from the model of "Jewish self-hatred" developed within the work of German and Austrian Jewish social scientists). Such a model of negation ignored the specific context of the African American and the potential for individual responses and reactions. It suppressed the power of the very institution that shaped and limited it, and also the resources of the multiple strands of identity on which virtually each of us can potentially draw. Its power arose from the sense that African American psychologists acquired status from the liberal academic world of psychology even if it implicitly meant calling their own psychological health into question. Were they too psychologically impaired because of the segregated world they lived in, or did the neutralizing force of their science enable them to transcend this potential disability?

Resistance to such stereotyping can take four identifiable forms of externalization.[12] It can take the form of an outright *rejection* of the categories applied to the group in which one is situated. This articulation that the labels applied to the group are false is rare in groups that see themselves as powerless and dependent on the toleration of the group in power. None of the Jewish physicians involved in the debate about the Jews' predisposition to disease were able to separate the premise of biological determinism from the arguments about the "Jewish race" and achieve an understanding of what "predisposition" implies as an ideological construct. There can be externalization in the form of a romantic *reversal* and resultant transvaluation of categories. Thus the representations of control applied to the stereotyped group are internalized and seen as positive attributes. Certainly there is no better fin-de-siècle example than Theodor Herzl's reversal of the pejorative sense associated with the label "Oriental" as applied to the Jews. There can be a *universalization* of the qualities. Here the qualities that are seen as attributes of a type or category are applied to all human beings. The rhetoric of psychoanalysis moves attributes associated with the category of Jew in the science of the time to the realm of the universal, but the very concept of the "universal" is colored by this displacement. And finally, there can be a *recontextualization* of such categories. The qualities are accepted as valid, but alternative explanations are sought. Some Jewish scientists, such as Cesare Lombroso, reinterpret the accepted "facts" of Jewish predisposition as having a social-psychological rather than a biological-physical cause. Biological explanations are often replaced by social explanations when liminal groups seek to explain the nature of their own identity in the late nineteenth century.

Yet the evocation of each of these models must reflect the historical context of the physician and the physician's sense of that localization. One example taken from Freud's own world must suffice. Earlier I cited a passage concerning the rampant anti-Semitism at the University of Vienna during the early 1930s. It was taken from the autobiography of Esther Menaker, a psychoanalyst who is an American of eastern European Jewish background. She went to Vienna in the early 1930s with her husband to undertake training in psychology and psychoanalysis. Her experiences there exemplify the complexity of understanding the implications of race as a category at that time. In Vienna she "misunderstood" the implications of the rhetoric of race for herself while quite clearly comprehending its implications for the world she had come to live in. She tells an anecdote about how she and her husband began to fill out the application for admission to the University in Vienna and were initially confronted with the question of their religion. This seemed to present a real conflict for her: "We were of Jewish origin and in the Vienna of that period, with its atmosphere of growing anti-Semitism, we had no wish to hide behind the category of *Confessionslos,* i.e., 'without religion,'"[13] So she boldly "wrote that she was of the Mosaic Faith" on her application to the university. But in the same application she was asked about the distinction between her "nationality" and "the country of which she was a citizen—a difference that, to this day, I fail to understand." So she wrote: Nationality—American, Citizenship—United States, Religion—Mosaic.

What Menaker could not articulate then or now is that the question of nationality was simultaneously a request for a designation of her "race." "What kind of American are you?" the official asked. "By now I had lost my composure and yelled back, 'All you want to know is whether I'm Jewish or not, and that is already clear from what I have written under "Religion." I refuse to be any special kind of American. It is terrible the way one is treated here.'" She seems initially to be torn between "being Jewish and being without religion, that is *Confessionslos,*" but the real question she cannot confront is her racial identification. For she had "been brought up without any formal religious affiliation or within the framework of a particular faith." Being Jewish, for her, was belonging to a religion, which one could practice or not practice, could accept or reject. It was not belonging to a race, a sign of an immutable identity. The anxiety of the Jews was that being seen as a race in the United States in the 1920s, the high point of Ku Klux Klan activity, meant one was branded as inexorably different, as different as the African American.[14] One could not opt for or against membership in a race—one simply belonged to a race and was so identified and so persecuted. Yet Menaker could not recognize this in a context seemingly so remote from her own experience. In Austria, where Jews are openly attacked, she fantasized, we are in a world in which being Jewish is only to be accepted as a label for a religion. Remember, she had rejected her religious identity as a Jew. But this restriction of the category of the Jew to the realm of religion was as little true for Austria as it was for the United States. "I expressed all this to my analyst. 'We have found,' she said, 'that it is better to be what one is.' In itself not a bad statement, yet she failed to address the conflict, the issue was who, indeed, was I 'really'? . . . My defiant answer on the University questionnaire did not represent a resolution of identity conflict. The response grew out of a counter-indication in the name of an ethical code that was indeed part of my identity" (44–45). But the true conflict, that of the racial identity of the Jew, was repressed and projected onto the world as a question of religious identity.

The power of the arguments about biological determinism in the psychology Menaker would have been exposed to cannot be underestimated. Often it was quite overt, as in the case of C. G. Jung's statements about the Jewish nature of Freudian psychoanalysis after his break with Freud. Jung stressed the differences between a Jewish and an Aryan psychology as early as 1918. He emphasized the rootlessness of the Jew, the fact that "he is badly at a loss for that quality in man which roots him to the earth and draws new strength from below."[15] This view of rootlessness made the Jew's creativity, especially in the sphere of psychology, of value only for the Jew: "Thus it is a quite unpardonable mistake to accept the conclusions of a Jewish psychology as generally valid" (7:149 n. 8). This statement, made in 1927, was repeated virtually verbatim in 1934, at which point Jung noted that it was "no deprecation of Semitic psychology, any more than it is a deprecation of the Chinese to speak of the peculiar psychology of the Oriental" (10:534). He further qualified his view of the psychology of the Jew (and the very meaning of a Semitic psychology) by paraphrasing Ernest Renan about the "Jew who is something of a nomad, has never yet created a cultural form of his own and as far as we can see never will, since all his instincts and talents require a more or less civilized nation to act as a host for their development" (10:165–66). Jung's private condemnation of the "essentially corrosive nature" of Freud and Alfred Adler's "Jewish gospel" in a 1934 letter reflected his general view of valuelessness of the "Jewish points of view" that constitute Freudian psychoanalysis.[16]

Jung based his views on a theory of racial memory that is part of early psychoanalysis. However, he presented this view of racial memory within a clearly anti-Semitic discourse about the Jews. For Jung, the male Jew is feminized. They "have this peculiarity in common with women; being physically weaker they have to aim at the chinks in the armor of their adversary, and thanks to this technique which has been forced on them through the centuries, the Jews themselves are best protected where others are most vulnerable" (10:165). It is this compensatory feminized psychology that has generated psychoanalysis:

> In my opinion it has been a grave error in medical psychology up till now to apply Jewish categories—which are not even binding on all Jews—

> indiscriminately to Germanic and Slavic Christendom. Because of this the most precious secret of the Germanic peoples—their creative and intuitive depth of soul—has been explained as a morass of banal infantilism, while my own warning voice has for decades been suspected of anti-Semitism. This suspicion emanated from Freud. He did not understand the Germanic psyche any more than did his Germanic followers. Has the formidable phenomenon of National Socialism, on which the whole world gazes with astonished eyes, taught them better? (10:166)

Jung's views stand in the light of the interrelation between the Jewish body (weak like the body of his essential woman) and the Jewish mind. The entire field of Freudian psychoanalysis is merely a further representation of that weakness, of that sexualized disease of soul, that "morass of banal infantilism." Jung's categories reflect the complex interrelation between the structure of gender and that of race. It is no wonder the Jews desire to, but cannot, become Christian Aryans: "Just as every Jew has a Christ complex, so every Negro has a white complex. . . . As a rule the colored man would give anything to change his skin, and the white man hates to admit that he has been touched by a black" (10:508). And the Jew? Jews cannot shed their Jewishness even though, to follow Jung's argument, they desperately desire to do so, and the Aryan cringes at any contact with the Jew. This cannot simply be dismissed as a return to a theory of different national psychologies.[17] Indeed, as was discussed in chapter 1, the very evocation of the concept of a national psychology is one means of evoking as well as combating the nineteenth-century scientific discourse about the inherent difference of the Jews. It is a pejorative continuation of the ancient view that sees the mind of the Jew as inherently different from that of the Christian or Aryan.

Freud's Jewish racial identity shaped Jung's reception of psychoanalysis, just as dealing with its implications shaped Freud's creation of psychoanalysis. It is Freud whom Jung in his fantasy would wish to psychoanalyze, to cure of his Jewish neurosis, but he cannot because of the inherent difference in their racial psychologies (10:164). This placed the Swiss psychoanalyst in a position to distance himself from Freud's stress on sexuality and move to the phylogenetic aspects of Freud's theory. Racial memory, an important aspect of Freud's self-understanding, is transmuted into the universal archetype. Jung thus creates a psychological space for himself and his own system in relation to Freudian ("Jewish") psychoanalysis. His Christian/Aryan identity, so vital to Freud in avoiding the charge that psychoanalysis was a Jewish science, becomes his means of distancing himself from Freud. Jewish psychologists, such as Esther Menaker, respond in no small measure to the inexorable rhetoric of Jewish psychological immutability as expressed in this tradition within the very "science" they have come to Vienna to study.

Throughout the late nineteenth century and the early twentieth the "scientific" claims about the Jew shaped the Jewish medical scientist's self-definition in light of the demands placed upon the medical scientist to be both objective and healthy. Science was to liberate the individual from the conservative world of religion and politics. It was to be a new universal discourse in which precisely those conflicts about racial identity that dominated the spheres of religious and political persecution were to be suspended. But of course this Enlightenment ideal of science conflicted with the simple and rather pedestrian reality that many of the older models of oppression were secularized into its rhetoric. The Christian view of the Jews as Christ killers and the conservative political opposition to the process of civil emancipation that built upon this rhetoric were easily transmogrified during the course of the nineteenth century into a rhetoric of racial difference and pathological predisposition. This could be done because the very rhetoric of religion and state had always evoked the biological ("essential") difference of the Jews as part of its anti-Semitic rhetoric. Whether it was in the sermons against the Jews by Saint John Chrysostom at the very beginning of the church or in the German philosopher Johann Fichte's diatribes at the beginning of the nineteenth century, the body of the Jew was always evoked as different.[18]

The biological difference of the Jews was not solely an invention of the anti-Semite. Jewish ritual practices, such as infant male circumcision, ritual bathing, and endogamous marriage, marked the Jews' awareness of their bodies as separate from the pattern of awareness that exists in Christian Europe. Yet it was not these religious practices that set the Jews apart, but the reading of these practices by those who needed to use the image of the inherent, innate, and immutable difference of the Jews as a boundary for their own identity. Placed in a position of powerlessness in the Diaspora, the Jews internalized, to one degree or another, this image of essential Jewish difference as part of their self-definition. For acculturated Jews whose self-definition was formed in no small part by the institutions in which they chose to function, this internalization of their own difference was even more clearly marked. It was therefore even more necessary for these Jews to distance themselves from this charge.

This is not to say that all Jews learned (and learn) from the Diaspora experience to question their bodies and their minds, to see themselves as damaged and damaging. The extent of the belief in this difference was largely determined by the historical and institutional context in which they found themselves. Thus Jewish physicians of the eighteenth and early nineteenth centuries who moved into the world of "real" medicine of the university from the folk medicine of the ghetto (whether this was accompanied by an improvement in medical knowledge may well be debated) saw themselves as acquiring a broader social status. And this status reflected the growing status of medicine at the time. The free profession of medicine acquired ever greater prestige among the general public as well as among liminal groups such as Jews during the nineteenth century with the development of major innovations in public health and therapeutic treatments (such as the introduction of antisepsis and anesthesia). The gradual civil emancipation of such groups as the Jews by the end of the century led to the sense that true social emancipation could be sought beyond those professions, such as finance and banking, traditionally open to and therefore associated with the Jews. But the traditional professions brought with them an image of the Jew against which the Jewish bankers of the late nineteenth century, such as Gerson von Bleichröder, could consciously react.[19] The new science of medicine was even more pernicious, since accepting the status of the scientist meant accepting (if also combating) the assumptions hidden in the statistics about Jewish illness as well as other images of the Jew in the medical literature of the period. No such link was made in the world of finance. On the contrary, Jewish bankers were able to distance themselves from the caricature of the Jewish financier, since they saw it as in no manner related to the new world in which they were able to function.

From the conflicts about the definition and implications of the image of the Jew in the science of his time, Sigmund Freud sought a complex answer that transcended the limitations of the debates about biological determinism and yet remained framed by them. It is this complexity that is to be found within the overall theory of psychoanalysis, as can be seen in the extraordinary adaptivity of the theory in our contemporary thought. When we look at the question of identity formation and medicine in fin-de-siècle culture, we already see the potential for extraordinary growth and development. Freud's project is an example of his positive reaction to the bind of race and science that he was placed in. His strong belief in the emancipating nature of science, his questioning of religion as a social institution and a psychological state, his refusal to disavow his sense of Jewish identity, his need to create a new and freer space for his intellectual pursuits are all creative responses to the constitution of the world in which he found himself.

NOTES

Introduction

1. *New York Times,* March 23, 1990, A17.

2. D. S. Greenberg, "Black Health: Grim Statistics," *Lancet* 335 (1990): 780–81, as well as Leith Mullings, "Inequality and African-American Health Status: Policies and Prospects," in *Race: Twentieth Century Dilemmas—Twenty-first Century Prognoses*, ed. W. Van Horne (Madison: University of Wisconsin Institute on Race and Ethnicity, 1989), 154–81.

3. Without a doubt, the best critique of this can be found in Vincente Navarro, "Race or Class versus Race and Class: Mortality Differentials in the United States," *Lancet* 336 (1990): 1238–40.

4. *New York Times,* September 25, 1990, C1, 10.

5. C. Loring Brace, "A Nonracial Approach toward the Understanding of Human Diversity," in *Man in Evolutionary Perspective,* ed. C. Loring Brace and James Metress (New York: John Wiley, 1973), 341–63, here 342.

6. On the use of medicine in the Third Reich see Robert Jay Lifton, *The Nazi Doctors: Medical Killing and the Psychology of Genocide* (New York: Basic Books, 1986). The sort of medicalization of race that ends in the death camps can be found in works such as Johannes Schottky, ed., *Rasse und Krankheit* (Munich: J. F. Lehmann, 1937). On the biological presupposition of such works see Änne Bäumer, ed., *NS-Biologie* (Stuttgart: S. Hirzel, 1990), which places the debates about race in Germany into the general biological tradition. On the use of medicine in the colonial world see Oliver Ransford, *"Bid the Sickness Cease": Disease in the History of Black Africa* (London: John Murray, 1983).

7. Theodosius Dobzhansky, "On Types, Genotypes, and the Genetic Diversity in Populations," in *Genetic Diversity and Human Behavior,* ed. J. N. Spuhler (Chicago: Aldine, 1967), 12.

8. Cited by William McDougall, *The Group Mind: A Sketch of the Principles of Collective Psychology with Some Attempt to Apply Them to the Interpretation of National Life and Character* (Cambridge: Cambridge University Press, 1920), 108.

9. See, for example, Peter A. Bochnik, *Die mächtigen Diener: Die Medizin und die Entwicklung von Frauenfeindlichkeit und Antisemitismus in der europäischen Geschichte* (Reinbek bei Hamburg: Rowohlt, 1985).

10. W. Petersen,"Jews as a Race," *Midstream,* February 1988, 35–37.

11. Henry Rothschild, "Diseases of the Jews," in his *Biocultural Aspects of Disease* (New York: Academic Press, 1981), 551. For an older bibliographic

tabulation of the meaning and extent of such "Jewish diseases" in the medical literature of the early twentieth century, see Emil Bogen,"Disease among the Jews," *Medical Leaves* 5 (1943): 151–59.

12. On the present state of the assumptions about the "diseases" attributed to the Jews see Usiel O. Schmelz and F. Keidanski, comps., *Jewish Health Statistics* (Jerusalem: Academon, 1966); Ailon Shiloh and Ida Cohen Selavan, eds., *Ethnic Groups of America: Their Morbidity, Mortality, and Behavior Disorders,* 2 vols. (Springfield, Ill.: Thomas, 1973–74), vol. 1, *The Jews;* Richard M. Goodman, *Genetic Disorders among the Jewish People* (Baltimore: Johns Hopkins University Press, 1979); Richard M. Goodman and Arno G. Motulsky, eds., *Genetic Diseases among Ashkenazi Jews* (New York: Raven Press, 1979); Rothschild, "Diseases of the Jews," 531–56; E. Stern, J. Blau, Y. Rusecki, M. Rafaelovsky, and M. P. Cohen, "Prevalence of Diabetes in Israel: Epidemiologic Survey," *Diabetes* 37 (1988): 297–302. On the history of this tradition see Michael Tschoetschel, "Die Diskussion über die Häufigkeit von Krankheiten bei den Juden bis 1920" (Diss., Mainz, 1990), and Marianne Turmann, "Jüdische Krankheiten (Historisch-kritische Betrachtungen zu einem medizinischen Problem)" (Diss., Kiel, 1968).

13. A parallel case can be made for the discussion of the relation between crime and "race"; see Carl E. Pope, "Race and Crime Revisited," *Crime and Delinquency* 25 (1979): 347–57.

14. Here I disagree with Edward Shorter's and Hannah Decker's reading of my earlier work. I certainly believe there were and are diseases that are to be found in specific groups for various reasons, including mental illnesses caused or manifested by intense anxiety. The creation and epidemiology of these illnesses is not at the center of my present investigation. Rather, I am interested in how the internalization of the assumption of risk (whether warranted or not) provides a vocabulary for the articulation of such anxiety. See Edward Shorter, "Women and Jews in a Private Nervous Clinic in Late Nineteenth-Century Vienna," *Medical History* 33 (1989): 149–83, and Hannah S. Decker, *Freud, Dora, and Vienna 1900* (New York: Free Press, 1990), 43–44.

15. Max Horkheimer, "Sociological Background of the Psychoanalytic Approach," in *Anti-Semitism: A Social Disease,* ed. Ernst Simmel (New York: International Universities Press, 1946), 1–11, here 4.

16. Bernhard Berliner, "On Some Religious Motives of Anti-Semitism," in Simmel, *Anti-Semitism,* 79–84, here 83.

17. Robert K. Merton, "The Normative Structure of Science," reprinted in his *The Sociology of Science: Theoretical and Empirical Investigations* (Chicago: University of Chicago Press, 1973), 267–78.

18. I am using the term "Jewish physician" to refer to those physicians who either label themselves as Jews or are so labeled in the standard reference works of the time. See, for example, the listing in Solomon R. Kagan, *Jewish Medicine* (Boston: Medico-Historical Press, 1952).

19. Londa Schiebinger, *The Mind Has No Sex? Women in the Origins of Modern Science* (Cambridge: Harvard University Press, 1989), 250–56.

20. See John Duffy, "Social Impact of Disease in the Late Nineteenth Century," *Bulletin of the New York Academy of Medicine* 47 (1971): 797–811.

21. Regina Markell Morantz-Sanchez, *Sympathy and Science: Women Physicians in American Medicine* (New York: Oxford University Press, 1985).

22. An extensive sample of the literature on this topic follows: Ulla Haselstein, "Poets and Prophets: The Hebrew and the Hellene in Freud's Cultural Theory," *German Life and Letters* 45 (1992): 50–65; Jacquy Chemouni, *Freud, la psychanalyse et le judaïsme: Un messianisme sécularisé* (Paris: Éditions Universitaires, 1991); Leon Botstein, *Judentum und Modernität: Essays zur Rolle der Juden in deutschen und österreichischen Kultur, 1848 bis 1938* (Cologne: Böhlau, 1991), 171–93; José Brunner, "The (Ir)relevance of Freud's Jewish Identity to the Origins of Psychoanalysis," *Psychoanalysis and Contemporary Thought* 14 (1991): 655–84; Harold Bloom, "Freud: Frontier Concepts, Jewishness, and Interpretation," *American Imago* 48 (1991): 135–52; Yosef Hayim Yerushalmi, *Freud's Moses: Judaism Terminable and Interminable* (New Haven: Yale University Press, 1991); Jerry V. Diller, *Freud's Jewish Identity: A Case Study in the Impact of Ethnicity* (Rutherford, N.J.: Fairleigh Dickinson University Press, 1991); Ilse 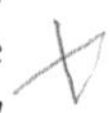 Grubich-Simitis, *Freuds Moses-Studie als Tagestraum: Ein biographischer Essay* (Weinheim: Verlag Internationale Psychoanalyse, 1991); Jacques Le Rider, *Modernité viennoise et crises de l'identité* (Paris: Presses Universitaires de France, 1990), 197–222; Gerard Haddad, *L'enfant illégitime: Sources talmudiques de la psychanalyse* (Paris: Point Hors Ligne, 1990); Ken Frieden, *Freud's Dream of Interpretation* (Albany: State University of New York Press, 1990); Emanuel Rice, *Freud and Moses: The Long Journey Home* (Albany: State University of New York Press, 1990); Jakob Hessing, "Jüdische Kritiken an Sigmund Freud," *Neue Deutsche Hefte* 36 (1989): 285–88; Y. H. Yerushalmi, "Freud on the 'Historical Novel': From the Manuscript Draft (1934) of *Moses and Monotheism*," *International Journal of Psychoanalysis* 70 (1989): 375–95; Erich Simenauer, "Freud und die jüdische Tradition," *Jahrbuch der Psychoanalyse* 24 (1989): 29–60. Renate Böschenstein, "Mythos als Wasserscheide: Die jüdische Komponente der Psychoanalyse. Beobachtungen zu ihrem Zusammenhang mit der Literatur des Jahrhundertbeginns," in *Conditio Judaica: Judentum, Antisemitismus und deutschsprachige Literatur vom 18. Jahrhundert bis zum Ersten Weltkrieg*, ed. Hans Otto Horch and Horst Denkler (Tübingen: Max Niemeyer, 1989), 287–310; Edward Shorter, "Women and Jews in a Private Nervous Clinic in Late Nineteenth-Century Vienna," *Medical History* 33 (1989): 149–83; Robert S. Wistrich, *The Jews of Vienna in the Age of Franz Joseph* (Oxford: Littman Library of Jewish Civilization/Oxford University Press, 1989), 537–82; Jakob Hessing, *Der Fluch des Propheten: Drei Abhandlung zu Sigmund Freud* (Rheda-Wiedenbrück: Daedalus, 1989); Mortimer Ostow, "Sigmund and Jakob Freud and the Philippson Bible (with an Analysis of the Birthday Inscription)," *International Review of Psychoanalysis* 16 (1989); 483–92; Jacquy Chemouni, "Au-delà de la psychoanalyse: L'identité juive," *Frénésie* 7 (1989): 99–124; Jerzy Strojonwski, "Polish-Jewish Background of Psychoanalysis," *XXX Congrès International d'Histoire de la Médecine, 1986* (Düsseldorf, 1988), 1224–30; Francine

Beddock, *L'héritage de l'oubli—de Freud à Claude Lanzmann,* Collection TRAMES (Nice: Z'éditions, 1988); Jacquy Chemouni, *Freud et le sionisme* (Paris: Solin, 1988); Paul C. Vitz, *Sigmund Freud's Christian Unconscious* (New York: Guilford Press, 1988); David S. Blatt, "The Development of the Hero: Sigmund Freud and the Reformation of the Jewish Tradition," *Psychoanalysis and Contemporary Thought* 11 (1988): 639–703; Susann Heenen-Wolff, *"Wenn ich Oberhuber hieße . . . ": Die Freudsche Psychoanalyse zwischen Assimilation und Antisemitismus* (Frankfurt am Main: Nexus, 1987); Peter Gay, *A Godless Jew: Freud, Atheism, and the Meaning of Psychoanalysis* (New Haven: Yale University Press, 1987); Mordechai Rotenberg, *Re-biographing and Deviance: Psychotherapeutic Narrativism and the Midrash* (New York: Praeger, 1987); Jacquy Chemouni, "Freud interprète de l'antisémitisme," *Frénésie* 4 (1987): 117–36; Jacquy Chemouni, "Freud et les associations juives: Contribution à l'étude de sa judéité," *Revue Française de Psychanalyse* 4 (1987): 1207–43; H. Bloom, "Grenzbegriffe, Interpretation und jüdisches Erbe bei Freud," *Psyche* 40 (1986): 600–616; L. J. Rather, "Disraeli, Freud, and Jewish Conspiracy Theories," *Journal of the History of Ideas* 47 (1986): 111–31; J. Kirsch, "Jung's Transference on Freud: Its Jewish Element," *American Imago* 41 (1984): 63–84; Elliott Oring, *The Jokes of Sigmund Freud: A Study in Humor and Jewish Identity* (Philadelphia: University of Pennsylvania Press, 1984); Stanley Rosenman, "A Psychohistorical Source of Psychoanalysis—Malformed Jewish Psyches in an Immolating Setting," *Israel Journal of Psychiatry and Related Sciences* 21 (1984): 103–16; H. Baruk, "Moïse, Freud et le veau d'or," *Revue Historique de la Médecine Hébraïque* 37 (1984): 19–23; Elaine Amado Lévy-Valensi, *Le Moïse de Freud ou la référence occulte* (Monaco: Editions Rocher, 1984); Stanley Rosenman, "The Late Conceptualization of the Self in Psychoanalysis: The German Language and Jewish Identity," *Journal of Psychohistory* 11 (1983): 9–42; Harold Bloom, "Jewish Culture and Jewish Memory," *Dialectical Anthropology* 8 (1983): 7–19; Mortimer Ostow, *Judaism and Psychoanalysis* (New York: Ktav, 1982); Avner Falk, "Freud und Herzl: Geschichte einer Beziehung in der Phantasie," *Zeitgeschichte* 9 (1982): 305–37; Susan A. Handelman, *The Slaying of Moses: The Emergence of Rabbinic Interpretation in Modern Literary Theory* (Albany: State University of New York Press, 1982), 129–52; Theo Pfrimmer, *Freud: Lecteur de la Bible* (Paris: Presses Universitaires de France, 1982); Max Kohn, *Freud et le Yiddish: Le préanalytique* (Paris: Christian Bourgois, 1982); Sigmund Diamond, "Sigmund Freud, His Jewishness, and Scientific Method: The Seen and the Unseen as Evidence," *Journal of the History of Ideas* 43 (1982): 613–34; Peter Gay, "Six Names in Search of an Interpretation: A Contribution to the Debate over Sigmund Freud's Jewishness," *Hebrew Union College Annual* 53 (1982): 295–308; Marie Balmery, *Psychoanalyzing Psychoanalysis: Freud and the Hidden Fault of the Father,* trans. Ned Lukacher (Baltimore: Johns Hopkins University Press, 1982); Dennis B. Klein, *Jewish Origins of the Psychoanalytic Movement* (New York: Praeger, 1981); Justin Miller, "Interpretations of Freud's Jewishness, 1924–1974," *Journal of the History of the Behavioral Sciences* 17 (1981): 357–74; David Aberbach, "Freud's Jewish Problem," *Commen-*

tary 69 (1980): 35–39; Carl Schorske, "Freud: The Psycho-archaeology of Civilizations," *Proceedings of the Massachusetts Historical Society* 92 (1980): 52–67; C. Musatti, "Freud e l'ebraismo," *Belfagor* 35 (1980): 687–96; Carl E. Schorske, *Fin-de-Siècle Vienna: Politics and Culture* (New York: Alfred A. Knopf, 1980), 181–207; Moshe Halevi Spero, *Judaism and Psychology: Halakhic Perspectives* (New York: Ktav, 1980); Marianne Krüll, *Freud und sein Vater: Die Entstehung der Psychoanalyse und Freuds ungelöste Vaterbindung* (Munich: C. H. Beck, 1979), published in English as *Freud and His Father,* trans. Arnold Pomerans (New York: W. W. Norton, 1986); Hugo Knoepfmacher, "Sigmund Freud and the B'nai B'rith," *Journal of the American Psychoanalytic Association* 27 (1979): 441–49; Fred Grubel, "Zeitgenosse Sigmund Freud," *Jahrbuch der Psychoanalyse* 11 (1979): 73–75; Avner Falk, "Freud and Herzl," *Contemporary Psychoanalysis* 14 (1978): 357–87; Avner Falk, "Freud and Herzl," *Haummah* 56 (1978): 57–75 (in Hebrew); Jeffrey Masson, "Buried Memories on the Acropolis: Freud's Response to Mysticism and Anti-Semitism," *International Journal of Psychoanalysis* 59 (1978): 199–208; Peter Gay, *Freud, Jews, and Other Germans* (New York: Oxford University Press, 1978), 29–92; N. K. Dor-Shav, "To Be or Not to Be a Jew? A Dilemma of Sigmund Freud?" *Acta Psychiatrica et Neurologica Scandinavica* 56 (1977): 407–20; O. Herz, "Sigmund Freud und B'nai B'rith," in *B'nai B'rith Wien, 1895–1975* (Vienna: B'nai B'rith, 1977), 50–56; Avner Falk, "Freud and Herzl," *Midstream* 23 (1977): 3–24; Martin S. Bergmann, "Moses and the Evolution of Freud's Jewish Identity," *Israeli Annals of Psychiatry and Related Disciplines* 14 (1976): 3–26; Paul Roazen, *Freud and His Followers* (New York: Alfred A. Knopf, 1975), 22–27; Reuben M. Rainey, *Freud as a Student of Religion* (Missoula, Mont.: American Academy of Religion, 1975); Léon Vogel, "Freud and Judaism: An Analysis in the Light of His Correspondence," trans. Murray Sachs, *Judaism* 24 (1975): 181–93; Robert Gordis, "The Two Faces of Freud," *Judaism* 24 (1975): 194–200; Stanley Rothman and Phillip Isenberg, "Men and Ideas: Freud and Jewish Marginality," *Encounter* 43 (1974): 46–54; Marthe Robert, *D'Oedipe à Moïse: Freud et la conscience juive* (Paris: Calmann-Levy, 1974), published in English as *From Oedipus to Moses: Freud's Jewish Identity,* trans. Ralph Manheim (Garden City, N.Y.: Anchor Books, 1976); John Murray Cuddihy, *The Ordeal of Civility: Freud, Marx, Lévi-Strauss, and the Jewish Struggle with Modernity* (New York: Basic Books, 1974); A. L. Merani, *Freud y el Talmud: Seguido de crítica de los fundamentos de la psicopatología* (Mexico City: Grijalbo, 1974); Max Schur, *Freud: Living and Dying* (New York: International Universities Press, 1972), 22–27; David Singer, "Ludwig Lewisohn and Freud: The Zionist Therapeutic," *Psychoanalytic Review* 58 (1971): 169–82; A. W. Szafran, "Aspects socio-culturels judaïques de la pensée de Freud," *Evolution Psychiatrique* 36 (1971): 89–107; Peter Loewenberg, "'Sigmund Freud as a Jew': A Study in Ambivalence and Courage," *Journal of the History of the Behavioral Sciences* 7 (1971): 363–69, as well as his "A Hidden Zionist Theme in Freud's 'My Son, the Myops . . .' Dream," *Journal of the History of Ideas* 31 (1970): 129–32; Donald Capps, "Hartmann's Relationship to Freud: A Reappraisal," *Journal of the History of the Behavioral Sciences*

6 (1970): 162–75; Robert Couzin, "Leibniz, Freud and Kabbala," *Journal of the History of the Behavioral Sciences* 6 (1970): 335–48; Ignaz Maybaum, *Creation and Guilt: A Theological Assessment of Freud's Father-Son Conflict* (London: Vallentine, Mitchell, 1969); M. S. Maravon, "Contribution à l'étude critique de la psychopathologie du juif: Psychoanalyse du juif" (Thesis, Paris, 1969), 25–51; Lary Berkower, "The Enduring Effect of the Jewish Tradition upon Freud," *American Journal of Psychiatry* 125 (1969): 103–9; Richard L. Rubenstein, "Freud and Judaism: A Review Article," *Journal of Religion* 47 (1967): 39–44; Earl A. Grollman, *Judaism in Sigmund Freud's World* (New York: Appleton-Century, 1965); David Bakan, *Sigmund Freud and the Jewish Mystical Tradition* (New York: Van Nostrand, 1958); Theodore Lewis, "Freud, the Jews, and Judaism," *Jewish Spectator,* March 1958, 11–14; Ernst Simon, "Sigmund Freud: The Jew," *Leo Baeck Institute Yearbook* 2 (1957): 270–305; Karl Menninger, "The Genius of the Jew in Psychiatry," *Medical Leaves* 1 (1937): 127–32, reprinted in *A Psychiatrist's World: The Selected Papers of Karl Menninger,* ed. Bernard H. Hall (New York: Viking Press, 1959); W. Aron, "Notes on Sigmund Freud's Ancestry and Jewish Contacts," *YIVO Annual of Jewish Social Sciences* 2 (1956): 286–95; Samuel Felix Mendelsohn, *Mental Healing in Judaism: Its Relationship to Christian Science and Psychoanalysis* (Chicago: Jewish Gift Shop, 1936); A. A. Roback, *Jewish Influence in Modern Thought* (Cambridge, Mass.: Sci-Art Publishers, 1929), 152–97; Charles E. Maylan, *Freuds tragischer Komplex* (Munich: E. Reinhardt, 1929) (in the Freud Library, London); Enrico Morselli, *La psicanalisi: Studii ed appunti critici,* 2 vols. (Turin: Bocca, 1926) (in the Freud Library, London); A. A. Roback, "Freud, Chassid or Humanist," *B'nai B'rith Magazine* 40 (1926): 118; A. A. Roback, "Is Psychoanalysis a Jewish Movement?" *B'nai B'rith Magazine* 40 (1926): 118–19, 129–30, 198–201, 238–39; Ludwig Braun, "Die Persönlichkeit Freuds und seine Bedeutung als Bruder: Festsitzung der 'Wien' anlässlich des 70. Geburtstages Br. Univ. Prof. Doktor Sigmund Freud. Wien 1926," (special issue of) *B'nai B'rith Mitteilung für Österreich* 26 (1926): 118–31; Arnold Kutzinki, "Sigmund Freud, ein jüdischer Forscher," *Der Jude* 8 (1924): 216–21.

23. Paul Weindling, *Health, Race and German Politics between National Unification and Nazism, 1870–1945* (Cambridge: Cambridge University Press, 1989), does discuss the question of Jewish physicians and their participation in the eugenics movement (482–84) but does not put this together with the discourse on Jewish disease. Michael H. Kater, *Doctors under Hitler* (Chapel Hill: University of North Carolina Press, 1989), has his primary focus after 1933. Gerrit Hohendorf and Achim Magull-Seltenreich, eds., *Von der Heilkunde zur Massentötung: Medizin im Nationalsozialismus* (Heidelberg: Wunderhorn, 1990); Robert Proctor, *Racial Hygiene: Medicine under the Nazis* (Cambridge: Harvard University Press, 1988); Peter Weingart, Jürgen Kroll, and Kurt Bayertz, *Rasse, Blut und Gene: Geschichte der Eugenik und Rassenhygiene in Deutschland* (Frankfurt am Main: Suhrkamp, 1988); Doris Byer, *Rassenhygiene und Wohlfahrtspflege: Zur Entstehung eines sozial-demokratistischen Machtdispositivs in Österreich bis 1934* (Frankfurt am Main: Campus, 1988); Hans-Walter

Schmuhl, *Rassenhygiene, Nationalsozialismus, Euthanasie: Von der Verhütung zur Vernichtung lebensunwerten Lebens, 1890–1945* (Göttingen, Vandenhoeck und Ruprecht, 1987), give little attention to this topic. Of interest given the importance of French science for the German medical tradition is the study of eugenics in France during this period by William H. Schneider, *Quality and Quantity: The Quest for Biological Regeneration in Twentieth-Century France* (New York: Cambridge University Press, 1990).

24. Philip Rieff, *Freud: The Mind of the Moralist* (New York: Viking Press, 1959), 258.

25. Paul Brienes, *Tough Jews: Political Fantasies and the Moral Dilemma of American Jewry* (New York: Basic Books, 1990), especially the chapter "Sigmund Freud's Tough Jewish Fantasy, Philip Roth's, and Mine," 1–75.

26. Isaiah Berlin, *Against the Current: Essays in the History of Ideas,* ed. Henry Hardy (New York: Viking Press, 1980), 258.

27. See the discussion by Carl E. Schorske, *Fin-de-Siècle Vienna: Politics and Culture* (New York: Alfred A. Knopf, 1980), 195.

28. Mikkel Borch-Jacobsen, *The Freudian Subject,* trans. Catherine Porter (Stanford: Stanford University Press, 1988), 47.

29. See his essay "To Look, to See, to Know" (1947), translated from the Polish in Robert S. Cohen and Thomas Schnelle, eds., *Cognition and Fact: Materials on Ludwik Fleck* (Dordrecht: D. Reidel, 1986), 129–51.

1. Psychoanalysis, Race, and Identity

1. MS., Nationalbibliothek Wien, Altenberg, Beilag zur 290/32-1.

2. On the creation of this concept see G. E. Allen, "Naturalists and Experimentalists: The Genotype and the Phenotype," *Studies in the History of Biology* 3 (1979): 179–209; F. B. Churchill, "William Johannsen and the Genotype Concept," *Journal of the History of Biology* 7 (1974): 5–30; J. H. Wanscher, "An Analysis of Wilhelm Johannsen's Genetical Term 'Genotype,' " *Hereditas* 79 (1975): 1909–26.

3. The shift from the antithesis "Jew/Christian" to "Jew/Aryan" in the German-speaking world takes place in the late 1870s and is most widely disseminated in the works of Wilhelm Marr, who coined the term "anti-Semitism" in 1879. See Paul R. Mendes-Flohr and Jehuda Reinharz, eds., *The Jew in the Modern World: A Documentary History* (New York: Oxford University Press, 1980), 271–73. For the broader scientific context see Louis Snyder, *Race: A History of Modern Ethnic Theories* (New York: Longmans, Green, 1939); Jacques Barzun, *Race: A Study in Superstition* (New York: Harper Torchbooks, 1965); George L. Mosse, *Toward the Final Solution: A History of European Racism* (New York: Howard Fertig, 1975); Léon Poliakov, *The Aryan Myth: A History of Racist and Nationalist Ideas in Europe,* trans. Richard Howard (New York: Basic Books, 1974); James C. King, *The Biology of Race* (Berkeley and Los Angeles: University of California Press, 1981); Nancy Stepan, *The Idea of*

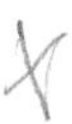

Race in Science: Great Britain, 1800–1960 (Hamden, Conn.: Archon Books, 1982); Paul Lawrence Rose, *Revolutionary Antisemitism in Germany from Kant to Wagner* (Princeton: Princeton University Press, 1990); Carl Degler, *In Search of Human Nature: The Decline and Revival of Darwinism in American Social Thought* (New York: Oxford University Press, 1991). After my initial work in this area I was sent the draft of a dissertation that comprehensively surveys the question of the racial anthropology of the Jews and the Jewish response: John Efron, "Defining the Jewish Race: The Self-Perceptions and Responses of Jewish Scientists to Scientific Racism in Europe, 1882–1933" (Ph.D. diss., Columbia University, 1991). I was also the primary reader on a dissertation by Laura Otis, "Organic Memory: Racial Memory in the Works of Émile Zola, Thomas Mann, Sigmund Freud, Miguel de Unamuno, and Thomas Hardy" (Ph.D. diss., Cornell University, 1991). I am indebted to both of these scholars.

4. This quote is attributed to Georg von Schönerer by Ernst Hiemer, *Der Jude im Sprichwort der Völker* (Nuremberg: Der Stürmer, 1942), 10. See also Raphael Patai and Jennifer Patai, *The Myth of the Jewish Race* (Detroit: Wayne State University Press, 1989), 406.

5. Adolf Hitler, *Mein Kampf,* trans. Ralph Manheim (Boston: Houghton Mifflin, 1943), 232.

6. In George L. Mosse's view the German Jews (and their Austrian contemporaries) of the fin de siècle were attempting to see themselves as members of the cultured middle class (no matter the strength of their religious identity). This self-identification comes profoundly into conflict with the view of the racialism of the Jew found in science. The scientists are thus Mosse's best examples. See George L. Mosse, *German Jews beyond Judaism* (Bloomington: Indiana University Press, 1985).

7. Max Marcuse, "Die christliche-jüdische Mischehe," *Sexual-Probleme* 7 (1912): 691–749, here 708.

8. The debate about the nature of race is reflected in the very use of the terms "Aryan" and "Jew," which reflect the ideology of the science of race. See Maurice Olender, *Les langues du paradis: Aryens et sémites—un couple providentiel* (Paris: Gallimard, 1989).

9. Cited in S. S. Prawer's translation from his *Heine's Jewish Comedy* (Oxford: Oxford University Press, 1983), 433. See my "Nietzsche, Heine, and the Rhetoric of Anti-Semitism," *London German Studies* 2 (1983): 76–93, and Shmuel Almog, "'Le judaïsme comme maladie'—Stéréotype et image de soi," *Parades* 13 (1991): 124–45.

10. Friedrich Nietzsche, *The Genealogy of Morals,* trans. Francis Golffing (New York: Doubleday/Anchor, 1956), 167–68.

11. *SE* 23:30–31. See the general context for this remark as discussed in the chapter "The Jewish Reader: Freud Reads Heine Reads Freud," in my *The Jew's Body* (New York: Routledge, 1991), 150–68.

12. Franz Alexander, "Sigmund Freud—the Man," *Medical Leaves* 3 (1940): 11–17, here 11.

13. Carl Heinrich Stratz, *Was sind Juden? Eine ethnographisch-anthropologische Studie* (Vienna: F. Tempsky, 1903), 5 (in the Freud Library, London).

14. See the discussion in Hannah S. Decker, *Freud in Germany: Revolution and Reaction in Science, 1893–1907* (New York: International Universities Press, 1977).

15. Wilhelm Griesinger, "Vorwort," *Archiv für Psychiatrie und Nervenkrankheiten* 1 (1868): iii–viii, here iii.

16. Richard Weinberg, "Über einige ungewöhnliche Befunde an Judenhirnen," *Biologisches Centralblatt* 23 (1903): 154–62, with a summary of the older literature beginning in 1882.

17. These arguments are well documented by Patai and Patai, *Myth of the Jewish Race,* 21–37. All the following undocumented references are to this discussion.

18. Francis Galton, *Inquiries into Human Faculty and Its Development* (New York: Macmillan, 1883), 305. See *SE* 4:139, 293; 5:494, 649.

19. Robert Knox, *The Races of Men: A Fragment* (Philadelphia: Lea and Blanchard, 1850), 131.

20. Friedrich Delitzsch, *Babel und Bibel* (Leipzig: J. C. Hinrich, 1902), 10–11.

21. This reading of the Assyrian beard as a sign of the Jew can be seen in contemporary references to Herzl's appearance collected at the Central Zionist Archive in Jerusalem. It permeated popular German consciousness. In his diary the German anti-Fascist Friedrich Percyval Reck-Malleczewen remembered the German Jewish anarchist Erich Mühsam as "looking not too unlike a winged Assyrian ox with his berry-brown beard" (*Diary of a Man in Despair,* trans. Paul Rubens [London: Macmillan, 1970], 115).

22. Anatole Leroy-Beaulieu, *Israel among the Nations: A Study of the Jews and Antisemitism,* trans. Frances Hellman (New York: G. P. Putnam's Sons, 1895), 178.

23. Georg Buschan, ed., *Illustrierte Völkerkunde,* 2 vols. (Stuttgart: Stercker und Schröder, 1922–26), 2, 2:299–304, here 299. The essay on the Jews was written by Michael Halberstadt and included Henry Ford's anti-Semitic diatribe *The International Jew* in its bibliography. See *SE* 22:187. Buschan was also the author of a widely cited popular account of the pathologies of the Jews, "Einfluss der Rasse auf die Form und Häufigkeit pathologischer Veränderungen," *Globus* 67 (1895):21–24, 43–47, 60–63, 76–80; on the Jews, 45–47, 60–62.

24. Stratz, *Was sind Juden?* 25.

25. On the background to these questions see Ina Spiegel-Rösing and Ilse Schwideltzky, *Maus und Schlange: Untersuchungen zur Lage der deutschen Anthropologie* (Munich: R. Oldenbourg, 1982); George W. Stocking, Jr., *Victorian Anthropology* (New York: Free Press, 1987), and Douglas Lorimer, "Theoretical Racism in Late-Victorian Anthropology," *Victorian Studies* 31 (1988): 405–30.

26. See the discussion of Karl Vogt, *Vorlesungen über den Menschen: Seine Stellung in der Schöpfung und in der Geschichte der Erde,* 2 vols. (Giessen: J. Ricker, 1863), 2:238.

27. Felix Ritter von Luschan, "Die anthropologische Stellung der Juden,"

Correspondenzblatt der Deutschen Gesellschaft für Anthropologie, Ethnologie und Urgeschichte 23 (1892): 94–102.

28. Raphael Isaacs, "The So-Called Jewish Type," *Medical Leaves* 3 (1940): 119–22, here 119.

29. An overview of the nineteenth-century discussion of the anthropological theories dealing with the Jews is offered by Maurice Fishberg, "Materials for the Physical Anthropology of the Eastern European Jew," *Memoirs of the American Anthropological Association* 1 (1905–7): 5–20.

30. Maurice Fishberg, *The Jews: A Study of Race and Environment* (New York: Walter Scott, 1911), 6, 324–25.

31. Leonard B. Glick, "Types Distinct from Our Own: Franz Boas on Jewish Identity and Assimilation," *American Anthropologist* 84 (1982): 544–65.

32. A. C. Haddon, Review of Maurice Fishberg, *The Jews*, in *Eugenics Review* 3 (1912): 65.

33. Friedrich Ratzel, *The History of Mankind*, trans. A. J. Butler, 3 vols. (London: Macmillan, 1896), 3:183. The German edition appeared between 1885 and 1888. For a more detailed discussion see my *Jewish Self-Hatred: Anti-Semitism and the Hidden Language of the Jews* (Baltimore: Johns Hopkins University Press, 1986; paperback edition, 1990), 216–17.

34. Houston Stewart Chamberlain, *Foundations of the Nineteenth Century*, trans. John Lees, 2 vols. (London: John Lane/Bodley Head, 1913), 1:354. On Freud's reading of Chamberlain see *GW*, Nachtragsband, 787.

35. Otto Jackmann, "Der Einfluss der Mikroben auf die Entstehung der Menschenrassen," *Archiv für Rassen- und Gesellschaftsbiologie* 6 (1909): 759–60. See also E. Below, "Rassen- und Zonenvergleichende Physiologie und Pathologie," *Allgemeine Medicinische Central-Zeitung* 66 (1897): 570–72.

36. See Michael Tschoetschel, "Die Diskussion über die Häufigkeit von Krankheiten bei den Juden bis 1920" (Diss., Mainz, 1990), and Marianne Turmann, "Jüdische Krankheiten (Historisch-kritische Betrachtungen zu einem medizinischen Problem" (Diss., Kiel, 1968).

37. Jacob Wassermann, *My Life as German and Jew* (London: George Allen and Unwin, 1933), 156.

38. "Beda" [Fritz Löhner], *Israeliten und andere Antisemiten* (Vienna: R. Löwit, 1919), 32–33. (By this edition the volume had sold 15,000 copies.)

39. On the cultural background for this concept see Jacob Katz, *Out of the Ghetto: The Social Background of Jewish Emancipation, 1770–1870* (Cambridge: Harvard University Press, 1973), and Rainer Erb and Werner Bergmann, *Die Nachtseite der Judenemanzipation: Der Widerstand gegen die Integration der Juden in Deutschland, 1780–1860* (Berlin: Metropol, 1989).

40. Johannes Buxtorf, *Synagoga Judaica . . .* (Basel: Ludwig Königs selige Erben, 1643), 620–22.

41. Johann Jakob Schudt, *Jüdische Merkwürdigkeiten* (Frankfurt am Main: S. T. Hocker, 1714–18), 2:369, trans. in Patai and Patai, *Myth of the Jewish Race*, 13. On the later ideological life of this debate see Wolfgang Fritz Haug, *Die Faschisierung des bürgerlichen Subjekts: Die Ideologie der gesunden Nor-*

malität und die Ausrottungspolitiken im deutschen Faschismus (West Berlin: Argument Verlag, 1986).

42. Bernardino Ramazzini, *The Diseases of Workers,* trans. Wilmer Cave Wright (New York: Hafner, 1964), 287.

43. Elcan Isaac Wolf, *Von den Krankheiten der Juden* (Mannheim: C. F. Schwan, 1777), 3. On Wolf's position in the medicine of the eighteenth century see Samuel Krauss, *Geschichte der jüdischen Ärzte vom frühsten Mittelalter bis zur Gleichberechtigung* (Vienna: A. S. Bettelheim-Stiftung, 1930), 154–55.

44. F. L. de La Fontaine, *Chirurgisch-medicinische Abhandlungen vershiedenen* [sic] *Inhalts Polen betreffend* (Breslau: Korn, 1792), 145–55.

45. See R. P. Neuman, "Masturbation, Madness, and the Modern Concepts of Childhood and Adolescence," *Journal of Social History* 8 (1975): 1–27.

46. Johann Pezzl, *Skizze von Wien: Ein Kultur- und Sittenbild aus der josephinischen Zeit,* ed. Gustav Gugitz and Anton Schlossar (Graz: Leykam-Verlag, 1923), 107–8.

47. On the meaning of this disease in the medical literature of the period see the following dissertations on the topic: Michael Scheiba, *Dissertatio inauguralis medica, sistens quaedam plicae pathologica: Germ. Juden-Zopff, Polon. Koltun: quam . . . in Academia Albertina pro gradu doctoris* (Regiomonti: Litteris Reusnerianis, [1739]), and Hieronymus Ludolf, *Dissertatio inauguralis medica de plica, vom Juden-Zopff . . .* (Erfordiae: Typis Groschianis [1724]).

48. Joseph Rohrer, *Versuch über die jüdischen Bewohner der österreichischen Monarchie* (Vienna: Verlag des Kunst- und Industrie-Comptoirs, 1804), 26. The debate about the special tendency of the Jews for skin disease, especially *plica polonica,* goes on well into the twentieth century. See Richard Weinberg, "Zur Pathologie der Juden," *Zeitschrift für Demographie und Statistik der Juden* 1 (1905): 10–11.

49. Wolfgang Häusler, *Das galizische Judentum in der Habsburgermonarchie im Lichte der zeitgenössischen Publizistik und Reiseliteratur von 1772–1848* (Vienna: Verlag für Geschichte und Politik, 1979). On the status of the debates about the pathology of the Jews in the East after 1919 see *Voprosy biologii i patologii evreev* (Leningrad: State Publishing House, 1926).

50. Arthur Schopenhauer, *Parerga and Paralipomena,* trans. E. F. J. Payne, 2 vols. (Oxford: Clarendon Press, 1973), 2:357.

51. Abbé Grégoire, *Essai sur la régénération physique, morale et politique des juifs* (Metz: Claude Lamort, 1789), 44–54. See also Richard H. Popkin, "Medicine, Racism, Anti-Semitism: A Dimension of Enlightenment Culture," in *The Language of Psyche: Mind and Body in Enlightenment Thought,* ed. George S. Rousseau (Berkeley and Los Angeles: University of California Press, 1990), 405–42.

52. Jacob Katz, *From Prejudice to Destruction: Anti-Semitism, 1700–1933* (Cambridge: Harvard University Press, 1980), 56–57.

53. Karl Wilhelm Friedrich Grattenauer, *Über die physische und moralische Verfassung der heutigen Juden* (Leipzig, 1791).

54. Dr. zum Tobel, "Mittheilungen über einige unter den hiesigen Israeliten

häufiger vorkommende Krankheiten," *Medizinisches Korrespondenzblatt für Württemberg* 6 (1836): 8–11.

55. Martin Engländer, *Die auffallend häufigen Krankheitserscheinung der jüdischen Rasse* (Vienna: J. L. Pollak, 1902), 46. Leo Sofer, also a physician in Vienna, provided a survey of the medical literature on the diseases of the Jewish race: "Zur Biologie und Pathologie der jüdischen Rasse," *Zeitschrift für Demographie und Statistik der Juden* 2 (1906): 85–92.

56. Nietzsche, *Genealogy of Morals*, 167–68.

57. On this theme see Mosse, *Final Solution*, 99, as well as Michael H. Kater, *Doctors under Hitler* (Chapel Hill: University of North Carolina Press, 1989), 177–83.

58. Letter of September 16, 1919, cited by Joachim C. Fest, *Hitler: Eine Biographie* (Frankfurt: Propyläen-Verlag, 1973), 167.

59. Hitler, *Mein Kampf*, 57–58.

60. Ludwig Wittgenstein, *Culture and Value*, ed. G. H. von Wright and Heikki Nyman (Oxford: Blackwell, 1980), 20.

61. Sigmund Freud, *Briefe, 1873–1939*, ed. Ernst und Lucie Freud (Frankfurt am Main: Fischer, 1960), 359; translation from *Letters of Sigmund Freud, 1873–1939*, ed. Ernst L. Freud, trans. Tania and James Stern (London: Hogarth Press, 1961), 346.

62. *Hippocrates*, trans. W. H. S. Jones, 6 vols. (Cambridge: Harvard University Press, 1959), 2:311.

63. George A. Aitken, ed., *The Tatler*, 4 vols. (London: Duckworth, 1899), 4:162 (for September 19, 1710).

64. All references to this hitherto unpublished essay are to the translation by Dennis Klein, published as appendix C of his *Jewish Origins of the Psychoanalytic Movement* (New York: Praeger, 1981), here 171.

65. Richard Andree, *Zur Volkskunde der Juden* (Leipzig: Velhagen und Klasing, 1881), 24–25; translation from Maurice Fishberg, "Materials for the Physical Anthropology of the Eastern European Jew," *Memoirs of the American Anthropological Association* 1 (1905–7): 6–7.

66. For a more detailed discussion of this aspect of Jewish difference see my *Jewish Self-Hatred*.

67. Andree, *Zur Volkskunde der Juden*, 117.

68. Otto Fenichel, "Elements of a Psychoanalytic Theory of Anti-Semitism," in *Anti-Semitism: A Social Disease*, ed. Ernst Simmel (New York: International Universities Press, 1946), 11–33, here 21.

69. Arthur de Gobineau, *The Inequality of Human Races*, trans. Adrian Collins (New York: Howard Fertig, 1967), 194–95. See Michael Biddis, *The Father of Racist Ideology: The Social and Political Thought of Count Gobineau* (London: Weidenfeld and Nicolson, 1970).

70. Johann Caspar Lavater, *Physiognomische Fragment zur Beförderung des Menschenkenntnis und Menschenliebe*, 4 vols. (Leipzig: Weidmann, 1775–78), 3:98 and 4:272–74. This reference is cited (and rebutted) in Paolo Mantegazza, *Physiognomy and Expression* (New York: Walter Scott, 1904), 239.

71. Buschan, *Illustrierte Völkerkunde,* 301.

72. Marie von Bülow, ed., *Hans von Bülow: Briefe und Schriften,* 8 vols. (Leipzig: Breitkopf und Härtel, 1895–1908), 7:254.

73. Diary entry for March 19, 1907. Cited from the unpublished diaries by Jacques Le Rider, *Der Fall Otto Weininger: Wurzeln des Antifeminismus und Antisemitismus,* trans. Dieter Hornig (Vienna: Löcker, 1985), 207.

74. See the discussion in Heinrich Loewe, *Die Sprachen der Juden* (Cologne: Jüdischer Verlag, 1911).

75. See the discussion of this in Ignaz Zollschan, *Das Rassenproblem unter besonderer Berücksichtigung der theoretischen Grundlagen der jüdischen Rassenfrage* (Vienna: Wilhelm Braumüller, 1911), 128 (in the Freud Library, London, with the dedication of the author). See Efron, "Defining the Jewish Race," 404–34. There is a powerful literature that attempts to debate the meaning of "race" as applied to the Jews. Some of these Jewish scientists accept the discourse of the pure Jewish race, others argue against any pure race at all. See Julius Goldstein, *Rasse und Politik* (Schlüchtern: Neuwerk, 1925), and Fritz Kahn, *Die Juden als Rasse und Kulturvolk* (Berlin: Welt-Verlag, 1921).

76. Theodor Lessing, "Eindrücke aus Galizien," *Allgemeine Zeitung des Judenthums* 73, nos. 49, 51, 52, 53 (1909): 587, 610–11, 620–22, and 634–35, respectively.

77. Binjamin Segel, *Die Entdeckungsreise des Herrn Dr. Theodor Lessing zu den Ostjuden* (Lemberg: Verlag "Hatiwka": 1910), 12–13.

78. Ludwig Woltmann, *Politische Anthropologie* (Leipzig: Justus Dörner, 1936), 161. On Woltmann see Jürgen Misch, *Die politische Philosophie Ludwig Woltmanns: Im Spannungsfeld von Kantianismus, historischem Materialismus und Sozialdarwinismus* (Bonn: Bouvier Verlag/Herbert Grundmann, 1975).

79. Adolf Bastian, *Das Beständige in den Menschenrasse und die Spielweite ihrer Veränderlichkeit* (Berlin: Dietrich Reimer, 1868), 204.

80. John Lubbock, *The Origin of Civilization and the Primitive Condition of Man* (1870; Chicago: University of Chicago Press, 1978), 275. See *SE* 13:13, 111.

81. M. J. Gutmann, *Über den heutigen Stand der Rasse- und Krankheitsfrage der Juden* (Berlin: Rudolph Müller und Steinecke, 1920), 10.

82. Reprinted as "Reindeutsche Sprache" in Heymann Steinthal, *Über Juden und Judentum: Vorträge und Aufsätze,* ed. Gustav Karpeles (Berlin: M. Poppelauer, 1910), 78–80.

83. See the discussion by Leo Metmann, "Die hebräische Sprache der Gegenwart," *Zeitschrift für Demographie und Statistik der Juden* 3 (1907): 129–34.

84. "Die Umgangssprache der Juden in Oesterreich," *Zeitschrift für Demographie und Statistik der Juden* 1 (1905): 13–14.

85. Gustav Jaeger, *Die Entdeckung der Seele* (Leipzig: Ernst Günther, 1880), 106–9 (in the Freud Collection, New York). For a catalog of the smell attributed to the Jew see Hans F. K. Günther, "Der rasseeigene Geruch der Hautausdünstung," *Zeitschrift für Rassenphysiologie* 2 (1930): 94–99, here 97–99. Günther strongly believes in the reality of the Jew's smell and offers his own as well as

historical testimony. This is repeated in summary in Hans F. K. Günther, *Rassenkunde des jüdischen Volkes* (Munich: J. F. Lehmann, 1931), 260–67.

86. Schudt, *Jüdische Merkwürdigkeiten,* 1:349.

87. Marcuse, "Mischehe," 714 n. 24.

88. Berhard Blechmann, *Ein Beitrag zur Anthropologie der Juden* (Dorpat: Wilhelm Just, 1882).

89. Erna Lesky, *The Vienna Medical School in the Nineteenth Century* (Baltimore: Johns Hopkins University Press, 1976), 107.

90. Theodor Reik, *Jewish Wit* (New York: Gamut Press, 1962), 31.

91. Otto Hauser, *Die Juden und Halbjuden in der deutschen Literatur* (Danzig: Verlag "Der Mensch," 1933), 12–13.

92. Theodor Adorno, Else Frenkel-Brunswik, Daniel J. Levinson, and R. Nevitt Sanford, *The Authoritarian Personality* (New York: Harper, 1950), 643.

93. Samuel Weissenberg, "Zur Anthropologie der deutschen Juden," *Zeitschrift für Ethnologie* 44 (1912): 269.

94. On the immutability of the body of the Eastern Jew see the 1939 dissertation written with Eugen Fischer in Berlin by Walter Dornfeldt, *Studien über Schädelform und Schädelveränderung von Berliner Ostjuden und ihren Kindern* (Stuttgart: E. Schweizerbart, 1940).

95. I see the scale of potential integration running from acculturation, the acquisition of the "external" trappings of a culture, which would include professional identity such as that of the scientist, but maintaining a primary group orientation to the original definition of the self, through to assimilation, the complete merging with that external identity as the primary group orientation of the individual. The individual variations along this scale are infinite and shift over time within each person's life experience. I follow loosely the guidelines sketched by Milton M. Gordon, *Assimilation in American Life—the Role of Race, Religion, and National Origin* (New York: Oxford University Press, 1964).

96. T. Maurer, "Medizinalpolizei und Antisemitismus: Die deutsche Politik der Grenzsperre gegen Ostjuden im ersten Weltkrieg," *Jahrbuch für die Geschichte Osteuropas* 33 (1985): 205–30, and Jack Wertheimer, *Unwelcome Strangers: East European Jews in Imperial Germany* (New York: Oxford University Press, 1987).

97. Erwin H. Ackerknecht, *Rudolf Virchow: Doctor, Statesman, Anthropologist* (Madison: University of Wisconsin Press, 1953), 123–45.

98. Cited by Ackerknecht, *Rudolf Virchow,* 127.

99. Heinrich Coudenhove-Kalergi, *Das Wesen des Antisemitismus* (Berlin: S. Calvary, 1901), 499. On Freud's reading of this text see *SE* 23:292. The 1929 revised edition is present in the Freud Library, London. For the context of this extraordinarily important philo-Semitic text see Erika Weinzierl, "Katholizismus in Österreich," in *Kirche und Synagoge: Handbuch zur Geschichte von Christen und Juden,* ed. Karl Heinrich Rengstorf and Siegfried von Kortzfleisch, 2 vols. (Stuttgart: Ernst Klett, 1970), 2:483–531, here 2:517–18.

100. Talcott Parsons, *Action Theory and the Human Condition* (New York: Free Press, 1978).

101. Joseph Ben-David, "Roles and Innovations in Medicine," *American Journal of Sociology* 65 (1960): 561–68.

102. Elias Auerbach, "Judenvolk und Weltkrieg," *Archiv für Rassen- und Gesellschaftsbiologie* 12 (1916–18): 65.

103. Philip Rieff, "The Authority of the Past: Sickness and Society in Freud's Thought," *Social Research* 51 (1984): 527–50, here 537 n. 17.

104. Karl Kautsky, *Rasse und Judentum,* 2d ed. (Stuttgart: Dietz, 1921), 62. This book was first published in 1914. On the general context of antiurbanism and its relation to protofascist thought see George L. Mosse, *The Crisis of German Ideology: Intellectual Origins of the Third Reich* (New York: Grosset and Dunlap, 1964).

105. Günther, *Rassenkunde des jüdischen Volkes,* 260 (first published in 1922). The other side of the debate about the meaning of the special language of the Jews as a purely social phenomenon was articulated by Matthias Mieses, *Die Entstehungsursache der jüdischen Dialekte* (Wiesbaden: R. Löwith, 1915). Mieses used ethnopsychological categories to describe the appropriateness of Yiddish as a vehicle for the expression of the Jewish psyche.

106. See the discussion "Sigmund Freud and the Jewish Joke" in *Difference and Pathology: Stereotypes of Sexuality, Race, and Madness,* by Sander L. Gilman (Ithaca, N.Y.: Cornell University Press, 1985), 175–90.

107. Freud uses the phrase "Kück des Rebben" in his essay "Psychoanalysis and Telepathy" (1921), *SE* 18:180; the joke this phrase is taken from is recorded in "Jokes and Their Relation to the Unconscious" (1905), *SE* 8:63. See Ken Frieden, *Freud's Dream of Interpretation* (Albany: State University of New York Press, 1990), 100–102.

108. Reik, *Jewish Wit,* 135.

109. Theodor Reik, *From Thirty Years with Freud,* trans. Richard Winston (New York: Farrar and Rinehart, 1940), 6.

110. Wilhelm Reich, *Reich Speaks of Freud* (Harmondsworth, England: Penguin, 1975), 63.

111. A. A. Brill, *Freud's Contribution to Psychiatry* (New York: Norton, 1944), 195.

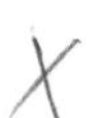

112. The translation is by Jack Zipes; Oskar Panizza, "The Operated Jew," *New German Critique* 21 (1980): 63–79. See also Jack Zipes, "Oscar Panizza: The Operated German as Operated Jew," *New German Critique* 21 (1980): 47–61.

113. On posthioplasty see Thomas J. S. Patterson, ed., trans., and rev., *The Zeiss Index and History of Plastic Surgery, 900 B.C.–1863 A.D.* (Baltimore: Williams and Wilkins, 1977), 250–54, and *The Patterson Index, 1864 A.D. to 1920 A.D.* (Baltimore: Williams and Wilkins, 1978), 427–28.

114. Panizza, "Operated Jew," 79.

115. Immanuel Kant, *Anthropology from a Pragmatic Point of View,* trans. Victor Lyle Dowdell (Carbondale: Southern Illinois University Press, 1978), 60. A German edition (edited by J. H. Kirchmann [Leipzig: E. Koschny, 1800]) is in the Freud Library, London.

116. The story is reproduced as an extended footnote to a reprint of Oskar Panizza's tale in Oskar Panizza, *Der Korsettenfritz: Gesammelte Erzählungen* (Munich: Matthes und Seitz, 1981), 279–92. On Panizza see Michael Bauer, *Oskar Panizza: Ein literarisches Porträt* (Munich: Hanser, 1984).

117. See Mynona, *Das Eisenbahnunglück, oder Der Anti-Freud* (Berlin: Elena Gottschalk Verlag, 1925). On Mynona see Peter Cardoff, *Friedlaender (Mynona) zur Einführung* (Hamburg: Ed. SOAK in Junius Verlag, 1988).

118. Karl Kraus, in *Die Fackel,* December 1924, 148–49. On Karl Kraus and psychoanalysis see Thomas Szasz, *Karl Kraus and the Soul-Doctors* (Baton Rouge: Louisiana State University Press, 1976); M. H. Sherman, ed., *Psychoanalysis and Old Vienna: Freud, Reik, Schnitzler, Kraus* (New York: Human Sciences Press, 1978), especially his "Prefatory Notes: Arthur Schnitzler and Karl Kraus," 5–13; E. Eben, "Karl Kraus und die Psychiatrie: Ein Essay," *Confinia Psychiatrica* 22 (1979): 9–18; Edward Timms, *Karl Kraus, Apocalyptic Satirist: Culture and Catastrophe in Habsburg Vienna* (New Haven: Yale University Press, 1986); and Leo Lensing, "'Geistige Väter' und 'Das Kindweib': Sigmund Freud, Karl Kraus und Irma Karczewska in der Autobiographie von Fritz Wittels," *Forum* 36 (1989): 62–71.

119. Ladislaw Klima, *Die Leiden des Fürsten Sternenhoch,* trans. Franz Peter Künziel (n.p.: Sirene, 1986), 113–15.

120. Mynona, "Operated Goy," 282.

121. Oskar Panizza, *The Council of Love,* trans. O. F. Pucciani (New York: Viking, 1979), 79. Panizza provided clinical descriptions of the various illnesses afflicting his characters. See his statement before the Munich court on December 1, 1895, reprinted in Kurt Boeser, ed., *Der Fall Oskar Panizza: Ein deutscher Dichter im Gefängnis* (Berlin: Hentrich, 1989), 46. See in this context the discussion of Panizza in Claude Quétel, *History of Syphilis,* trans. Judith Braddock and Brian Pike (London: Polity Press, 1990), 45–49.

122. *SE* 4:217. See in this context Didier Anzieu, *Freud's Self-Analysis,* trans. Peter Graham (London: Hogarth Press, 1986), 349–50, and Alexander Grinstein, *Sigmund Freud's Dreams* (New York: International Universities Press, 1980), 151–56.

123. *Protokolle der Wiener Psychoanalytischen Vereinigung,* ed. Herman Nunberg and Ernst Federn, 4 vols. (Frankfurt am Main: Fischer, 1976–81), 1:225; translation in *Minutes of the Vienna Psychoanalytic Society,* trans. M. Nunberg, 4 vols. (New York: International Universities Press, 1962–75), 1:239.

124. On the general questions raised by this argument see the essay by Nancy Stepan and Sander L. Gilman, "Appropriating the Idioms of Science: Some Strategies of Resistance to Biological Determinism," in *The Bounds of Race,* ed. Dominick La Capra (Ithaca, N.Y.: Cornell University Press, 1991), 72–103. On a model of modern science that is useful in writing this type of the history of psychoanalysis see Lewis S. Feuer, *The Scientific Intellectual: The Psychological and Sociological Origins of Modern Science* (New Brunswick, N.J.: Transaction Books, 1992) (with a new introduction on the critical reception of this book).

125. See Lesky, *Vienna Medical School,* 146, as well as William M. Johnston,

The Austrian Mind: An Intellectual and Social History, 1848–1938 (Berkeley and Los Angeles: University of California Press, 1972), 228.

126. Schudt, *Jüdische Merkwürdigkeiten,* 2:368.

127. Johann Friedrich Blumenbach, *Decas collectionis suae craniorum diversarum genitum illustrata* (Göttingen: J. C. Dietrich, 1790), 10.

128. Peter Camper, *Der natürliche Unterschied der Gesichtszüge in Menschen verschiedener Gegenden und verschiedenen Alters,* trans. S. Th. Sömmering (Berlin: Voss, 1792), 7.

129. Charles Darwin, *The Descent of Man, and Selection in Relation to Sex* (Princeton: Princeton University Press, 1981), 242.

130. Cited (with photographs) in Joseph Jacobs, *Studies in Jewish Statistics* (London: D. Nutt, 1891), xl. These plates were reproduced from scholarly journals in *Photographic News* 29 (April 17, 1885, and April 24, 1885) as unnumbered insets and as the frontispiece to vol. 16 (1886) of the *Journal of the Anthropological Institute,* which included the first publication of Joseph Jacobs, "On the Racial Characteristics of Modern Jews," 23–63, as well as A. Neubauer, "Notes on the Race Types of the Jews," 17–22). See Nathan Roth, "Freud and Galton," *Comprehensive Psychiatry* 3 (1962): 77–83. On the tradition of photographic evidence in the history of anthropology see Alan Sekula, "The Body and the Archive," *October* 39 (1986): 40–55, and Joanna Cohan Scherer, ed., *Picturing Cultures: Historical Photographs in Anthropological Inquiry, Visual Anthropology* (special issue) 3 (1990): 2–3. It is also in the work of Lombroso that the image of race plays a major role. See F. Bazzi and R. Bèttica-Giovannini, "L'atlante fisiognomonico e frenologico del sig: Ysabeau tra quelli di Lavater e di Fall e quello di Lombroso," *Annali dell Ospedale Maria Vittoria di Torino* 23 (1980): 343–416, and A. T. Caffaratto, "La raccolta di fotografie segnaletiche del Museo di Antropologia Criminale di Torino: La fotografia come documento e testimonianza dell'opera di Cesare Lombroso," *Annali dell Ospedale Maria Vittoria di Torino* 23 (1980): 295–332. The tradition of fixing the racial gaze continues into the world of the scientific motion picture in the 1890s, such as the chronophotograph. See Elizabeth Cartwright, "Physiological Modernism: Cinematography as a Medical Research Technology" (Ph.D. diss., Yale University, 1991), 38.

131. Francis Galton, "Photographic Composites," *Photographic News* 29 (April 17, 1885): 243–46, here 243.

132. See Hervé Huot, *Du sujet à l'image: Une histoire de l'oeil chez Freud* (Paris: Éditions Universitaires, 1987).

133. Stratz, *Was sind Juden?* 7. Stratz is citing Joseph Deniker, *Races of Man* (London: W. Scott, 1900), 423.

134. Günther, *Rassenkunde des jüdischen Volkes,* 70 (on the physiology of the Jewish eye); 210–11 (on Galton's photographs); 217 (on the Jewish gaze).

135. Robert Burton, *The Anatomy of Melancholy,* ed. Holbrook Jackson (New York: Vintage, 1977), 211–12 (a 1938 edition is in the Freud Library, London).

136. Redcliffe N. Salaman, "Heredity and the Jew," *Eugenics Review* 3 (1912): 190.

137. S. Seligmann, *Der Böse Blick und Verwandtes: Ein Beitrag zur Geschichte des Aberglaubens aller Zeiten und Völker,* 2 vols. (Berlin: Hermann Barsdorf, 1910–11), 1:86.

138. Jacobs, *Studies in Jewish Statistics,* xxxiii.

139. Poliakov, *Aryan Myth,* 155–82.

140. Gobineau, *Inequality,* 122.

141. Carl Huter, *Menschenkenntnis: Körperform- und Gesichts-Ausdruckskunde* (1904; Schwaig bei Nuremberg: Verlag für Carl Huters Werke, 1957). See the partisan discussion in Fritz Aerni, *Carl Huter (1861–1912): Leben und Werk* (Zurich: Kalos, 1986), and his *Huter und Lavater: Von der Gefühlsphysiognomik zur Psychologie und Psycho-Physiognomik* (Zurich: Kalos, 1984).

142. Maurice Fishberg and Joseph Jacobs, "Anthropological Types," in *The Jewish Encyclopedia,* 12:294.

143. Leroy-Beaulieu, *Israel among the Nations,* 172.

144. Gutmann, *Über den heutigen Stand,* 17.

145. Zollschan, *Das Rassenproblem,* 44.

146. Leo Goldhammer, "Herzl and Freud," in *Theodor Herzl Jahrbuch* (Vienna, 1937), 266–68; reprinted and translated in the *Herzl Year Book,* vol. 1 (New York, 1958), 194–96, here 195.

147. Freud, *Briefe, 1873–1939,* 318; translation from *Letters of Sigmund Freud, 1873–1939,* 313.

148. William J. McGrath, *Freud's Discovery of Psychoanalysis: The Politics of Hysteria* (Ithaca, N.Y.: Cornell University Press, 1986), 285.

149. W[illiam] O[sler], "Letters from Berlin," *Canada Medical and Surgical Journal* 12 (1884): 721–28, here 728.

150. See L. Chertok, "On Objectivity in the History of Psychotherapy: The Dawn of Dynamic Psychology (Sigmund Freud, J. M. Charcot)," *Journal of Nervous and Mental Diseases* 153 (1971): 71–80, as well as Charles Coulston Gillispie, *The Edge of Objectivity: An Essay in the History of Scientific Ideas* (Princeton: Princeton University Press, 1960). On the relationship between the narrative forms of "science" and of "fiction" see Steven E. Goldberg, *Two Patterns of Rationality in Freud's Writings* (Tuscaloosa: University of Alabama Press, 1988).

151. George Herbert Mead, *Movements of Thought in the Nineteenth Century* (Chicago: University of Chicago Press, 1936), 176.

152. Karl Pearson, *The Grammar of Science* (London: Adam and Charles Black, 1911), v (in the Freud Library, London; passage underlined by Freud).

153. H[ilde] D[oolittle], *Tribute to Freud* (New York: New Directions, 1956), 71.

154. Hanns Sachs, *Freud: Master and Friend* (Cambridge: Harvard University Press, 1946), 130.

155. Lou Andreas-Salomé, *The Freud Journal,* trans. Stanley A. Leavy (New York: Basic Books, 1964), 74.

156. *Protokolle der Wiener Psychoanalytischen Vereinigung,* 4:166; translation from *Minutes of the Vienna Psychoanalytic Society,* 4:178.

157. Chamberlain, *Foundations of the Nineteenth Century,* 1:389.

158. See the discussion in Anzieu, *Freud's Self-Analysis,* 213–18.

159. *SE* 4:293. See also the mentions of this technique on 4:494 and 4:649 as well as 15:172 n. 1 and 23:10.

160. Maurice Fishberg, "Hair," in *The Jewish Encyclopedia,* 6:157–60. See also his "Zur Frage der Herkunft des blonden Elements im Judentum," *Zeitschrift für Demographie und Statistik der Juden* 4 (1907): 7–12, 25–30.

161. Hitler, *Mein Kampf,* 325.

162. Karl Marx was also nicknamed the "Moor" because of his perceived coloration.

163. Zollschan, *Das Rassenproblem,* 120.

164. Otto Fenichel, "Elements of a Psychoanalytic Theory of Anti-Semitism," in Simmel, *Anti-Semitism,* 11–33, here 16.

165. Ray Monk, *Ludwig Wittgenstein: The Duty of Genius* (New York: Free Press, 1990), 279. The German text is reproduced in Monk's notes.

166. *Sigmund Freud–Karl Abraham, Briefe, 1907–1926,* ed. Hilda C. Abraham and Ernst L. Freud (Frankfurt am Main: Fischer, 1980), 269; translation from *A Psycho-Analytic Dialogue: The Letters of Sigmund Freud and Karl Abraham, 1907–1926,* ed. Hilda C. Abraham and Ernst L. Freud, trans. Bernard Marsh and Hilda C. Abraham (London: Hogarth Press, 1965), 286. On Pötzl see H. Hoff, "In Memoriam Otto Pötzl," *Wiener Klinische Wochenschrift* 72 (1962): 369–70.

167. *Sigmund Freud–Karl Abraham,* 254; translation from *Psycho-Analytic Dialogue,* 270.

168. Cited in a letter from Pötzl to Freud on November 15, 1937, in the appendix to *The Diary of Sigmund Freud, 1929–1939: A Record of the Final Decade,* ed. and trans. Michael Molnar (New York: Charles Scribner's Sons, 1992), 281.

169. Molnar, 98.

170. Richard F. Sterba, *Reminiscences of a Viennese Psychoanalyst* (Detroit: Wayne State University Press, 1982), 161–63. See also the discussion of Pötzl and his role in the psychiatric treatment of shell-shocked soldiers in World War I in Helene Deutsch, *Confrontations with Myself: An Epilogue* (New York: W. W. Norton, 1973), 111.

171. Otto Pötzl, "Experimentell erregte Traumbild in ihren Beziehung zum indirekten Sehen," *Zeitschrift für die gesamte Neurologie und Psychiatrie* 37 (1917): 278–339, here 300–311.

172. Such as the following discussion: "Castration has a place too in the Oedipus legend, for the blinding with which Oedipus punishes himself after the discovery of his crime is, by the evidence of dreams, a symbolic substitute for castration. The possibility cannot be excluded that a phylogenetic memory-trace may contribute to the extraordinarily terrifying effect of the threat—a memory trace from the pre-history of the primal family, when the jealous father actually

robbed his son of his genitals if the latter became troublesome to him as a rival with a woman. The primeval custom of circumcision, another symbolic substitute for castration, can only be understood as an expression of submission to the father's will. (Cf. the puberty rites of primitive peoples.) No investigation has yet been made of the form taken by the events described above among peoples and in civilizations which do not suppress masturbation in children" (*SE* 23:190). See Stephen Kern, "The Prehistory of Freud's Theory of Castration Anxiety," *Psychoanalytic Review* 62 (1975): 309–14. On the cross-cultural dimensions see Orphan M. Ozturk, "Ritual Circumcision and Castration Anxiety," *Psychiatry* 36 (1973): 49–60.

173. Anton Edler von Rosas, "Über die Quellen des heutigen ärtzlichen Missbehagens, und die Mittel um demselben wirksam zu steuern," *Medizinische Jahrbücher des Kaiserlichen Königlichen Österreichischen Staates* 40 (1842): 16–19.

174. See the detailed accusations in Georg Pictorius, *Von zernichten Artzten: Clarer Bericht ob die Christen von den jüdischen Artzten, vertrewlich Artzney gebrauchen mögen* (Strassburg: Hans Knoblauch, 1557) (especially on the false cures for venereal diseases); Ludwig von Hornigk, *Medicaster apella; oder, Juden Artzt* (Strasbourg: Mary von der Heiden, 1631); and Christian Trewmundt, *Dess Christiani Trewmundts Gewissen-loser Juden-Doctor in Welchem Erstlich Das wahre Conterfeit eines Christlichen Medici, und dessen nothwendige Wissenschafften, wie auch gewissenhaffte Praxis, zweytens Die hingegen abscheuliche Gestalt* . . . (Freiburg, 1698). The last two authors call upon the work of the convert Anthonius Margaritha, *Der gantz Jüdisch glaub* (Augsburg: Heinrich Steyner, 1530), and his comments on the "Jewish quack." On the self-defense of Jewish physicians against these charges see Harry Friedenwald, *The Jews and Medicine: Essays,* 2 vols. (Baltimore: Johns Hopkins Press, 1944), 1:31–68. Freud's own 1926 defense of Theodor Reik against the accusation of quackery (*SE* 20:179–258, as well as *GW,* Nachtragsband, 715–17) should be read in this context. See my *Disease and Representation: Images of Illness from Madness to AIDS* (Ithaca, N.Y.: Cornell University Press, 1988), 182–201. On Reik see Jean-Marc Alby, *Theodor Reik: Le trajet d'un psychanalyste de Vienne "fin de siècle" aux États-Unis* (Paris: Clancier-Guenaud, 1985).

175. Rosas, *Über die Quellen,* 19.

176. It was Mannheimer who officiated at the marriage of Sigmund Freud's parents Jacob Freud and Amalia Nathanson on July 29, 1855.

177. Isaac Noah Mannheimer, "Einige Worte über Juden und Judenthum . . . ," *Oesterreichische Medicinische Wochenschrift* (1842), Ausserordentliche Beilage zur Wochenschrift 34:1–10. A further fifteen-page rebuttal by a self-labeled Jewish physician Dr. J. Hayne appeared as a supplement to volume 38 of the same journal.

178. Anton Edler von Rosas, "Erwiederung auf Herrn Mannheimer's Einrede, bezüglich auf den Andrang der Israeliten zur Medicin," *Oesterreichische Medicinische Wochenschrift* (1842), Ausserordentliche Beilage zur Wochenschrift 34:11–16. Rosas admits to being overinclusive with his condemnation of Jewish

doctors as quacks. In a classical act of self-defense, he calls on his own Jewish students as witnesses to his lack of prejudice; and he closes his piece with a bit of late Enlightenment rhetoric evoking Lessing's *Nathan der Weise,* the epitome of toleration—all in all, an object lesson that overt, public anti-Semitism was not quite acceptable in the Viennese medical establishment of the 1840s.

179. Leopold von Sacher-Masoch, "Zwei Ärtze," in his *Jüdisches Leben in Wort und Bild* (Mannheim: J. Bensheimer, 1892), 287–98. See David Biale, "Masochism and Philosemitism: The Strange Case of Leopold von Sacher-Masoch," *Journal of Contemporary History* 17 (1982): 305–24, and Hans Otto Horch, "Der Aussenseiter als 'Judenraphael': Zu den Judengeschichten Leopolds von Sacher Masoch," in *Conditio Judaica: Judentum, Antisemitismus und deutschsprachige Literatur vom 18. Jahrhundert bis zum Ersten Weltkrieg,* ed. Hans Otto Horch and Horst Denkler (Tübingen: Max Niemeyer, 1989), 258–86.

180. See David Lawrence Preston, "Science, Society, and the German Jews, 1870–1933" (Ph.D. diss., University of Illinois, 1971); Monika Richarz, *Der Eintritt der Juden in die akademischen Berufe* (Tübingen: Mohr, 1974); and T. Schlich, "Der Eintritt von Juden in das Bildungsburgertum des 18. und 19. Jahrhunderts: Die jüdisch-christliche Arztfamilie Speyer," *Medizinhistorisches Jahrbuch* 25 (1990): 129–42.

181. On the historical context of the Jews of Vienna see Dirk Van Arkel, "Antisemitism in Austria" (Diss., Leiden, 1966); Alfred Schick, "The Vienna of Sigmund Freud," *Psychoanalytic Review* 55 (1968–69): 529–51; John Reginald Peter Theobold, "The Response of the Jewish Intelligentsia in Vienna to the Rise of Anti-Semitism, with Special Reference to Karl Kraus" (Diss., University of Southampton, 1975); Peter Schmidtbauer, "Households and Household Forms of Viennese Jews in 1857," *Journal of Family History* 5 (1980): 375–89; Eric Fischer, "Seven Viennese Jewish Families: From the Ghetto to the Holocaust and Beyond," *Jewish Social Studies* 42 (1980): 345–60; John W. Boyer, *Political Radicalism in Late Imperial Vienna: Origins of the Christian Social Movement, 1848–1897* (Chicago: University of Chicago Press, 1981); George Clare, *Last Waltz in Vienna: The Rise and Destruction of a Family, 1842–1942* (New York: Holt, Reinhart, and Winston, 1982); Marsha L. Rozenblit, *The Jews of Vienna, 1867–1914: Assimilation and Identity* (Albany: State University of New York Press, 1983); Ezra Mendelsohn, *The Jews of East Central Europe between the World Wars* (Bloomington: Indiana University Press, 1983); Léon Poliakov, *The History of Anti-Semitism,* vol. 4, *Suicidal Europe, 1870–1933,* trans. George Klim (Oxford: Oxford University Press, 1985); Norbert Leser, ed., *Theodor Herzl und das Wien des Fin de Siècle* (Vienna: Böhlau, 1987); Ivar Oxaal, Michael Pollak, and Gerhard Botz, eds., *Jews, Antisemitism, and Culture in Vienna* (New York: Routledge and Kegan Paul, 1987); Michael Mitterauer, ed., *Gelobt sei, der dem schwächen Kraft verlieht: Zehn Generationen einer jüdischen Familie im alten und neuen Österreich* (Vienna: Böhlau, 1987); George E. Berkley, *Vienna and Its Jews: The Tragedy of Success, 1880–1980s* (Cambridge, Mass.: Abt/Madison, 1988); William O. McCagg, Jr., *A History of Habsburg Jews,*

1670–1918 (Bloomington: Indiana University Press, 1989); Robert Wistrich, *The Jews of Vienna in the Age of Franz Joseph* (Oxford: Littman Library of Jewish Civilization/Oxford University Press, 1989); Steven Beller, *Vienna and the Jews, 1867–1938: A Cultural History* (Cambridge: Cambridge University Press, 1989); Harriet Pass Freidenreich, *Jewish Politics in Vienna, 1918–1938* (Bloomington: Indiana University Press, 1991); Michael P. Steinberg, "'Fin-de-Siècle Vienna' Ten Years Later, 'Viel Traum, Wenig Wirklichkeit,'" *Austrian History Yearbook* 22 (1991): 151–62.

182. See the discussion of Du Bois-Reymond and Billings in Fielding H. Garrison, *John Shaw Billings: A Memoir* (New York: G. P. Putnam's Sons, 1915), 234–35.

183. All quotations are from the English translation, Otto Weininger, *Sex and Character* (London: William Heinemann, 1906), 315. On Weininger see my *Jewish Self-Hatred,* 244–51; Le Rider, *Der Fall Otto Weininger;* Jacques Le Rider and Norbert Leser, eds., *Otto Weininger: Werk und Wirkung* (Vienna: Österreichischer Bundesverlag, 1984); Peter Heller, "A Quarrel over Bisexuality," in *The Turn of the Century: German Literature and Art, 1890–1915,* ed. Gerald Chapple and Hans H. Schulte (Bonn: Bouvier, 1978), 87–116; Franco Nicolino, *Indagini su Freud e sulla psicoanalisi* (Naples: Liguori Editore, n.d.), 103–10.

184. Hermann Schneider, *Kultur und Denken der Babylonier und Juden* (Leipzig: J. C. Hinrich, 1910), 663 (in the Freud Library, London).

185. Julius Moses, "Die Hetze gegen die jüdischen Ärzte," *Kassenarzt* 9 (1932): 1–7, here 1. See Susanne Hahn, "Antisemitismus in der Wissenschafts- und Gesundheitspolitik der Weimarer Republik—Zum besonderen Gedächtnis an Julius Moses (1868–1942)," *Zeitschrift für die Gesamte Innere Medizin* 44 (1989): 313–16.

186. William F. Bynum, "The Great Chain of Being after Forty Years: An Appraisal," *History of Science* 13 (1975): 1–28.

187. Kurt Danziger, *Constructing the Subject: Historical Origins of Psychological Research* (Cambridge: Cambridge University Press, 1990), 193.

2. Conversion, Circumcision, and Discourse

1. Sander L. Gilman, *Jewish Self-Hatred: Anti-Semitism and the Hidden Language of the Jews* (Baltimore: Johns Hopkins University Press, 1986; paperback edition, 1990), 177. See also Peter Heinegg, "Heine's Conversion and the Critics," *German Life and Letters* 30 (1976): 45–51.

2. Ernest Jones, *The Life and Work of Sigmund Freud,* 3 vols. (New York: Basic Books, 1953–57), 1:101.

3. Theodor Mommsen, *Auch ein Wort über unser Judentum* (Berlin: Weidmann, 1880), 15–16.

4. Heinrich Treitschke, *Deutsche Geschichte im 19. Jahrhundert* (Leipzig: S. Hirzel, 1889), 455.

5. *Ein Wort zur Judenfrage* (Berlin: F. Heinicke, 1880), 17.

6. A. A. Brill, *Freud's Contribution to Psychiatry* (New York: W. W. Norton, 1944), 197.

7. Quoted in the translation from Joseph B. Maier, Judith Marcus, and Zoltán Tarr, eds., *German Jewry, Its History and Sociology: Selected Essays by Werner Cahnman* (New Brunswick, N.J.: Transaction Books, 1989), 162–63. For the broader implications see Jacques Le Rider, "La 'lutte des races' selon Ludwig Gumplowicz," *Lignes* 12 (1990): 220–36.

8. Erika Weinzierl, "Katholizismus in Österreich," in *Kirche und Synagoge: Handbuch zur Geschichte von Christen und Juden,* ed. Karl Heinrich Rengstorf and Siegfried von Kortzfleisch, 2 vols. (Stuttgart: Ernst Klett, 1970), 2:483–531, here 2:525 n. 19.

9. Helen Walker Puner, *Freud: His Life and His Mind* (New York: Dell, 1959), 194, 191.

10. Jones, *Life and Work,* 2:17.

11. Cited in the chapter "Difficult to Baptize" in Theodor Reik, *Jewish Wit* (New York: Gamut Press, 1962), 92.

12. Jacob Wassermann, *My Life as German and Jew* (London: George Allen and Unwin, 1933), 72.

13. Reik, *Jewish Wit,* 90.

14. "Beda" [Fritz Löhner], *Israeliten und andere Antisemiten* (Vienna: R. Löwit, 1919), 25.

15. Gerson Wolf, *Judentaufen in Oesterreich* (Vienna: Herzfeld und Bauer, 1863).

16. Gerson Wolf, *Geschichte der Juden in Wien (1156–1875)* (1876; Vienna: Geyer, 1974), 194.

17. N. Samter, *Judentaufen im neunzehnten Jahrhundert* (Berlin: M. Poppelauer, 1906), 146.

18. In Vienna 4.5 Jews out of a thousand converted, while in Berlin the figure was 1.0 per thousand and in Hamburg 2.0. Arthur Ruppin, "Der Verlust des Judentums durch Taufe und Austritt," *Zeitschrift für Demographie und Statistik der Juden* 26 (1930): 24. A detailed account of the breakdown of conversions in Vienna for the first decade of the twentieth century is presented by Horator, "Die Bevölkerungsbewegung der Stadt Wien von 1900 bis 1911 mit besonderer Berücksichtigung der Juden," *Zeitschrift für Demographie und Statistik der Juden* 10 (1914): 10.

19. One of the powerful fantasies of Jewish racial arguments at the fin de siècle was the specter of Christian conversion to Judaism as a threat of thinning the blood of the Jews. See Heinrich Loewe, *Proselyten: Ein Beitrag zur Geschichte der jüdischen Rasse* (Berlin: Soncino, 1926).

20. Arthur Landsberger, ed., *Judentaufe* (Munich: Georg Müller, 1912), 7–8. Sombart here is also quoting from his own *Die Zukunft der Juden* (Leipzig: Duncker und Homblot, 1912), 52.

21. On Sombart's view of the Jews see Arthur Mitzman, *Sociology and Estrangement: Three Sociologists of Imperial Germany* (New York: Knopf, 1973), 251–55; Freddy Raphael, *Judaïsme et capitalisme: Essai sur la controverse entre*

Max Weber et Werner Sombart (Paris: Presses Universitaires de France, 1982); Werner Krause, *Werner Sombarts Weg vom Kathedersozialismus zum Faschismus* (Berlin: Rutten und Loening, 1962).

22. Werner Sombart, *The Jews and Modern Capitalism,* trans. M. Epstein (Glencoe, Ill.: Free Press, 1951), 322.

23. Hans F. K. Günther, *Rassenkunde des jüdischen Volkes* (1922; Munich: J. F. Lehmann, 1931), 14–15.

24. Anatole Leroy-Beaulieu, *Israel among the Nations: A Study of the Jews and Antisemitism,* trans. Frances Hellman (New York: G. P. Putnam's Sons, 1895), 122.

25. Theodor Gomperz, *Griechische Denker,* 3 vols. (Leipzig: Veit, 1896–1909), 1:39 (in the Freud Library, London).

26. Sombart, *Jews and Modern Capitalism,* 272.

27. Landsberger, *Judentaufe,* 45, 134–35.

28. Ibid., 76.

29. Ludwig Braun, "Die Persönlichkeit Freuds und seine Bedeutung als Bruder": "Festsitzung der 'Wien' anlässlich des 70. Geburtstages Br. Univ. Prof. Doktor Sigmund Freud. Wien 1926," (special issue of) *B'nai B'rith Mitteilung für Österreich* 26 (1926): 118–31, here 127.

30. Jones, *Life and Work,* 1:13, 119, 2:17.

31. Jeffrey Moussaieff Masson, ed., *The Complete Letters of Sigmund Freud to Wilhelm Fliess, 1887–1904* (Cambridge: Harvard University Press, 1985), 272. Hereafter cited as *Freud-Fliess.*

32. *Freud-Fliess,* 272. On the relationship between Freud and Fliess see the astute analysis by Madelon Sprengnether, *The Spectral Mother: Freud, Feminism, and Psychoanalysis* (Ithaca, N.Y.: Cornell University Press, 1990), 22–38.

33. *Freud-Fliess,* 268. I follow here the suggestion of Josef Sajner and Peter Swales that the nursemaid was Theresa "Resi" Wittek rather than the older view that she was Monika Zajíc. See Marianne Krüll, *Freud and His Father,* trans. Arnold J. Pomerans (New York: W. W. Norton, 1986), 119.

34. The discussion of the Oedipus myth and its structure relies on the account given in *Pauls Real-Encyclopädie der classischen Altertumswissenschaft,* 34 vols. (Stuttgart: J. B. Metzler, 1894–1972), vol. 17, 2, cols. 2103–17.

35. See the discussion in Paul C. Vitz, *Sigmund Freud's Christian Unconscious* (New York: Guilford Press, 1988), 3–29. On Freud and religion see C. Kolbe, *Heilung oder Hindernis: Religion bei Freud, Adler, Fromm, Jung und Frankl* (Stuttgart: Kreuz, 1985).

36. See the discussion in Natalie Isser and Lita Linzer Schwartz, *The History of Conversion and Contemporary Cults* (New York: Peter Lang, 1988), 48–50.

37. *Freud-Fliess,* 272.

38. Martin Freud, *Glory Reflected: Sigmund Freud—Man and Father* (London: Angus and Robertson, 1957), 36. See the discussion of the attraction of such childhood exposure to Christian servants and their ritual practices in the autobiography of the Galician Jewish psychoanalyst Helene Deutsch, *Confrontations with Myself: An Epilogue* (New York: W. W. Norton, 1973), 65.

39. Cited from the oral history recorded in Neil M. Cowan and Ruth Schwartz Cowan, *Our Parents' Lives: The Americanization of Eastern European Jews* (New York: Basic Books, 1989), 16.

40. On the need for later psychoanalysts to deny the relation between these two pathological states, see the detailed rebuttal by Ernst Harms, *Psychologie und Psychiatrie der Conversion* (Leiden: A. W. Sijthoff, 1939), 11–12. Freud carefully uses the term *Bekehrung* for religious conversion and *Konversion* for symptom conversion, even though the term *Konversion* can be used for both. See *GW* 1:215 for the use of *Konversion* in the sense of the conversion of symptoms and *GW* 14:396 for *Bekehrung* in the sense of religious conversion.

41. See the discussion of this episode in William J. McGrath, "Freud as Hannibal: The Politics of the Brother Band," *Central European History* 7 (1974): 31–57; Sebastiano Timpanaro, "Freud's 'Roman Phobia,'" trans. Kate Soper and M. H. Ryle, *New Left Review* 147 (1984): 4–31; J. N. Isbister, *Freud: An Introduction to His Life and Work* (London: Polity Press, 1985), 77–82; and Alexander Grinstein, *Sigmund Freud's Dreams* (New York: International Universities Press, 1980), 69–91.

42. On the sociological background see Isser and Linzer Schwartz, *History of Conversion,* which does not reflect much on the German situation; Todd M. Endelman, ed., *Jewish Apostasy in the Modern World* (New York: Holmes and Meier, 1987); and Guido Kisch, *Judentaufen: Eine historisch-biographisch-psychologisch-soziologische Studie besonders für Berlin und Königsberg* (Berlin: Colloquium Verlag, 1973). Of the older literature see Hans Jörg Weitbrecht, *Beiträge zur Religionspsychopathologie insbesondere zur Psychopathologie der Bekehrung* (Heidelberg: Scherer, 1948).

43. Christian Heinrich Spiess, *Biographien der Wahnsinnigen,* ed. Wolfgang Promies (Cologne: Luchterhand, 1966), 88–180.

44. Elcan Issac Wolf, *Von den Krankheiten der Juden* (Mannheim: C. F. Schwan, 1777), 13–14.

45. Peter Joseph Schneider, "Medizinisch-polizeiliche Würdigung einiger Religionsgebräuche und Sitten des israelitischen Volkes rücksichtlich ihres Einflusses auf den Gesundheitszustand desselben," *Zeitschrift für die Staatsarzneikunde* 10 (1825): 213–301, here 250–51.

46. Karl Wilhelm Ideler, *Der religiöse Wahnsinn erläutert durch Krankengeschichte: Ein Beitrag zur Geschichte der religiösen Wirren der Gegenwart* (Halle: C. A. Schwetschke, 1847). Ideler's work was well known to Freud. It also provided an important antithesis to the traditional late nineteenth-century case study. Ideler's cases are expansive and detailed, and at least one of the case studies relies on the written autobiographical account of a patient (case 18, 197–211).

47. Ernst Meumann, *Vorlesungen zur Einführung in die experimentelle Pädagogik und ihre psychologische Grundlagen,* 3 vols. (Leipzig: W. Engelmann, 1911–14), 1:614 ff.

48. Edwin Diller Starbuck, *The Psychology of Religion* (London: Walter Scott, 1901).

49. William James, *The Varieties of Religious Experience,* ed. John E. Smith (Cambridge: Harvard University Press, 1985), 28. On the early and positive reception of James in Germany see Johannes Bresler, *Religionshygiene* (Halle: Carl Marhold, 1907), 31–35 (in the Freud Collection, New York). On the general background see John O. King, *The Iron of Melancholy: Structures of Spiritual Conversion in America from the Puritan Conscience to Victorian Neurosis* (Middletown, Conn.: Wesleyan University Press, 1983).

50. Philip Rieff, *Freud: The Mind of the Moralist* (New York: Viking Press, 1959), 65.

51. Sante de Sanctis, *La conversione religiosa* (Bologna: Zanichelli, 1924) (in the Freud Library, London, with marginalia on 39, on adolescence; 41–43, on the affective moment of conversion; 52, on types of conversion; 81, on the mental process of conversion; 133, on Cardinal Newman's autobiography); translated as *Religious Conversion: A Bio-Psychological Study* by Helen Augur (New York: Harcourt, Brace, 1927). See *SE* 21:171–72. In Freud's London library there is also a copy of David Forsyth, *Psychology and Religion: A Study by a Medical Psychologist* (London: Watts, 1936), which summarizes this view.

52. *SE* 18:74, and Gustave Le Bon, *The Crowd: A Study of the Popular Mind* (New York: Viking Press, 1960), 72–78. Freud owned the translation of Le Bon by Rudolph Eisler (*Psychologie der Massen* [Leipzig: W. Klinkhardt, 1912]) (in the Freud Library, London).

53. Havelock Ellis, *Man and Woman: A Study of Human Secondary Sexual Characters* (New York: Scribner, 1904), 292 (in the Freud Library, London).

54. Francis E. Anstie, "Lectures on Disease of the Nervous System," *Lancet,* January 11, 1873, 41.

55. Francis Galton, *Inquiries into Human Faculty and Its Development* (London: Eugenics Society, 1951). See *SE* 4:139, 293; 5:494, 649.

56. Thomas King Chambers, "Ecstasy," in *System of Medicine,* ed. J. Russell Reynolds, 2 vols. (Philadelphia: J. B. Lippincott, 1872), 2:110.

57. Ellis, *Man and Woman,* 295.

58. Nathan G. Hale, Jr., ed., *James Putnam and Psychoanalysis: Letters between Putnam and Sigmund Freud, Ernest Jones, William James, Sándor Ferenczi, and Morton Prince, 1877–1917,* trans. Judith Bernays Heller (Cambridge: Harvard University Press, 1971), 189. Putnam also believed that "psychoneuroses in general are particularly common to . . . the Hebrew race." See Alfred Loomis and William Thompson, eds., *A System of Practical Medicine,* 4 vols. (New York: Lea Brothers, 1897–98), 4:553.

59. Jones, *Life and Work,* 2:49.

60. Max Nordau, *Degeneration* (1892–93; London: William Heinemann, 1913), 22.

61. A. A. Brill, *Freud's Contribution to Psychiatry* (New York: W. W. Norton, 1944), 195.

62. Ernest Jones, *Free Associations: Memories of a Psycho-Analyst* (New York: Basic Books, 1959), 210.

63. Landsberger, *Judentaufe,* 127.

64. Heinrich Coudenhove-Kalergi, *Das Wesen des Antisemitismus* (Vienna: Paneuropa, 1929), 258 (in the Freud Library, London).

65. Richard Krafft-Ebing, *Text-Book of Insanity,* trans. Charles Gilbert Chaddock (Philadelphia: F. A. Davis, 1905), 143 (in the Freud Library, London, in the 1888 and 1893 editions). A detailed summary of these views can be found in the work of Freud's colleague at the University of Vienna, Alexander Pilcz, *Beitrag zur vergleichenden Rassen-Psychiatrie* (Leipzig: Deuticke, 1906), 26–32.

66. Leroy-Beaulieu, *Israel among the Nations,* 163.

67. Krafft-Ebing, *Text-Book of Insanity,* 143.

68. David Friedrich Strauss, *Der alte und der neue Glaube: Ein Bekenntnis* (Leipzig: G. Hirzel, 1872), 71.

69. H. Knöpfmacher, "Sigmund Freud in High School," *American Imago* 36 (1979): 287–300, as well as Robert R. Holt, "Freud's Adolescent Reading: Some Possible Effects on His Work," in *Freud: Appraisals and Reappraisals,* ed. Paul Stepansky, 3 vols. (Hillsdale, N.J.: Analytic Press, 1988), 3:167–92, here 185–88.

70. See William Provine, "Geneticists and the Biology of Race Crossing," *Science* 182 (1973): 790–97, as well as his "Geneticists and Race," *American Zoologist* 26 (1986): 857–87.

71. Ernst Lissauer, "Deutschtum und Judentum," *Kunstwart* 25 (1912): 6–12, here 8 n.

72. Fritz Wittels, *Der Taufjude* (Vienna: Breitenstein, 1904). See my *Jewish Self-Hatred,* 293–94.

73. Lissauer, "Deutschtum und Judentum," 8.

74. Leroy-Beaulieu, *Israel among the Nations,* 209.

75. Harms, *Psychologie und Psychiatrie,* 46.

76. *Protokolle der Wiener Psychoanalytischen Vereinigung,* ed. Herman Nunberg and Ernst Federn, 4 vols. (Frankfurt am Main: Fischer, 1976–81), 2:66–67; translated as *Minutes of the Vienna Psychoanalytic Society* by M. Nunberg, 4 vols. (New York: International Universities Press, 1962–75), 2:60–61.

77. Rudolf Kleinpaul, *Das Leben der Sprache und ihre Weltstellung,* 3 vols., vol. 1, *Sprache ohne Worte* (Leipzig: Wilhelm Friedrich, 1893), 128–29 (in the Freud Library, London).

78. Felix Goldmann, *Taufjudentum und Antisemitismus* (Frankfurt am Main: J. Kaufmann, 1913).

79. *Freud-Fliess,* 311.

80. The diagnosis and description of the syndrome of "pseudologia fantastica" is taken from the third edition of Alexander Pilcz, *Lehrbuch der speziellen Psychiatrie für Studierende und Ärzte* (Leipzig: Franz Deuticke, 1912), 272–73 (the 1904 edition is in the Freud Library, London).

81. Emil Kraepelin, *Psychiatrie: Ein Lehrbuch für Studierende und Ärzte,* 3 vols. (Leipzig: Johann Ambrosius Barth, 1909–15), 3:2043–69 (in the Freud Library, London).

82. See the discussion of this diagnosis by Max Sichel, "Über die Geistesstörungen bei den Juden," *Neurologisches Centralblatt,* 1908, 351–67.

83. It is not of child abuse that Freud frees his own father in the letter to Fliess of September 21, 1897, but rather of transmitting the taint of Jewishness. This is the intent of universalizing the role of the father, rather than any hidden indicator that Freud himself had been abused. See Larry Wolff, *Postcards from the End of the World: An Investigation into the Mind of Fin-de-Siècle Vienna* (London: Collins, 1989), 197–204.

84. An excellent overview of Freud's attraction to Christianity is provided by Vitz, *Sigmund Freud's Christian Unconscious.* Vitz's readings and facts are a detailed presentation of the attraction and ambiguity that Christianity held for Freud. What is not addressed is why Freud did not convert. Omitted from Vitz's argument is that the very concept of "conversion" is a medicalized one by the turn of the century. This topic seems first to have been addressed in a polemical manner in Charles E. Maylan, *Freuds tragischer Komplex* (Munich: Ernst Reinhardt, 1929) (in the Freud Library, London).

85. Max Graf, "Reminiscences of Professor Sigmund Freud," *Psychoanalytic Quarterly* 11 (1942): 473.

86. Sigmund Freud, *Brautbriefe: Briefe an Martha Bernays aus den Jahren 1882–1886,* ed. Ernst L. Freud (Frankfurt am Main: Fischer, 1988), 137.

87. *SE* 21:170. In this context Freud cites the detailed study by Sante de Sanctis, *La conversione religiosa.*

88. *SE* 21:64.

89. Compare Jean-François Lyotard, "Jewish Oedipus," *Genre* 10 (1977): 395–411.

90. Theodor Reik, *From Thirty Years with Freud,* trans. Richard Winston (New York: Farrar and Rinehart, 1940), 145.

91. *SE* 4:136–37. I do not wish to engage here in the debate over whether Freud's reading of his professional situation was correct. It is clear that he associates his status as an academic physician and the difficulty of his faculty appointment with his Jewish identity. See Josef Glicklhorn and Renée Glicklhorn, *Sigmund Freuds akademische Laufbahn im Lichte der Dokumente* (Vienna: Urban und Schwarzenberg, 1960).

92. Peter Stephan Jungk, *Franz Werfel: A Life in Prague, Vienna, and Hollywood,* trans. Anselm Hollo (New York: Fromm, 1991), 112–13.

93. Leonid Grossman, ed., *Die Beichte seines Juden in Briefen an Dostojewski,* trans. René Fülöp-Miller and Friedrich Eckstein (Munich: R. Piper, 1927) (in the Freud Library, London, well chewed by one of the Freud chows). On the background of this exchange see David I. Goldstein, *Dostoyevsky and the Jews* (Austin: University of Texas Press, 1981), 88–116.

94. The original paper was published anonymously in the *Internationale Zeitschrift für Ärztliche Psychoanalyse* 2 (1914): 327–53; the translation is taken from Theodor Reik, "On the Effect of Unconscious Death Wishes," trans. Harry Zohn, *Psychoanalytic Review* 65 (1978): 38–67; these quotations are primarily from the notes on 49–50.

95. Theodor Reik, *Fragment of a Great Confession: A Psychoanalytic Autobiography* (New York: Farrar, Straus, 1949), 230.

96. S. Ehrmann, in the "Festsitzung der 'Wien' anlässlich des 70. Geburtstages Br. Univ. Prof. Doktor Sigmund Freud. Wien 1926," 101–38, here 102–3.

97. Joseph Wortis, *Fragments of an Analysis with Freud* (New York: Jason Aronson, 1984), 144.

98. See Peter Amacher, *Freud's Neurological Education and Its Influence on Psychoanalytic Theory* (New York: International Universities Press, 1965); Kenneth Levin, *Freud's Early Psychology of the Neurosis: A Historical Perspective* (Pittsburgh, Pa.: University of Pittsburgh Press, 1978); M. Solms and M. Saling, "On Psychoanalysis and Neuroscience: Freud's Attitude to the Localizationist Tradition," *International Journal of Psychoanalysis* 67 (1986): 397–416; P. Juignet, *De la neuropathologie à la psychopathologie* (Paris: Findakly, 1986).

99. *Freud-Fliess,* 306.

100. Frank J. Sulloway, *Freud, Biologist of the Mind: Beyond the Psychoanalytic Legend* (New York: Basic Books, 1979), 152, 148–50.

101. G. Valentin, *Handbuch der Entwickelungsgeschichte der Menschen* (Berlin: Rücker, 1835).

102. Wilhelm His, *Anatomie menschlicher Embryonen,* 3 vols. (Leipzig: F. C. W. Vogel, 1880–85). See Stephen Jay Gould, *Ontogeny and Phylogeny* (Cambridge: Belknap Press of Harvard University Press, 1977), 189–93.

103. Eduard Fuchs, *Die Juden in der Karikatur* (Munich: Langen, 1921), and Judith Vogt, *Historien om et image: Antisemitisme og antizionisme i karikaturer* (Copenhagen: Samieren, 1978).

104. Friedrich Nietzsche, *Beyond Good and Evil,* trans. Marianne Cowan (Chicago: Henry Regnery, 1955), 184–88.

105. Hanns Bächtold-Stäubli, ed., *Handwörterbuch des deutschen Aberglaubens,* vol. 6 (Berlin and Leipzig: W. de Gruyter, 1934–35), "Nase," 970–79.

106. The meaning of the hair color of the Jews, especially of the "blond Jews," is one focus of the debates about the mutability of the Jews and the status of their mixed or pure racial status. See Maurice Fishberg, "Zur Frage der Herkunft des blonden Elements im Judentum," *Zeitschrift für Demographie und Statistik der Juden* 3 (1907): 7–9, 25–27, as well as the rebuttal by Elias Auerbach, "Bermerkungen zu Fishbergs Theorie," *Zeitschrift für Demographie und Statistik der Juden* 3 (1907): 92–94.

107. Oskar Hovorka, *Die äussere Nase: Eine anatomisch-anthropologische Studie* (Vienna: Alfred Hölder, 1893), 130–40. On the pathological meaning of the nose in German science for the later period see Hans Leichner, *Die Vererbung anatomischer Variationen der Nase, ihre Nebenhöhlen und des Gehörorgans* (Munich: J. F. Bergmann, 1928), 81.

108. On the symbolic value of this manifestation see Herbert Ian Hogbin, *The Island of Menstruating Men: Religion in Wogeo, New Guinea* (Scranton, Pa.: Chandler, 1970), and James L. Brain, "Male Menstruation in History and Anthropology," *Journal of Psychohistory* 15 (1988): 311–23.

109. *Freud-Fliess,* 256.

110. See, for example, F. A. Forel, "Cas de menstruation chez un homme," *Bulletin de la Société Médicale de la Suisse Romande* (Lausanne), 1869, 53–61, and W. D. Halliburton, "A Peculiar Case," *Weekly Medical Review and Journal of Obstetrics* (Saint Louis, Mo.), 1885, 392.

111. Paolo Albrecht, "Sulla mestruazione ne maschio," *L'Anomalo* 2 (1890): 33.

112. Paul Näcke, "Kritisches zum Kapitel der normalen und pathologischen Sexualität," *Archiv für Psychiatrie und Nervenkrankheiten* 32 (1899): 356–86, here 364. See *SE* 14:73; 16:416. On Freud and Näcke see Helmut Gröger, "Sigmund Freud an Paul Näcke, Erstveröffentlichung zweier Freud-Briefe," *Luzifer Amor* 3 (1990): 144–62.

113. Magnus Hirschfeld, *Sexualpathologie,* 2 vols. (Bonn: A. Marcus und E. Weber, 1917–18), 2:1–92.

114. The irony is that the image of male menstruation among the Jews probably has a pathological origin. Even today in parts of Africa "male menstruation," in the form of urethral bleeding, seems to be an indicator of "sexual maturation." What actually happens is that, for reasons not completely understood, a parasite, *Schistosoma haematobium,* which lives in the veins surrounding the bladder, becomes active during the early teenage years. See E. P. Eckholm, *The Picture of Health: Environmental Sources of Disease* (New York: W. W. Norton, 1977). One can imagine that Jews infected with schistosomiasis, giving the appearance of menstruation, would have reified the sense of difference that northern Europeans, not prone to this snail-borne parasite, would have felt.

115. Thomas de Cantimpré, *Miraculorum et exemplorum memorabilium sui temporis libro duo* (Duaci: Baltazris Belleri, 1605), 305–6.

116. Heinrich Kormann, *Opera Curiosa I: Miracula vivorum* (1614; Frankfurt: Genschiana, 1694), 128–29; Thomas Calvert, *The Blessed Jew of Marocco; or, A Blackmoor Made White: Being a Demonstration of the True Messias out of the Law and Prophets by Rabbi Samuel* (York: Thomas Broad, 1649), 20–21.

117. Leroy-Beaulieu, *Israel among the Nations,* 166–67.

118. D. Chwolson, *Die Blutanklage und sonstige mittelalterliche Beschuldigungen der Juden: Eine historische Untersuchung nach den Quellen* (Frankfurt am Main: J. Kauffmann, 1901), 7, 207–10.

119. On Franco da Piacenza see Léon Poliakov, *The History of Anti-Semitism,* trans. Richard Howard, 4 vols. (New York: Vanguard, 1965–75), vol. 1, *From the Time of Christ to the Court Jews,* 143 n.

120. F. L. de La Fontaine, *Chirurgisch-medicinische Abhandlungen vershiedenen* [sic] *Inhalts Polen betreffend* (Breslau: Korn, 1792). See also J. A. Elie de la Poterie, "Questo medica: An viris lex eadem quä mulieribus, periodicas evacuationes pati?" (Diss., Paris, 1764).

121. Chrysostomus Dudulaeus, *Gründliche und Warhafftige Relation von einem Juden auss Jerusalem mit Nahmen Ahassverus* [1602], fol. Diiir; reprinted as *Evangelischer Bericht vom den Leben Jesu Christi . . .* (Stuttgart: J. Scheible, 1856), 126.

122. Theodor Fritsch, *Handbuch der Judenfrage* (Leipzig: Hammer, 1935), 409 (with a further discourse on psychoanalysis as a sign of Jewish degeneracy).

123. *Freud-Fliess,* 30.

124. *Freud-Fliess,* 19.

125. A good survey of the various readings of this dream is given by Didier Anzieu, *Freud's Self-Analysis,* trans. Peter Graham (London: Hogarth Press, 1986), 131–40.

126. On the identity of the persons appearing in the dream see Alexander Grinstein, *On Sigmund Freud's Dreams* (Detroit: Wayne State University Press, 1989), 21–24.

127. On the complexity of reading this dream see Jeffrey Mehlman, "Trimethylamin: Notes on Freud's Specimen Dream," in *Untying the Text: A Post-Structuralist Reader,* ed. Robert Young (Boston: Routledge and Kegan Paul, 1981), 177–88.

128. Letter from Abraham to Freud, January 8, 1908: *Sigmund Freud–Karl Abraham, Briefe, 1907–1926,* ed. Hilda C. Abraham and Ernst L. Freud (Frankfurt am Main: Fischer, 1980), 32; translation here is from *A Psycho-Analytic Dialogue: The Letters of Sigmund Freud and Karl Abraham, 1907–1926,* trans. Bernard Marsh and Hilda Abraham (London: Hogarth, 1965), 18.

129. *Abraham-Freud,* January 9, 1908, 34; translation from *Psycho-Analytic Dialogue,* 20.

130. J. Aguayo, "Charcot and Freud: Some Implications of Late Nineteenth-Century French Psychiatry and Politics for the Origins of Psychoanalysis," *Psychoanalysis and Contemporary Thought* 9 (1986): 223–60.

131. Toby Gelfand, " 'Mon Cher Docteur Freud': Charcot's Unpublished Correspondence to Freud, 1888–1893," *Bulletin of the History of Medicine* 62 (1988): 563–88, here 571.

132. *SE* 26:29–43. Although this paper was published only in 1893, it was conceptualized if not written before Freud left Paris in 1886.

133. Toby Gelfand, "Charcot's Response to Freud's Rebellion," *Journal of the History of Ideas* 50 (1989): 293–307. See also his essay on the medicalization of anti-Semitism in Paris: "Le Professeur Germain Sée (1818–1896) et le 'problème juif' dans la médecine à Paris," *Revue d'Histoire de la Médecine Hébraïque* 38 (1985): 23–27.

134. K. H. Pribram and M. M. Gill, *Freud's "Project" Re-assessed: Preface to Contemporary Cognitive Theory and Neuropsychology* (New York: Basic Books, 1976); M. Sirkin and M. Fleming, "Freud's 'Project' and Its Relationship to Psychoanalytic Theory," *Journal of the History of the Behavioral Sciences* 18 (1982): 230–41; J. Friedman and J. Alexander, "Psychoanalysis and Natural Science: Freud's 1895 Project Revisited," *International Review of Psychoanalysis* 10 (1983): 303–18; I. F. Knight, "Freud's 'Project': A Theory for Studies on Hysteria," *Journal of the History of the Behavioral Sciences* 20 (1984): 340–58.

135. *SE* 21:71. See Gould, *Ontogeny and Phylogeny,* 157.

136. Samson Raphael Hirsch, *The Collected Writings,* vol. 3, *Basic Guidelines for a Jewish Symbolism* (New York: Feldheim, 1956).

137. See A. Momigliano, *Jacob Bernays* (Amsterdam: North-Holland, 1969).

138. E. M. Butler, *The Tyranny of Greece over Germany* (Cambridge: Cambridge University Press, 1935). See also Henry C. Hatfield, *Aesthetic Paganism in German Literature from Winckelmann to the Death of Goethe* (Cambridge: Harvard University Press, 1964). Of central importance to the argument about the relation of the nineteenth-century image of the classical world to the idea of race is Martin Bernal, *Black Athena: The Afroasiatic Roots of Classical Civilization,* vol. 1, *The Fabrication of Ancient Greece, 1785–1985* (London: Free Associations, 1987).

139. Sander L. Gilman, "Pforta zur Zeit Nietzsches," *Nietzsche-Studien* 8 (1979): 398–426, on Nietzsche's schooling, which, even though it was "German" rather than "Austrian" and occurred somewhat earlier in the century than Freud's, stressed a "Latin" reading of the classics.

140. The original is published by Viktor Tausk, "Zur Psychopathologie des Alltagsleben," *Internationale Zeitschrift für Ärztliche Psychoanalyse* 4 (1916–17): 158. A further case of the confusion conversion leads to in his patients is recounted by Karl Abraham in a letter to Freud in March 1908. See *Sigmund Freud–Karl Abraham, Briefe, 1907–1926,* 43.

141. Karl Abraham, *Traum und Mythus: Eine Studie zur Völkerpsychologie,* Schriften zur angewandten Seelenkunde 4 (1909; Nendeln: Kraus Reprint, 1970) (original, in the Freud Library, London); the translation is taken from Karl Abraham, *Dreams and Myths: A Study in Race Psychology,* trans. William A. White (New York: Journal of Nervous and Mental Disease Publishing, 1913), here 36 (in the Freud Library, London).

142. *Sigmund Freud–Karl Abraham, Briefe, 1907–1926,* 249; translation from *Psycho-Analytic Dialogue,* 264.

143. Theodor Reik, "Die Unheimlichkeit fremder Götter und Kulte," in his *Der Eigene und der fremde Gott* (Leipzig: Internationaler Psychoanalytischer Verlag, 1923), 161–86, here 166.

144. Alvin E. Rodin and Jack D. Key, *Medicine, Literature, and Eponyms: An Encyclopedia of Medical Eponyms Derived from Literary Characters* (Malabar, Fla.: Robert E. Krieger, 1989). The term "sadism" is documented as early as 1834. It was Krafft-Ebing who linked this concept with "masochism" in 1874 within a medical context. See the discussion of the history of this term in David Coward, "Porncrat or Libertarian: The Moral Darwinism of the Marquis de Sade," *Times Literary Supplement* (London), February 15, 1990, 5.

145. Stanley Rosenman, "A Psychohistorical Source of Psychoanalysis—Malformed Jewish Psyches in an Immolating Setting," *Israel Journal of Psychiatry and Related Sciences* 21 (1984): 103–16, here 113.

3. The Degenerate Foot and the Search for Oedipus

1. Carl Claus, *Grundzüge der Zoologie* (Marburg: N. G. Elwert, 1872), 1123. On Freud and the biology of his day see Frank J. Sulloway, *Freud, Biologist of*

the Mind: Beyond the Psychoanalytic Legend (New York: Basic Books, 1979); Stephen Jay Gould, *Ontogeny and Phylogeny* (Cambridge: Belknap Press of Harvard University Press, 1977), 155–64; Lucille B. Ritvo, *Darwin's Influence on Freud: A Tale of Two Sciences* (New Haven: Yale University Press, 1990). See also her earlier studies (all of which are summarized or included in her book): "The Impact of Darwin on Freud," *Psychoanalytic Quarterly* 43 (1974): 177–92; "Freuds neo-Lamarckistische Darwin-Interpretation," *Psyche* 27 (1973): 460–74; "Carl Claus, Freud und die Darwinsche Biologie," *Psyche* 27 (1973): 475–86; "Carl Claus as Freud's Professor of the New Darwinian Biology," *International Journal of Psychoanalysis* 53 (1972): 277–83. See also S. Yearley, "Imputing Intentionality: Popper, Demarcation and Darwin, Freud and Marx," *Studies in the History and Philosophy of Science* 16 (1985): 337–50. None explores the racial implications of this theory for Freud, even though Gould discusses these questions in detail elsewhere in his book.

2. Carl Heinrich Stratz, *Was sind Juden? Eine ethnographisch-anthropologische Studie* (Vienna: F. Tempsky, 1903), 19 (in the Freud Library, London).

3. Felix Langer, *Die Protokolle der Weisen von Zion: Rassenhass und Rassenhetze* (Vienna: Saturn, 1934), 15 (in the Freud Library, London).

4. *SE* 19:72–105. The text is available in English as *Schizophrenia 1677: A Psychiatric Study of an Illustrated Autobiographical Record of Demonical Possession,* ed. and trans. Ida Macalpine and Richard A. Hunter (London: William Dawson, 1956).

5. Oskar Panizza, *The Council of Love,* trans. O. F. Pucciani (New York: Viking, 1979), 79, 91–92. On the general background see Joshua Trachtenberg, *The Devil and the Jews: The Medieval Conception of the Jew and Its Relation to Modern Antisemitism* (New Haven: Yale University Press, 1943), 46–48.

6. Robert Burton, *The Anatomy of Melancholy,* ed. Holbrook Jackson (New York: Vintage, 1977): 211–12 (present in a 1938 edition in the Freud Library, London).

7. Johann Jakob Schudt, *Jüdische Merkwürdigkeiten* (Frankfurt am Main: S. T. Hocker, 1714–18), 2:369.

8. Johann Caspar Lavater, *Physiognomische Fragment zur Beförderung des Menschenkenntnis und Menschenliebe,* 4 vols. (Leipzig: Weidmann, 1775–78), 2:53.

9. That the Jewish woman had a special place in the debate about the nature of the Jewish body is without a doubt true, but it was not in regard to her role as a member of the body politic. In the context of nineteenth-century science it was assumed that she could not function in this manner. See Moriz Lazarus's introduction to Nahida Remy [Nahida Ruth Lazarus], *Das jüdische Weib* (Leipzig: Gustav Fock, [1891]), iii–vi. On the general background to this image see Livia Bitton Jackson, *Madonna or Courtesan? The Jewish Woman in Christian Literature* (New York: Seabury Press, 1982).

10. See the discussion in Léon Poliakov, *The History of Anti-Semitism,* trans. Miriam Kochan, 4 vols. (New York: Vanguard, 1965–75), vol. 3, *From Voltaire to Wagner,* 177.

11. Joseph Rohrer, *Versuch über die jüdischen Bewohner der österreichischen Monarchie* (Vienna: Verlag des Kunst- und Industrie-Comptoirs, 1804), 25–26.

12. Hermann Schaaffhausen, "Die Physiognomik," *Archiv für Anthropologie* 17 (1888): 309–38, here 337.

13. On the medical debate in the late nineteenth century about the difference between "weak feet" and "flat feet" see Edgar M. Bick, *Source Book of Orthopaedics* (Baltimore: Williams and Wilkins, 1948), 450–51. See also the general discussion of these historical figures in Stephan Mencke, *Zur Geschichte der Orthopädie* (Munich: Michael Beckstein, 1930), 68–69, and Bruno Valentin, *Geschichte der Orthopädie* (Stuttgart: Georg Thieme, 1961).

14. Theodor Fontane, *Der deutsche Krieg von 1866* (Berlin: Verlag der Königlichen Geheimen Ober-Hofbuchdruckerei, 1870), vol. 1, *Der Feldzug in Böhmen und Mähren,* 413. On the Jewish role in the German army see Rolf Vogel, *Ein Stück von uns: Deutsche Juden in deutschen Armeen, 1813–1976. Eine Dokumentation* (Mainz: Von Hase und Koehler, 1977), and Werner T. Angress, "Prussia's Army and the Jewish Reserve Officer Controversy before World War I," *Leo Baeck Yearbook* 17 (1972): 19–42.

15. Mark Twain, *Concerning the Jews* (Philadelphia: Running Press, 1985), 29.

16. Cesare Lombroso, "Atavismus und Civilisation," *Politisch-Anthropologische Revue* 3 (1904): 152–56, here 156.

17. All of these comments are made in a review of Ernest Renan, *Nouvelles considérations sur le caractère général des peuples sémitiques* (1859), *Zeitschrift für Völkerpsychologie* 1 (1860): 328–45, here 334–35.

18. Steven Beller, *Vienna and the Jews, 1867–1938: A Cultural History* (Cambridge: Cambridge University Press, 1989), 189.

19. István Deák, *Jewish Soldiers in Austro-Hungarian Society,* Leo Baeck Memorial Lecture 34 (New York: Leo Baeck Institute, 1990), 14.

20. Cited by Max Grunwald, *Vienna* (Philadelphia: Jewish Publication Society of America, 1936), 408.

21. Cited by Grunwald, *Vienna,* 177.

22. Wilhelm Busch, *Gesamtausgabe,* ed. Friedrich Bohne, 4 vols. (Wiesbaden: Emil Vollmer, n.d.), 2:204; the English translation, which is very accurate to the tone, but not to the order of the parts of the Jew's body, is from Walter Arndt, comp. and trans., *The Genius of Wilhelm Busch* (Berkeley and Los Angeles: University of California Press, 1982), 42. Freud cites this text in *Civilization and Its Discontents* (*SE* 21:75).

23. See Hans Lobner, "Some Additional Remarks on Freud's Library," *Sigmund Freud House Bulletin* 1 (1975): 18–29.

24. H. Naudh [H. Nordmann], *Israel im Heere* (Leipzig: Hermann Beyer, 1893). On the background see Horst Fischer, *Judentum, Staat und Heer in Preussen im frühen 19. Jahrhundert: Zur Geschichte der staatlichen Judenpolitik* (Tubingen: J. C. B. Mohr, 1968).

25. At the fin de siècle a postcard showing an ill-formed "little Mr. Kohn" showing up for his induction into the military was in circulation in Germany

(reprinted in Dietz Bering, *Der Name als Stigma: Antisemitismus im deutschen Alltag, 1812–1933* [Stuttgart: Klett/Cotta, 1987], 211). And in the Viennese fin-de-siècle anti-Semitic magazine *Kikeriki,* the flat and malformed feet of the Jew served as an indicator of the Jewish body almost as surely as the shape of the nose (Eduard Fuchs, *Die Juden in der Karikatur* [Munich: Langen, 1921], 200). By the 1930s the image of the Jew's feet had become ingrained in the representation of the Jewish body. The Nazi caricaturist Walter Hofmann, who drew under the name of Waldl, presented a series of images of the construction of the Jewish body in a cartoon strip ironically titled "What Can Sigismund Do about the Fact That He Is So Pretty?" (Walter Hofmann, *Lacht ihn tot! Ein tendenziöses Bilderbuch von Waldl* [Dresden: Nationalsozialistischer Verlag für den Gau Sachsen, n.d.], 23). The body of Sigismund, the archetypal Jew, was literally constructed, like that of Adam or the golem, from wet clay, but the Jew disobeyed the divine order and arose before his body was truly formed: "Since the clay was still damp and soft, the smarty developed after the first few steps extraordinarily bandy legs, but also flat feet."

26. Otto Fenichel, "Elements of a Psychoanalytic Theory of Anti-Semitism," in *Anti-Semitism: A Social Disease,* ed. Ernst Simmel (New York: International Universities Press, 1946), 11–33, here 25.

27. *Die Juden als Soldaten* (Berlin: Sigfried Cronbach, 1897).

28. See Joachim Petzold, *Die Dolchstosslegende: Eine Geschichtsfälschung im Dienst des deutschen Imperialismus und Militarismus* ([East] Berlin: Akademie Verlag, 1963), which discusses the statistical arguments.

29. Otto Armin [Alfred Roth], *Die Juden im Heere, eine statistische Untersuchung nach amtlichen Quellen* (Munich: Deutsche Volks-Verlag, 1919).

30. Jacob Segall, *Die deutschen Juden als Soldaten im Kriege, 1914–1918* (Berlin: Philo Verlag, 1922).

31. Franz Oppenheimer, *Die Judenstatistik des preussischen Kriegsministeriums* (Munich: Verlag für Kulturpolitik, 1922).

32. Elias Auerbach, "Die Militärtauglichkeit der Juden," *Jüdische Rundschau* 50 (December 11, 1908): 491–92.

33. See John M. Hoberman, *Sport and Political Ideology* (Austin: University of Texas Press, 1984), as well as his "Why Jews Play Sports," *Moment,* April 1991, 34–42.

34. Heinrich Singer, *Allgemeine und spezielle Krankheitslehre der Juden* (Leipzig: Benno Konegen, 1904), 14.

35. Gustav Muskat, "Ist der Plattfuss eine Rasseneigentümlichkeit?" *Im Deutschen Reich,* 1909, 354–58. Compare J. C. Dagnall, "Feet and the Military System," *British Journal of Chiropody* 45 (1980): 137.

36. In other contexts the atavistic foot is taken to be a sign of insanity. See Charles L. Dana, "On the New Use of Some Older Sciences: A Discourse on Degeneration and Its Stigmata," *Transactions of the New York Academy of Medicine* 11 (1894): 471–89, here 484–85, and J. Park Harrison, "On the Relative Length of the First Three Toes of the Human Foot," *Journal of the Anthropological Institute* 13 (1884): 258–72. See also my discussion in *Difference and*

Pathology: Stereotypes of Sexuality, Race, and Madness (Ithaca, N.Y.: Cornell University Press, 1986), 155.

37. George L. Mosse, *Germans and Jews: The Right, the Left, and the Search for a "Third Force" in Pre-Nazi Germany* (Detroit: Wayne State University Press, 1987), 14–15.

38. Moritz Alsberg, *Militäruntauglichkeit und Grossstadt-Einfluss: Hygienisch-volkswirtschaftliche Betrachtungen und Vorschläge* (Leipzig: B. G. Teubner, 1909), 10. Compare the discussion of the rate of military readiness of the various sections of Vienna during this period: Victor Noach, "Militärdiensttauglichkeit und Berufstätigkeit, soziale Stellung und Wohnweise in Österreich-Ungarn, insbesondere in Wien," *Archiv für Soziale Hygiene und Demographie* 10 (1915): 77–128.

39. See my discussion in *Difference and Pathology*, as well as in my *Disease and Representation: Images of Illness from Madness to AIDS* (Ithaca, N.Y.: Cornell University Press, 1988). Compare with D. B. Larson et al., "Religious Affiliations in Mental Health Research Samples as Compared with National Samples," *Journal of Nervous and Mental Disease* 177 (1989): 109–11.

40. Gustav Muskat, "Die Kosmetik des Fusses," in *Handbuch der Kosmetik*, ed. Max Joseph (Leipzig: Veit, 1912), 646–64, here 662.

41. Leopold Boehmer, "Fussschäden und schwingedes Schuhwerk," in *Zivilizationsschäden am Menschen*, ed. Heinz Zeiss and Karl Pintschovius (Munich: J. F. Lehmann, 1940), 180. Compare J. Swann, "Nineteenth-Century Footwear and Foot Health," *Cliopedic Items* 3 (1988): 1–2.

42. *SE* 1:39, 58. See also the autobiographical statement in *SE* 20:18.

43. A. Villaret, *Handwörterbuch der Gesamten Medizin*, 2 vols. (Stuttgart: Ferdinand Enke, 1891), 2:805 (in the Freud Library, London).

44. Hoffa is the author of the authoritative study *Die Orthopädie im Dienst der Nervenheilkunde* (Jena: Gustav Fischer, 1900), and the compiler (with August Blencke) of the standard overview of the orthopedic literature of the fin de siècle, *Die orthopädische Literatur* (Stuttgart: Enke, 1905).

45. M. J. Gutmann, *Über den heutigen Stand der Rasse- und Krankheitsfrage der Juden* (Munich: Rudolph Müller und Steinicke, 1920), 38.

46. Conrad Rieger, *Die Castration in rechtlicher, socialer und vitaler Hinsicht* (Jena: Gustav Fischer, 1900), 18–19.

47. Günther Just, ed., *Handbuch der Erbbiologie des Menschen: I. Erbbiologie und Erbpathologie Körperlicher Zustände und Funktionen: Stützgewebe, Haut, Auge*, 3 vols. (Berlin: Julius Springer, 1939–40), 39.

48. The translation is by Jack Zipes; Oskar Panizza, "The Operated Jew," *New German Critique* 21 (1980): 63–79, here 64. See also Jack Zipes, "Oscar Panizza: The Operated German as Operated Jew," *New German Critique* 21 (1980): 47–61, and Michael Bauer, *Oskar Panizza: Ein literarisches Porträt* (Munich: Hanser, 1984).

49. Hans F. K. Günther, *Rassenkunde des jüdischen Volkes* (1922; Munich: J. F. Lehmann, 1931), 215, 252.

50. Erwin Baur, Eugen Fischer, and Fritz Lenz, eds., *Menschliche Erblehre*

und Rassenhygiene: I. Menschliche Erblehre (Munich: J. F. Lehmann, 1936), 396.

51. Otmar Freiherr von Verschuer, *Erbpathologie: Ein Lehrbuch für Ärtze und Medizinstudierende* (Dresden: Theodor Steinkopff, 1945), 87.

52. Benjamin Ward Richardson, *Diseases of Modern Life* (New York: Bermingham, 1882), 98.

53. Max Nordau, *Zionistische Schriften* (Cologne: Jüdischer Verlag, 1909), 379–81. This call, articulated at the second Zionist congress, followed his address on the state of the Jews that keynoted the first congress. There he spoke on the "physical, spiritual and economic status of the Jews." In July 1902 Nordau recapitulated his views in an essay in the *Jüdische Turnzeitung* titled "Was bedeutet das Turnen für uns Juden?" (*Zionistische Schriften,* 382–84). On Nordau see P. M. Baldwin, "Liberalism, Nationalism, and Degeneration: The Case of Max Nordau," *Central European History* 13 (1980): 99–120, and Hans-Peter Söder, "A Tale of Dr. Jekyll and Mr. Hyde? Max Nordau and the Problem of Degeneracy," in *Disease and Medicine in Modern German Cultures,* ed. Rudolf Käser and Vera Pohland (Ithaca, N.Y.: Western Societies Program/Cornell University Press, 1990), 56–70.

54. Hermann Jalowicz, "Die körperliche Entartung der Juden, ihre Ursachen und ihre Bekämpfung," *Jüdiche Turnzeitung* 2 (1901): 57–65.

55. Richard Lichtbaum, *Die Geschichte des deutschen Zionismus* (Jerusalem: Rubin Mass, 1954), 121.

56. Isidor Wolff, ed., *Die Verbreitung des Turnens unter den Juden* (Berlin: Verlag der Jüdischen Turnzeitung, 1907).

57. M. Jastrowitz, "Muskeljuden und Nervenjuden," *Jüdische Turnzeitung* 9 (1908): 33–36.

58. His first paper on this topic is Jean-Martin Charcot, "Sur la claudication intermittente," *Comptes rendus des séances et mémoires de la Société de biologie* (Paris), 1858, Mémoire 1859, 2d ser., 5, 25–38. While this is not the first description of the syndrome, it is the one that labels it as a separate disease entity. It is first described by Benjamin Collins Brodie, *Lectures Illustrative of Various Subjects in Pathology and Surgery* (London: Longman, 1846), 361. Neither Brodie nor Charcot attempted to provide an etiology for this syndrome. Compare M. S. Rosenbloom et al., "Risk Factors Affecting the Natural History of Intermittent Claudication," *Archives of Surgery* 123 (1989): 867–70.

59. The work, dated as early as 1831, is cited in detail by Charcot, "Sur la claudication," 25–26.

60. See my *Difference and Pathology,* 155, and Toby Gelfand, "Charcot's Response to Freud's Rebellion," *Journal of the History of Ideas* 50 (1989): 304.

61. Gutmann, "Über den heutigen Stand," 39. Compare Dr. M. Kretzmer, "Über anthropologische, physiologische und pathologische Eigenheiten der Juden," *Die Welt* 5 (1901): 3–5, and Dr. Hugo Hoppe, "Sterblichkeit und Krankheit bei Juden und Nichtjuden," *Ost und West* 3 (1903): 565–68, 631–38, 775–80, 849–52, collected as Hugo Hoppe, *Krankheiten und Sterblichkeit bei Juden und Nichtjuden* (Berlin: S. Calvary, 1903). See also Michael Tschoetschel,

"Die Diskussion über die Häufigkeit von Krankheiten bei den Juden bis 1920" (Diss., Mainz, 1990), 118–42.

62. G. Steiner, "Klinik der Neurosyphilis," in *Handbuch der Haut- und Geschlechtskrankheiten,* ed. Josef Judassohn et al., vol. 17, 1, ed. Gustav Alexander (Berlin: Springer, 1929), 230.

63. See "The Jewish Psyche: Freud, Dora, and the Idea of the Hysteric," in my book *The Jew's Body* (New York: Routledge, 1991), 60–103.

64. H. Higier, "Zur Klinik der angiosklerotischen paroxysmalen Myasthenie ('claudication intermittente' Charcot's) und der sog. spontanen Gangrän," *Deutsche Zeitschrift für Nervenheilkunde* 19 (1901): 438–67.

65. P. Olivier and A. Halipré, "Claudication intermittente chez un homme hystérique atteint de pouls lent permanent," *La Normandie Médicale* 11 (1896): 21–28.

66. Louis Basile Carré de Montgeron, *La vérité des miracles opérés par l'intercession de M. de Pâris et autres appellans démontrée contre M. l'archevêque de Sens . . .*, 3 vols. (Cologne: Librairies de la Campagnie, 1745–47).

67. Compare J. H. Baker and J. R. Silver, "Hysterical Paraplegia," *Journal of Neurology, Neurosurgery and Psychiatry* 50 (1987): 375–82, and J. R. Keane, "Hysterical Gait Disorders: Sixty Cases," *Neurology* 39 (1989): 586–89.

68. H. Idelsohn, "Zur Casuistik und Aetiologie des intermittierenden Hinkens," *Deutsche Zeitschrift für Nervenheilkunde* 24 (1903): 285–304.

69. Singer, *Allgemeine und spezielle Krankheitslehre,* 124–25.

70. Gustav Muskat, "Über Gangstockung," *Verhandlungen des Deutschen Kongresses für Innere Medizin* 27 (1910): 45–56.

71. Samuel Goldflam, "Weiteres über das intermittierende Hinken," *Neurologisches Centralblatt* 20 (1901): 197–213. See also his "Über intermittierende Hinken ('claudication intermittente' Charcot's) und Arteritis der Beine," *Deutsche Medizinische Wochenschrift* 21 (1901): 587–98.

72. See Enfemiuse Herman, "Samuel Goldflam (1852–1932)," in *Grosse Nervenärtze,* ed. Kurt Kolle, 3 vols. (Stuttgart: Thieme, 1963), 3:143–49.

73. Samuel Goldflam, "Zur Ätiologie und Symptomatologie des intermittierenden Hinkens," *Neurologisches Zentralblatt* 22 (1903): 994–96. On tobacco misuse as a primary cause of illness see the literature overview by Johannes Bresler, *Tabakologia Medizinalis: Literarische Studie über den Tabak in medizinischer Beziehung,* 2 vols. (Halle: Carl Marhold, 1911–13).

74. Toby Cohn, "Nervenkrankheiten bei Juden," *Zeitschrift für Demographie und Statistik der Juden,* n.s., 3 (1926): 76–85.

75. Kurt Mendel, "Intermitterendes Hinken," *Zentralblatt für die Gesamt Neurologie und Psychiatrie* 27 (1922): 65–95.

76. Wilhelm Erb, "Über das 'intermittirende Hinken' und andere nervöse Störungen in Folge von Gefässerkrankungen," *Deutsche Zeitschrift für Nervenheilkunde* 13 (1898): 1–77.

77. Wilhelm Erb, "Über Disbasia angiosklerotika (intermittierendes Hinken)," *Münchener Medizinische Wochenschrift* 51 (1904): 905–8.

78. Compare P. C. Waller, S. A. Solomon, and L. E. Ramsay, "The Acute

Effects of Cigarette Smoking on Treadmill Exercise Distances in Patients with Stable Intermittent Claudication," *Angiology* 40 (1989): 164–69.

79. Hermann Oppenheim, "Zur Psychopathologie und Nosologie der russisch-jüdischen Bevölkerung," *Journal für Psychologie und Neurologie* 13 (1908): 7.

80. This discussion is based on the chapter "Professor Lubarsch und die Juden," in Gerhard Jaeckel, *Die Charité: Die Geschichte eines Weltzentrums der Medizin* (Berlin: Ullstein, 1991), 488–99.

81. Sigmund Freud, *Jugendbriefe an Eduard Silberstein, 1871–1881,* ed. Walter Boehlich (Frankfurt am Main: Fischer, 1989), 194.

82. Ernest Jones, *The Life and Work of Sigmund Freud,* 3 vols. (New York: Basic Books 1953–57), 1:23.

83. Martin Freud, *Glory Reflected: Sigmund Freud—Man and Father* (London: Angus and Robertson, 1957), 22–23.

84. Jones, *Life and Work,* 1:23.

85. The debate about the "Jewish" content of this story, recounted by Freud in *The Interpretation of Dreams,* was joined in the 1920s. See Edgar Michaelis, *Die Menschheitsproblematik der Freudschen Psychoanalyse: Urbild und Maske* (Leipzig: Johann Ambrosius Barth, 1931), 73–76, and Charles E. Maylan, *Freuds tragischer Komplex: Eine Analyse der Psychoanalyse* (Munich: Ernest Reinhardt, 1929), 27–36. Maylan, citing an earlier edition of Michaelis, argues for a strongly "Jewish" interpretation of this incident, with the equation between the father and the Jew being an integral part of the formative imagery of psychoanalysis. He notes that "Freud kept his promise: to revenge his insulted/raped father on Christian Rome" by "a scientific detour," that is, psychoanalysis. Michaelis responded to Maylan's view by stressing the father's role and not mentioning anti-Semitism in his interpretation at all.

86. Paul Brienes, *Tough Jews: Political Fantasies and the Moral Dilemma of American Jewry* (New York: Basic Books, 1990), 41, stresses how important it is that Freud, in 1930, appended a note to this passage questioning Masséna's Jewish origin. He notes that it is the "power of wish and image, especially bodily image, over fact" that is vital here.

87. Freud, *Glory Reflected,* 70–71.

88. Beller, *Vienna and the Jews,* 188, presents quite the opposite image.

89. Francis L. Cohen, "Army," in *The Jewish Encyclopedia* (New York: Funk and Wagnalls, 1904), 2:127.

90. Deák, *Jewish Soldiers,* 17.

91. See Heinz Politzer's comment on this aspect of the story in the edition published by S. Fischer in 1967, 45.

92. Deák, *Jewish Soldiers,* 12.

93. *Monatsschrift der Österreichisch-Israelitischen Union* 16, 4 (April 1904): 2.

94. Sigmund Freud, *Briefe, 1873–1939,* ed. Ernst und Lucie Freud (Frankfurt am Main: Fischer, 1960), 135–36; translation from *Letters of Sigmund Freud, 1873–1939,* ed. Ernst L. Freud, trans. Tania Stern and James Stern (London: Hogarth Press, 1961), 143.

95. Amos Elon, *Herzl* (New York: Holt, Rinehart, and Winston, 1975), 63.

96. Felix von Luschan, *Völker, Rasse und Sprachen* (Berlin: Welt Verlag, 1922), 170.

97. Ernst Brücke, *Schönheit und Fehler der menschlichen Gestalt* (Vienna: Wilhelm Braumüller, 1891), 141–44.

98. See the discussion of this topos in Liliane Weissberg, "Stepping Out: The Writing of Difference in Rahel Varnhagen's Letters," in *Anti-Semitism in Times of Crisis,* ed. Sander L. Gilman and Steven T. Katz (New York: New York University Press, 1991), 140–53.

99. Gustav Jaeger, *Die Entdeckung der Seele* (Leipzig: Ernst Günther, 1880), 106–9. For a catalog of the smell attributed to the Jew see Hans F. K. Günther, "Der rasseeigene Geruch der Hautausdünstung," *Zeitschrift für Rassenphysiologie* 2 (1930): 94–99, here 97–99. Günther strongly believes in the reality of the Jew's smell and offers his own as well as historical testimony.

100. See especially Peter L. Rudnytsky, *Freud and Oedipus* (New York: Columbia University Press, 1987), as well as the following studies: J. Swan, "Mater and Nannie: Freud's Two Mothers and the Discovery of the Oedipus Complex," *American Imago* 31 (1974): 1–64; A. Bernstein, "Freud and Oedipus: A New Look at the Oedipus Complex in the Light of Freud's Life," *Psychoanalytic Review* 63 (1976): 393–407; R. C. Calogeras and F. X. Schupper, "Origins and Early Formulations of the Oedipus Complex," *Journal of the American Psychoanalytic Association* 20 (1972): 751–75; J. Dalma, "Comprobación etimológica de la hipotesis freudiana del tabu del incesto," *Acta Psiquiatrica y Psicológica de America Latina* 20 (1974): 253–60.

101. Marianne Krüll, *Freud and His Father,* trans. Arnold Pomerans (New York: W. W. Norton, 1986), 61–63.

102. "There is a tradition that Laius pierced the infant's feet with a spike of iron; and another source notes that this is the source of Oedipus's name." L. Constans, *La légende d'Oedipe* (Paris: Maisonneuve, 1881), 25 (in the Freud Library, London, with many underlinings and notes).

103. Karl Abraham, "Vaterrettung und Vatermord in den neurotischen Phantasiegebilden," *International Zeitschrift für Psychoanalyse* 8 (1922): 71–77.

104. *Sigmund Freud–Arnold Zweig: Briefwechsel,* ed. Ernst L. Freud (Frankfurt am Main: Fischer, 1968), 108; translation from *The Letters of Sigmund Freud and Arnold Zweig,* ed. Ernst L. Freud, trans. Elaine Robson-Scott and William Robson-Scott (New York: Harcourt, Brace, and World, 1970), 97.

105. *SE* 13:216. See Jacques Le Rider, "Sigmund Freud et Theodor Herzl: Les deux 'hommes Moïse' du début de siècle," in his *Modernité viennoise et crises de l'identité* (Paris: Presses Universitaires de France, 1990), 273–97; S. A. Karpowitz, "'The Love-Child': Freud's Essay on the Moses of Michelangelo," *Psychoanalytic Review* 74 (1987): 333–45; Martin S. Bergmann, "Moses and the Evolution of Freud's Jewish Identity," *Israel Annals of Psychiatry and Related Disciplines* 14 (1976): V. Spruiell, "The Joke in 'The Moses of Michelangelo': Imagination and Creativity," *Psychoanalytic Study of the Child* 40 (1985): 473–92; Jean Jofen, "A Freudian Interpretation of Freud's *Moses and Monotheism,*"

Michigan Academician 12 (1979–80): 231–40; David Bakan, "Moses in the Thought of Freud: An Ambivalent Interpretation," *Commentary* 26 (1958): 322–31; Kate Victorius, "Der 'Moses des Michelangelo' von Sigmund Freud: Eine Studie," *Psyche* 10 (1956): 1–10.

106. Th. Gsell Fels, *Rom und die Campagna* (Leipzig: Bibliographisches Institut, 1912), 752–53 (in the Freud Library, London).

107. Carlo Ginzburg, "Morelli, Freud and Sherlock Holmes: Clues and Scientific Method," *History Workshop* 9 (1980): 5–36.

108. On this interpretation see Sarah Kofman, *Quatre romans analytiques* (Paris: Éditions Galilée, 1974), 101–37; Jean Bellemin-Noel, *Gradiva au pied de la lettre: Relecture du roman de W. Jensen dans une nouvelle traduction* (Paris: Presses Universitaires de France, 1983); Nora Crow Jaffe, "A Second Opinion on Delusions and Dreams: A Reading of Freud's Interpretation of Jensen," *Literature and Medicine* 2 (1983): 101–17; George Favier, "Le savoir des poètes: Freud lecteur de Jensen," *Cahiers d'Études Germaniques* 10 (1986): 55–107; Ingrid Haag, "La Gradiva de Jensen: Quelques notes de lecture," *Cahiers d'Études Germaniques* 10 (1986): 109–21; Peter Henninger, "Autour de la Gradiva," *Cahiers d'Études Germaniques* 10 (1986): 123–49; Harry Slochower, "Freud's Gradiva, *Mater Nuda Rediviva:* A Wish-Fulfillment of the 'Memory' on the Acropolis," *Psychoanalytic Quarterly* 40 (1971): 646–62. On the general context see Michael Worbs, *Nervenkunst: Literatur und Psychoanalyse im Wien der Jahrhundertwende* (Frankfurt am Main: Europäische Verlagsanstalt, 1983). On Freud's marginalia and reading of this text see Edward Timms, "Freud's Library and His Private Reading," in Edward Timms and Naomi Segal, eds., *Freud in Exile: Psychoanalysis and Its Vicissitudes* (New Haven: Yale University Press, 1988), 65–79.

109. Patrick Mahoney, *Freud as a Writer* (New York: International Universities Press, 1982), as well as his "Towards the Understanding of Translation in Psychoanalysis," *Metapsychology* 27 (1982): 63–71; "Further Consideration on Freud as a Writer" (1984), unpublished paper; and *Cries of the Wolf Man* (New York: International Universities Press, 1984).

110. Giovanni Papini, "A Visit to Freud," in *Freud as We Knew Him,* ed. Hendrik Ruitenbeck (Detroit: Wayne State University Press, 1973), 99–101.

111. In Freud's London library there is a detailed study of the ethnology of the foot by Siegmar von Schultze-Gellera writing as "Dr. Aigremont," *Fuss- und Schuh-Symbolik und Erotik: Folkloristische und sexualwissenschaftliche Untersuchungen* (Leipzig: Deutsche Verlags A.G., 1909).

112. Wilhelm Jensen, "Gradiva: A Pompeiian Fancy," translated by Helen M. Downey in Sigmund Freud, *Delusion and Dream and Other Essays,* ed. Philip Rieff (Boston: Beacon Press, 1956), 148. This translation was made in 1917. The German original, Wilhelm Jensen, *Gradiva* (Dresden: C. Reissner, 1903), is in the Freud Library, London, and is extensively annotated.

113. Freud owned at least three volumes of Arthur Schnitzler's works. Two were presented to him by Schnitzler and bear dedications from him (*Fräulein Else* [Vienna: Zsolnay, 1924]; *Buch der Sprüche und Bedenken* [Vienna: Phaidon,

1927]). The one volume Freud purchased seems to have been Schnitzler's extraordinary evocation of the link between the world of medicine and the power of anti-Semitism in fin-de-siècle Vienna, *Professor Bernardi* (Berlin: Fischer, 1912), with Freud's name inscribed on the flyleaf. All are in a private collection in London.

114. Wilhelm Jensen, "Drei unveröffentliche Briefe: Zur Geschichte von Freuds Gradiva-Analyse," *Die Psychoanalytische Bewegung* 1 (1929): 207. Jensen published a spirited attack on anti-Semitism in a major collection of such statements made by leading public figures of the turn of the century. See *Freiheit, Liebe, Menschlichkeit! Ein Manifest des Geistes von hervorragenden Zeitgenossen* (Berlin: J. van Groningen, 1893), 71.

115. Eckhardt Meyer-Krentler, "Stopfkuchen—Ein Doppelgänger: Wilhelm Raabe erzählt Theodor Storm," *Jahrbuch der Raabe-Gesellschaft,* 1987, 179–204.

116. Concerning the meaning of the signs of goiter see B. S. Hetzel, "The History of Goiter and Cretinism," in his *The Story of Iodine Deficiency: The Challenge of Prevention* (New York: Oxford University Press, 1989), 3–20; A. Giampalmo and E. Fulcheri, "An Investigation of Endemic Goiter during the Centuries in Sacral Figurative Arts," *Zentralblatt für Allgemeine Pathologie* 134 (1988): 297–307; F. Merke, *History and Iconography of Endemic Goiter and Cretinism* (Boston: MTP Press, 1984), and G. M. Wilson, "Early Photography, Goiter, and James Inglis," *British Medical Journal,* April 14, 1973, 104–5; as well as my *Seeing the Insane* (New York: John Wiley, 1976). Although there is a clinical difference between endemic goiter, usually the result of iodine insufficiency, and Graves' or Basedow's disease, the external signs and symptoms (except for cretinism) overlap. See A. Leovey, "A Basedow-Graves kor termeszetrajzarol," *Orv Hetil* 129 (1988): 1083–87, and J. G. Ljunggren, "Vem var mannen bakom syndromet: Ismail al-Jurjani, Testa, Flagani, Parry, Graves eller Basedow?" *Lakartidningen* 80 (1983): 2902.

117. *SE* 1:140. Freud is drawing on the work of P. J. Möbius, "Ueber die Basedow'sche Krankheit," *Deutsche Zeitschrift für Nervenheilkunde* 1 (1891): 400–444, here 424–27. Möbius supplies a detailed report of the literature on the hereditary transmission of Graves' disease.

118. Georg Buschan, *Die Basedow'sche Krankheit (Goître exothalmique, Graves' Disease, Morbo di Flajani)* (Leipzig: Franz Deuticke, 1894), 61. Buschan's views dominate the discussion of the period. See Michael Tschoetschel, "Die Diskussion über die Häufigkeit von Krankheiten bei den Juden bis 1920" (Diss., Mainz, 1990), 187–88.

119. *SE* 9:95. Freud's views were seconded by Otto Rank, in a review of *Fremdling unter den Menschen,* Jensen's last novel, in *Imago* 1 (1912): 537–38, in which he too stressed the incest motif and the role the sibling plays as a displaced image of the parent.

120. Jensen, "Briefe," 210.

121. Eva Gräfin Baudissin, Review of Wilhelm Jensen, *Fremdlinge unter den Menschen, Die Zeit* (Vienna), February 11, 1912, 31.

122. *The Freud/Jung Letters: The Correspondence between Sigmund Freud and C. G. Jung,* ed. William McGuire, trans. Ralph Mannheim and R. F. C. Hull (Princeton: Princeton University Press, 1974), 85.

123. Nathan G. Hale, Jr., *James Putnam and Psychoanalysis: Letters between Putnam and Sigmund Freud, Ernest Jones, William James, Sándor Ferenczi, and Morton Prince, 1877–1917,* trans. Judith Bernays Heller (Cambridge: Harvard University Press, 1971), 189.

124. January 17, 1909, *Freud/Jung Letters,* 93.

125. R. Andrew Pasauskaus, "Freud's Break with Jung: The Crucial Role of Ernest Jones," *Free Associations* 11 (1988): 7–34.

126. William J. McGrath, *Freud's Discovery of Psychoanalysis: The Politics of Hysteria* (Ithaca, N.Y.: Cornell University Press, 1986), 299–302.

127. On the context see Alexander Grinstein, *Sigmund Freud's Dreams* (New York: International Universities Press, 1980), 394–421, and Sandra M. Gilbert, "Rider Haggard's Heart of Darkness," in *Coordinates: Placing Science Fiction and Fantasy,* ed. George E. Slusser, Eric S. Rabkin, and Robert Scholes (Carbondale: Southern Illinois University Press, 1983), 124–38.

128. See the relation between this discussion and the idea of the Jewish quack in Eric Jameson, *The Natural History of Quackery* (London: Michael Joseph, 1961), 17.

129. Harry Friedenwald, *The Jews and Medicine: Essays* (Baltimore: Johns Hopkins University Press, 1944), 527.

130. Elcan Isaac Wolf, *Von den Krankheiten der Juden* (Mannheim: C. F. Schwan, 1777), 84.

131. Maurice Fishberg, "Cancer," in *The Jewish Encyclopedia,* 3:531, and Sigismund Peller, "Über Krebssterblichkeit der Juden," *Zeitschrift für Krebsforschung* 34 (1931): 128–47, here 134.

132. Maurice Fishberg, "Morbidity," in *The Jewish Encyclopedia,* 9:4.

133. Ignaz Bernstein, *Jüdische Sprichwörter und Redensarten* (Warsaw: For J. Kauffmann, Frankfurt am Main, 1908). The role of Bernstein's proverb collections in providing a source for the Western understanding of the sexuality of the Eastern Jews is documented in A. A. Roback's letter of March 10, 1930, to Freud. See A. A. Roback, *Freudiana* (Cambridge, Mass.: Sci-Art Publishers, 1957), 31. On the centrality of the proverb for an understanding of the image of the Eastern Jew in psychoanalysis see Theodor Reik, "The Echo of the Proverb," in his *From Thirty Years with Freud,* trans. Richard Winston (New York: Farrar and Reinhart, 1940), 228–41. On the negative use of these proverbs see Wolfgang Mieder, "Proverbs in Nazi Germany: The Promulgation of Anti-Semitism and Stereotypes through Folklore," *Journal of American Folklore* 95 (1982): 435–64, on Bernstein, 437.

134. Gutmann, *Über das heutigan Stand,* 38.

135. George W. Pickering, *Creative Malady: Illness in the Lives and Minds of Charles Darwin, Florence Nightingale, Mary Baker Eddy, Sigmund Freud, Marcel Proust, and Elizabeth Barrett Browning* (London: George Unwin, 1974), 222, and Jones, *Life and Work,* 2:101, 118, 206, 436.

136. W. Watkiss Lloyd, *The Moses of Michelangelo: A Study of Art History and Legend* (London: Williams and Norgate, 1863), 12 (in the Freud Library, London, dated October 25, 1912, on the flyleaf).

137. Lloyd, *Moses,* 12; "contemptuous indignation" underlined by Freud.

138. Arnold Kutzinski, "Über nervöse Entartung bei den Juden," *Ost und West* 12 (1912): cols. 905–10.

139. Max Jungmann, "Ist das jüdische Volk degeneriert?" *Die Welt* 6 (1912): 3–4.

140. On the medicalization of the idea of the "perversion" see Georges Lanteri-Laura, *Lecture des perversions: Histoire de l'appropriation médicale* (Paris: Masson, 1979).

141. Hermann Glaser, "Die 'kulturelle' Sexualmoral und die moderne Nervosität," in his *Sigmund Freuds Zwanzigstes Jahrhundert* (Munich: Carl Hanser, 1976), 51–168; Alexander Schusdek, "Freud's 'Seduction Theory': A Reconstruction," *Journal of the History of the Behavioral Sciences* 2 (1966): 159–66; Heinz Schott, "Traum und Geschichte: Zur Freudschen Geschichtsauffassung im Kontext der Traumdeutung," *Sudhoffs Archiv* 64 (1980): 298–312; Samuel Jaffe, "Freud as Rhetorician: Elocutio and the Dream-Work," *Rhetorik* 1 (1980): 42–69. Of little use, despite its title, is the speculative essay by Jean-Marc Dupen, "Freud and Degeneracy: A Turning Point," *Diogenes* 97 (1977): 43–64. The longer work announced in the essay has evidently not appeared.

142. See Emanuel Radl, *Geschichte der biologischen Theorien seit dem Ende des siebzehnten Jahrhunderts* (Leipzig: Engelmann, 1905), and Roderick Stackelberg, *Idealism Debased: From Völkisch Ideology to National Socialism* (Kent, Ohio: Kent State University Press, 1981).

143. The appearance of the hybrid theory in Chamberlain's *Die Grundlagen des neunzehnten Jahrhunderts* (Munich: Bruckmann, 1899), 1:406–9, as a way of denying the Jews the label of a "pure race" by labeling them as a hybrid with blacks, continues an identification between blackness and otherness that has very old historical roots in Germany but that is here given biological form. See my *On Blackness without Blacks: Essays on the Image of the Black in Germany* (Boston: G. K. Hall, 1982). Chamberlain cites "Siegmund" Freud in his discussion of the nature of sexual repression in the formation of neurosis in a virulently anti-Catholic discussion of Loyola. On the context see Geoffrey G. Field, *Evangelist of Race: The Germanic Vision of Houston Stewart Chamberlain* (New York: Columbia, 1981).

144. Paul Julius Möbius, *Geschlecht und Entartung* (Halle: Carl Marhold, 1903), is a typical summary of these earlier views. See Esther Fischer-Homburger, *Krankheit Frau: Zur Geschichte der Einbildungen* (Darmstadt: Luchterhand, 1984), 32–48, on the image of the hysteric, and Patricia Meyer Spacks, *The Adolescent Idea: Myths of Youth and the Adult Imagination* (New York: Basic Books, 1981).

145. Hermann Smidt, "Über das Vorkommen der Hysterie bei Kindern" (Diss., Strasbourg, 1880). See K. Codell Carter, "Infantile Hysteria and Infantile

Sexuality in Late Nineteenth-Century German Language Medical Literature," *Medical History* 26 (1983): 186–96.

146. Sigmund Freud, *Die infantile Cerebrallähmung* (Vienna: Alfred Hölder, 1897), 255–86. (This was also published as part of volume 9 of Hermann Nothnagel, ed., *Specielle Pathologie und Therapie,* 24 vols. [Vienna: Alfred Hölder, 1894–1908].)

147. See *SE* 2:87, 104, 294, 3:21, 46, 51, 249, 11:21, 12:207.

148. *SE* 12:207; but compare 7:254 and 263.

149. Jeffrey Moussaieff Masson, ed., *The Complete Letters of Sigmund Freud to Wilhelm Fliess, 1887–1904* (Cambridge: Harvard University Press, 1985), 76–78.

150. See Iwan Bloch's *Beiträge zur Aetiologie der Psychopathia sexualis* (Dresden: H. R. Dohrn, 1902–3) and his *Das Sexualleben unserer Zeit in seinen Beziehungen zur modernen Kultur* (Berlin: Marcus, 1907), as well as the work of Magnus Hirschfeld. These volumes are part of an attempt to achieve a political solution to the question of homosexuality by recruiting science onto the side of liberalism.

151. Richard Krafft-Ebing, *Psychopathia sexualis mit besonderer Berücksichtigung der konträren Sexualempfindungen* (1886; reprint Munich: Matthes und Seitz, 1984), 3 (in the Freud Library, London, in the German editions of 1892, 1894, and 1901). A translation is available as Richard von Krafft-Ebing, *Psychopathia Sexualis: A Medico-Forensic Study,* rev. trans. Harry E. Wedeck (New York: Putnam, 1956), 25.

152. See the discussion in Alain Corbin, "L'hérédosyphilis ou l'impossible rédemption: Contribution à l'histoire de l'hérédité morbide," *Romantisme* 31 (1981): 131–49.

153. *SE* 4:300–301. See the discussion in Grinstein, *Sigmund Freud's Dreams,* 221–44, and Didier Anzieu, *Freud's Self-Analysis,* trans. Peter Graham (London: Hogarth Press, 1986), 394–96.

154. Eduard Reich, *Die Nervosität bei den Frauen: Ihre Ursache und Verhütung* (Berlin: A. Zimmer, 1882), 109.

155. The great debate about prostitution in the nineteenth century was between the economic determinists, who relied on the work of Alexandre Jean Baptiste Parent-Duchatelet, *De la prostitution dans la ville de Paris . . .* (Paris: Baillière, 1836), and the biological determinists, represented by Lombroso. On Lombroso see Klaus Hofweber, "Die Sexualtheorien des Cesare Lombroso" (Diss., Munich, 1969).

156. *SE* 18:47. For the context of these remarks see Frederick B. Churchill, "Sex and the Single Organism: Biological Theories of Sexuality in Mid-Nineteenth Century," *Journal of the History of Biology* 12 (1979): 139–77.

157. Leopold Löwenfeld, *Über den National-Charakter der Franzosen und dessen krankhafte Auswüchse (Die Psychopathia gallica) in ihren Beziehung zum Weltkrieg* (Wiesbaden: Bergmann, 1914).

158. Wilfred Trotter, *Instincts of the Herd in Peace and War, 1916–1919*

(London: Keynes Press, 1985), 127–28 (in the Freud Library, London, in the 1921 edition).

4. Seduction, Parricide, and Crime

1. On Freud and *The Robbers* see William J. McGrath, *Freud's Discovery of Psychoanalysis: The Politics of Hysteria* (Ithaca, N.Y.: Cornell University Press, 1986), 21, 66–68.

2. See my essay "The Indelibility of Circumcision," *Koroth* 9 (1991): 806–17.

3. See, for example, C. P. T. Schwenken, *Notizen über die berüchtigsten jüdischen Gauner und Spitzbuben . . .* (Marburg: Johann Christian Krieger, 1820), and Karl Stuhlmüller, *Vollständige Nachrichten über eine polizeiliche Untersuchung gegen jüdischen, durch ganz Deutschland und dessen Nachbarstaaten verbreitete Gaunerbanden* (1823). An anti-Semitic summary of the historical literature on the Jews as criminals available to the readers through the 1930s is to be found in *Das Judentum in der Rechtswissenschaft* (Berlin: Deutscher Rechts-Verlag, 1936), 57–60. On the medicalization of this theme in the Third Reich see Michael H. Kater, *Doctors under Hitler* (Chapel Hill: University of North Carolina Press, 1989), 180. On the image of the Jew and the language of the thieves in the eighteenth century see my *Jewish Self-Hatred: Anti-Semitism and the Hidden Language of the Jews* (Baltimore: Johns Hopkins University Press, 1986; paperback edition, 1990, 68–87). On the medicalization of this topos in the United States see Max H. Weinberg, "Jewish Criminals: A Psychologic-Psychiatric Study of Jewish Prisoners in Penal Institutions of Western Pennsylvania," *Medical Leaves* 2 (1939): 174–94.

4. Hans Kurella, *Naturgeschichte des Verbrechers* (Stuttgart: Ferdinand Enke, 1893), 138–39 (on atavism); 180–85 (on the physiognomy of criminal and Jew); 220–35 (on the Jews' language and the language of thieves).

5. Erich Wulffen, *Kriminalpsychologie und Psychopathologie in Schillers "Räubern"* (Halle: Carl Marhold, 1907). See in this regard the study by G. von Rohden, "Schiller und die Kriminalpsychologie," *Monatsschrift für Kriminalpsychologie und Strafrechtsreform* 2 (1906): 81–88.

6. Albert Édouard Brutus Gilles de la Tourette, *Études cliniques et physiologiques sur la marche* (Paris: Delahaye, 1886).

7. Cesare Lombroso, *Der Verbrecher (Homo delinquens) in anthropologischer, ärztlicher und juristischer Beziehung,* trans. M. O. Fraenkel, 2 vols. (Hamburg: Verlags und Druckerei Actien-Gesellschaft, 1890), 2:343–44 (in the Freud Collection, New York).

8. Davydd Greenwood, *The Taming of Evolution: The Persistence of Nonevolutionary Views in the Study of Humans* (Ithaca, N.Y.: Cornell University Press, 1984).

9. Ernst Kretschmer, *Körperbau und Charakter: Untersuchungen zum Konstitutionsproblem und zur Lehre von den Temperamenten* (Berlin: Springer, 1922).

See also Gerhard Koch, *Die Gesellschaft für Konstitutionsforschung: Anfang und Ende, 1942–1965* (Erlangen: Palm und Enke, 1985).

10. Ludwig Stern-Piper, "Zur Frage der Bedeutung der psycho-physischen Typen," *Zeitschrift für die Gesamte Neurologie und Psychiatrie* 84 (1923): 408–14.

11. Ernst Kretschmer, "Konstitution und Rasse," *Zeitschrift für die Gesamte Neurologie und Psychiatrie* 82 (1923): 139–47. One can note that Kretschmer was refused a chair in psychiatry at Tübingen in January 1945 because of his "political world view," that is, because of his refusal to accept the arguments of racial science. See the letter of Stickl, rector of the University of Tübingen, in Kretschmer's "Personalnotizen" (1945), from "Der Bevollmächtigte für das Sanitäts- und Gesundheitswesen" at the Berlin Documentation Center.

12. Ludwig Stern-Piper, "Konstitution und Rasse," *Zeitschrift für die Gesamte Neurologie und Psychiatrie* 86 (1923): 265–73.

13. M. J. Gutmann, "Geisteskrankheiten bei Juden," *Zeitschrift für Demographie und Statistik der Juden,* n.s., 3 (1926): 103–17, here 109.

14. Lombroso, *Der Verbrecher,* 1:131.

15. Cited by Erich Wulffen, *Psychologie des Verbrechers: Ein Handbuch für Juristen, Ärzte, Pädagogen und Gebildete aller Stände,* 2 vols. (Berlin: P. Lagenscheidt, 1908), 1:264 (in the Freud Library, London, in the 1910 edition). On the context see Franziska Lamott, "Die Kriminologie und das Andere: Versuch über die Geschichte der Ausgrenzung," *Kriminalogisches Journal* 20 (1988): 168–90.

16. Lombroso, *Der Verbrecher,* 1:234, 233.

17. Moritz Benedickt, *Anatomical Studies upon Brains of Criminals,* trans. E. P. Fowler (New York: Wm. Wood, 1881).

18. Lombroso, *Der Verbrecher,* 1:236.

19. Cesare Lombroso, *Criminal Man,* briefly summarized by his daughter Gina Lombroso-Ferrero (New York: G. P. Putnam's Sons, 1911), 140.

20. Cesare Lombroso, *Die Ursachen und Bekämpfung des Verbrechens,* trans. Hans Kurella and E. Jentsch (Berlin: Hugo Bermühler, 1902), 31–34.

21. Max Sichel, *Die Geistesstörungen bei den Juden: Eine klinisch-historische Studie* (Leipzig: Kaufmann, 1909).

22. Carl Heinrich Stratz, *Was sind Juden? Eine ethnographisch-anthropologische Studie* (Vienna: F. Tempsky, 1903), 25 (on the face as a sign of degeneracy); 26–27 (on the Jewish type as degenerate); 29 (on inbreeding) (in the Freud Library, London).

23. Erich Wulffen, *Der Sexualverbrecher* (Berlin: P. Langenscheidt, 1910), 302. This was considered one of the major innovative contributions to criminology of the day. See the review in the *Jahrbuch für sexuelle Zwischenstufen,* n.s., 3 (1911): 376–78.

24. John S. Billings, "Vital Statistics of the Jews," *North American Review* 153 (1891): 70–84, here 84.

25. All of these fin-de-siècle sources are cited by Havelock Ellis, *Studies in the*

Psychology of Sex, 7 vols. (Philadephia: F. A. Davis, 1900–1928), 5:185–86 (in the Freud Library, London).

26. Hanns Sachs, *Freud: Master and Friend* (Cambridge: Harvard University Press, 1946), 19.

27. Leopold Löwenfeld, *Über die sexuelle Konstitution und andere Sexualprobleme* (Wiesbaden: J. F. Bergmann, 1911), 75–76 (in the Freud Library, London).

28. *Protokolle der Wiener Psychoanalytischen Vereinigung,* ed. Herman Nunberg and Ernst Federn, 4 vols. (Frankfurt am Main: Fischer, 1976–81), 2:41; translation from *Minutes of the Vienna Psychoanalytic Society,* trans. M. Nunberg, 4 vols. (New York: International Universities Press, 1962–75), 2:45.

29. The overall literature on this topic is available in M. L. Rodrigues de Areia and A. M. Elias Abade, eds., *Consangüínidade: Bibliografia* (Coimbra: Instituto de Antropologia, Universidade de Coimbra, 1983).

30. Cecil F. Beadles, "The Insane Jew," *Journal of Mental Science* 46 (1900): 732.

31. Maurice Fishberg, *The Jews: A Study of Race and Environment* (New York: Walter Scott, 1911), 349.

32. Rudolf Virchow, "Über Erblichkeit: I. Die Theorie Darwins," *Deutsche Jahrbücher für Politik und Literatur* 6 (1863): 339–58, here 354.

33. Houston Stewart Chamberlain, *Foundations of the Nineteenth Century,* trans. John Lees, 2 vols. (London: John Lane/Bodley Head, 1913), 1:366. On Freud's reading of Chamberlain see *GW,* Nachtragsband, 787.

34. On the question of Jews and crime, and the anxiety about violence in the nineteenth century see Paul Brienes, *Tough Jews: Political Fantasies and the Moral Dilemma of American Jewry* (New York: Basic Books, 1990), 106–12.

35. Wulffen, *Der Sexualverbrecher,* 302.

36. D. Ackner, "The Crime of Incest," *Medical and Legal Journal* 48 (1980): 79–91.

37. See the discussion in "The Jewish Murderer: Jack the Ripper, Race, and Gender," in my book *The Jew's Body* (New York: Routledge, 1991), 104–27.

38. Martin L. Friedland, *The Trials of Israel Lipski: A True Story of a Victorian Murder in the East End of London* (New York: Beaufort, 1984). Friedland believes, in spite of Lipski's confession on the eve of his hanging, that he was innocent of the crime.

39. Peter Pulzer, *The Rise of Political Anti-Semitism in Germany and Austria* (London: Peter Halban, 1988), 6.

40. B. Goldberg, "Zur Kriminalität der Juden in Russland," *Zeitschrift für Demographie und Statistik der Juden* 8 (1912): 127–30.

41. Rafael Becker, "Die Häufigkeit jüdischer Krimineller unter den geisteskranken Verbrecher in Polen," *Psychiatrische-Neurologische Wochenschrift* 33 (1931): 362–64.

42. Walter Pötsch, *Die jüdische Rasse im Lichte der Straffälligkeit: Zuchstätten der Minderrassigkeit* (Ratibor: Hans W. Pötsch, 1933).

43. Joachim Duckart, *Die Juden von Betsche: Ein Beitrag zum "Wirken" der*

Juden im deutschen Osten, Veröffentlichungen des Rassenpolitischen Amtes der NSDAP, vol. 1 (Meseritz: P. Matthias, 1939).

44. See Edward Bristow, *Prostitution and Prejudice: The Jewish Fight against White Slavery, 1870–1939* (New York: Schocken, 1983), as well as his essay "History versus Memory: Jews and White Slavery," *Moment* 9 (1984): 44–49, which has an overview of the critical literature on this topic.

45. Franz Alexander and Hugo Staub, *Der Verbrecher und seine Richter: Eine psychoanalytischer Einblick in die Welt der Paragraphen* (Vienna: Internationaler Psychoanalytischer Verlag, 1929) (in the Freud Library, London); translated by Gregory Zilboorg as *The Criminal, the Judge, and the Public: A Psychological Analysis* (New York: Macmillan, 1931) (in the Freud Library, London).

46. Paul Näcke, "Über den Wert der sog: Degenerationszeichen," *Monatsschrift für Kriminalpsychologie und Strafrechtsreform* 1 (1904): 99–111, here 110–11.

47. See Sander L. Gilman, *Sexuality: An Illustrated History* (New York: Wiley, 1989), 231–62.

48. See the discussion by Alain Corbin, "Commercial Sexuality in Nineteenth-Century France: A System of Images and Regulations," *Representations* 14 (1986): 209–19.

49. All references to this hitherto unpublished essay are to the translation by Dennis Klein, published as appendix C of his *Jewish Origins of the Psychoanalytic Movement* (New York: Praeger, 1981), 170–72.

50. Otto Rank, *Das Inzest-Motif in Dichtung und Sage: Grundzüge einer Psychologie des dichterischen Schaffens* (Leipzig: Deuticke, 1912). This has recently been translated as Otto Rank, *The Incest Theme in Literature and Legend: Fundamentals of a Psychology of Literary Creation,* trans. Gregory C. Richter (Baltimore: Johns Hopkins University Press, 1992).

51. Willy Helpach, "Berufspsychosen," *Die Zukunft* 14 (1906): 179–88.

52. Wilhelm Reutlinger, "Über die Häufigkeit der Verwandtenehen bei den Juden in Hohenzollern und über Untersuchungen bei Deszendten aus jüdischen Verwandtenehen," *Archiv für Rassen- und Gesellschaftsbiologie* 14 (1922): 301–5.

53. Robert Gaupp, "Die klinische Besonderheiten der Seelenstörungen unserer Grossstadtbevölkerung," *Münchener Medizinische Wochenschrift* 53 (1906): 1250–1312.

54. Richard Krafft-Ebing, *Psychopathia Sexualis: A Medico-Forensic Study,* rev. trans. Harry E. Wedeck (New York: Putnam, 1956), 27 (in the Freud Library, London, in the German editions of 1892, 1894, and 1901).

55. Adolf Hitler, *Mein Kampf,* trans. Ralph Manheim (Boston: Houghton Mifflin, 1943), 248.

56. Auguste Forel, *Die sexuelle Frage* (Munich: Ernst Reinhardt, 1906), 172, 179; translated as *The Sexual Question* by C. F. Marshall (New York: Medical Art Agency, 1922), 166 (in the Freud Library, London, in the 1905 edition).

57. J. G. Frazer, *Totemism and Exogamy: A Treatise on Certain Early Forms*

of Superstition and Society, 4 vols. (1910; London: Dawsons of Pall Mall, 1968), 4:108.

58. See Peter de Mendelssohn, *Der Zauberer: Das Leben des deutschen Schriftstellers Thomas Mann* (Frankfurt am Main: Fischer, 1975), 1:662–73, and Marie Walter, "Concerning the Affair Wälsungenblut," *Book Collector* 13 (1964): 463–72. On a parallel but illuminating representation of "Brothers and Sisters" see the discussion in William J. McGrath, *Freud's Discovery of Psychoanalysis: The Politics of Hysteria* (Ithaca, N.Y.: Cornell University Press, 1986), 276–312.

59. See the tabulation of literary sources on incest as a literary theme in Max Marcuse, "Inzest," *Zeitschrift für Sexualwissenschaft* 9 (1923), 1:171–77.

60. Hitler, *Mein Kampf,* 306.

61. Kurt Münzer, *Der Weg nach Zion* (Berlin: A. Juncker, 1907), 240–45, 380–87, 600–604. See the discussion, with liberal quotations, in Rank, *Das Inzest-Motif,* 666–67. The theme of brother-sister incest is evoked in the Torah, as, for example, in Abraham's ambiguous representation of his relationship to Sarah. Through a process of Christianization and then secularization, this charge is made an aspect of the essence of the Jew.

62. *Der Juden Antheil am Verbrechen: Auf Grund der amtlichen Statistik über die Thätigkeit der Schwurgerichte, in vergleichender Darstellung mit den christlichen Confessionen* (Berlin: Otto Henze, 1881).

63. S. Löwenfeld, *Die Wahrheit über der Juden Antheil am Verbrechen* (Berlin: Stuhr, 1881).

64. Ludwig Fuld, *Das jüdische Verbrecherthum: Eine Studie über den Zusammenhang zwischen Religion und Kriminalität* (Leipzig: Theodor Huth, 1885), 24–25. He also notes that the number of convictions for incest in the census is for Catholics, 25 convictions; Protestants, 31; and Jews, 1.

65. *Archives Israélites: Recueil Politique et Religieux Hebdomadaire* 46 (August 13, 1885): 260–61.

66. *Die Kriminalität der Juden in Deutschland* (Berlin: Siegfried Cronbach, 1896). This is followed up by *Die wirtschaftliche Lage, soziale Gliederung und die Kriminalstatistik der Juden* (Berlin: Verlag des Vereins zur Abwehr des Antisemitismus, 1912).

67. Arthur Ruppin, "Die Kriminalität der Christen und Juden in Deutschland, 1899–1902," *Zeitschrift für Demographie und Statistik der Juden* 1 (1905): 6–9.

68. Arthur Ruppin, *Die Juden der Gegenwart* (Berlin: S. Calvary, 1904), chap. 15.

69. Bruno Blau, *Die Kriminalität der deutschen Juden* (Berlin: Louis Lamm, 1906).

70. Wulffen, *Der Sexualverbrecher,* 303.

71. Richard Weinberg, "Psychische Degeneration, Kriminalität und Rasse," *Monatsschrift für Kriminalpsychologie und Strafrechtsreform* 2 (1906): 720–30.

72. Arthur de Gobineau, *The Inequality of Human Races,* trans. Adrian Collins (New York: Howard Fertig, 1967), 168–80.

73. Emil Kraepelin, *Psychiatrie: Ein Lehrbuch für Studierende und Ärzte,* 4 vols. (Leipzig: Johann Ambrosius Barth, 1909), 1:189 (in the Freud Library, London). See Kurt Kolle, *Kraepelin und Freud: Beitrag zur neueren Geschichte der Psychiatrie* (Stuttgart: Georg Thieme, 1957).

74. Simon Scherbel, *Über Ehen zwischen Blutsverwandten* (Berlin: Gustav Schade, 1883), 8.

75. Scherbel, *Über Ehen zwischen Blutsverwandten,* 12, 27 (deaf-mutism); 40–42 (mental illness).

76. Felix A. Theilhaber, "Blutverwandte, Ehen unter," in *Jüdisches Lexikon,* ed. Georg Herlitz and Bruno Kirschner, 4 vols. in 5 (Berlin: Jüdischer Verlag, 1927–30): 1:1088–92 (in the Freud Library, London).

77. Bruno Blau, "Die Kriminalität der Juden in Deutschland während der Jahre 1903–1906," *Zeitschrift für Demographie und Statistik der Juden* 5 (1909):49–53.

78. R. B. de Roos, "Über die Kriminalität der Juden," *Monatsschrift für Kriminalpsychologie und Rechtsreform* 6 (1909–10): 193–205.

79. Rudolf Wassermann, "Ist die Kriminalität der Juden Rassenkriminalität?" *Zeitschrift für Demographie und Statistik der Juden* 7 (1911): 36–39.

80. "Die Kriminalität deutschen Juden," *Ost und West* 12 (1912): 713–16.

81. Franz von Liszt, *Das Problem der Kriminalität der Juden* (Giessen: Alfred Töpelmann, 1907).

82. Magnus Hirschfeld, *Geschlecht und Verbrechen* (Leipzig: Verlag für Sexualwissenschaft, 1930).

83. Hirschfeld, *Geschlecht und Verbrechen,* 325.

84. Herbert Maisch, *Incest,* trans. Colin Bearne (London: André Deutsch, 1973), 11–64. Compare Jack Goody, "A Comparative Approach to Incest and Adultery," *British Journal of Sociology* 7 (1956): 286–305.

85. Hirschfeld, *Geschlecht und Verbrechen,* 326.

86. Christina von Braun, "Die 'Blutschande'—Wandlung eines Begriffs: Vom Inzesttabu zu den Rassengesetzen," in *Die schamlose Schönheit des Vergangenen: Zum Verhältnis von Geschlecht und Geschichte* (Frankfurt am Main: Verlag Neue Kritik, 1989), 81–112.

87. Hermann Rohleder, *Monographien über die Zeugung beim Menschen,* 7 vols. (Leipzig: Thieme, 1911–21), vol. 2, *Die Zeugung unter Blutsverwandten,* 3–8.

88. Hirschfeld, *Geschlecht und Verbrechen,* 329.

89. Isser Yehuda Unterman, *Shevet mi-Yehudah: Berure Sugyot, Hidusche Torah ve-Hikre Halakhah be-a Rba ah Helka Shulhan Arukh* (Jerusalem: Mosad ha-Rab Kook, 1983).

90. Johann Christoph Wagenseil, *Belehrung der Jüdisch-Teutschen Red- und Schreibart* (Königsberg: Paul Friedrich Rhode, 1699). See my *Jewish Self-Hatred,* 74.

91. *Yebamot,* 39b, 109a.

92. Edvard Westermarck, *The History of Marriage,* 3 vols. (London: Macmillan, 1921), 3:216 (in the Freud Library, London, in the translation by L. Katscher

and R. Grazer [Berlin: H. Barsdorf, 1902]). Of interest in this context is Westermarck's response to Freud, *Freuds Teori um Oedipuskomplexen* (Stockholm: Albert Bonnier, 1934). On the function of this tradition within the anthropological literature see Howard Eilberg-Schwartz, *The Savage in Judaism: An Anthropology of Israelite Religion and Ancient Judaism* (Bloomington: Indiana University Press, 1990), 36. On Westermarck see Timothy Stroup, ed., *Edward Westermarck: Essays on His Life and Works* (Helsinki: Societas Philosophica Fennica, 1982).

93. See the discussion of this theme in Hjalmar J. Nordin, "Die eheliche Ethik der Juden zur Zeit Jesu," trans. W. A. Kastner and Gustave Lewié in *Beiwerke zum Studium der Anthropophyteia* 4 (1911): 99–104, a periodical Freud both contributed to and used extensively (see *SE* 10:215 n. 1, 11:233–35, 12:177–203, 21:106–7). On the political implications of this theme see N. F. Anderson, "The 'Marriage with a Deceased Wife's Sister Bill' Controversy: Incest Anxiety and the Defense of Family Purity in Victorian England," *Journal of British Studies* 21 (1982): 67–86.

94. See the discussion in McGrath, *Freud's Discovery of Psychoanalysis,* 280.

95. Hirschfeld, *Geschlecht und Verbrechen,* 326.

96. Max Marcuse, ed., *Handwörterbuch der Sexualwissenschaft* (Bonn: A. Marcus und E. Webers, 1926), 311 (in the Freud Library, London).

97. Heinrich Singer, *Allgemeine und spezielle Krankheitslehre der Juden* (Leipzig: Benno Konegen, 1904), 22–23.

98. Albert Reibmayr, *Inzucht und Vermischung beim Menschen* (Leipzig: Franz Deuticke, 1897), 128–29 (on the negative effects of inbreeding on culture), 175–211 (on inbreeding and interbreeding among the ancient Jews), 238–44 (on inbreeding in the mountains).

99. Hermann Runge, "Ich glaube, es liegt im Blut," *Die Arche* 13 (October 28, 1925): 1–7.

100. Rudolf Wassermann, *Beruf, Konfession und Verbrechen: Eine Studie über die Kriminalität der Juden in Vergangenheit und Gegenwart* (Munich: Ernst Reinhardt, 1907).

101. Hugo Hoppe, *Alkohol und Kriminalität in allen ihren Beziehungen* (Wiesbaden: J. F. Bergmann, 1906); idem, "Die Kriminalität der Juden und der Alkohol," *Zeitschrift für Demographie und Statistik der Juden* 2 (1907): 38–41.

102. Émile Zola, *Nana,* trans. George Holden (Harmonsworth: Penguin, 1972), 221.

103. Wassermann, *Beruf,* 55.

104. Rudolf Wassermann, "Die Kriminalität der Juden in Deutschland in den letzten 25 Jahren (1882–1906)," *Monatsschrift für Kriminalpsychologie und Rechtsreform* 6 (1909): 609–19.

105. Felix A. Theilhaber, "Alkoholgenuss der jüdischen Jugend," *Zeitschrift für Demographie und Statistik der Juden,* n.s., 3 (1926): 128–34.

106. Louis A. Berman, *Jews and Intermarriage: A Study in Personality and Culture* (New York: Thomas Yoseloff, 1968).

107. Curt Michaelis, "Die jüdische Auserwählungsidee und ihre biologische

Bedeutung," *Zeitschrift für Demographie und Statistik der Juden* 1 (1905): 1–4, here 3.

108. So the Viennese physician Ignaz Zollschan, *Das Rassenproblem unter besonderer Berücksichtigung der theoretischen Grundlagen der jüdischen Rassenfrage* (Vienna: Wilhelm Braumüllers Verlag, 1911) (in the Freud Library, London, with the dedication of the author).

109. Alfred Nossig, "Die Auserwähltheit der Juden im Lichte der Biologie," *Zeitschrift für Demographie und Statistik der Juden* 1 (1905): 20–23.

110. Prof. Dr. Hanauer, "Zur Soziologie und Psychologie der jüdischen Ehen," *Zeitschrift für Sexualwissenschaft* 13 (1927): 175–81, here 177.

111. Adolf Brüll, *Die Mischehe im Judentum im Lichte der Geschichte: Vortrag* (Frankfurt am Main: A. J. Hofmann, 1905), 2.

112. Westermarck, *History of Marriage,* 3:172, 177.

113. Carl Claus, *Grundzüge der Zoologie zum Gerbrauche an Universitäten und höheren Lehranstalten sowie zum Selbststudium,* 2 vols. (Marburg: N. G. Elwerts Universitäts-Buchhandlung, 1872), 1:90–91, in the translation from Lucille B. Ritvo, *Darwin's Influence on Freud: A Tale of Two Sciences* (New Haven: Yale University Press, 1990), 145.

114. August Weismann, *Das Keimplasma: Eine Theorie der Vererbung* (Jena: Gustav Fischer, 1892), 340–55. See *SE* 18:45–46, 56.

115. August Weismann, *Amphimixis, oder Die Vermischung der Individuen* (Jena: Gustav Fischer, 1891), 135–47.

116. Wilhelm Wundt, *Völkerpsychologie: Eine Untersuchung der Entwicklungsgesetze von Sprache, Mythus und Sitte,* section 1, *Die Sprache,* 2 vols. (Leipzig: Wilhelm Engelmann, 1904), 1:393–401, 481–83, 2:639–47. See *SE* 6:60–61, 81, 131–32. See Christina Maria Schneider, *Wilhelm Wundts Völkerpsychologie: Entstehung und Entwicklung eines in Vergessenheit geratenen, wissenschafts-historisch relevanten Fachgebietes* (Bonn: Bouvier, 1990).

117. William McDougall, *The Group Mind: A Sketch of the Principles of Collective Psychology with Some Attempt to Apply Them to the Interpretation of National Life and Character* (Cambridge: Cambridge University Press, 1920), 110 (in the Freud Library, London).

118. See the discussion in Kaufman Kohler, "Intermarriage," in *The Jewish Encyclopedia,* 12 vols. (New York: Funk and Wagnalls, 1904), 6:610–12. Compare Raymond Pearl and Celeste Franklin, "Jewish and Christian Intermarriages in Budapest: A Footnote to Recent Social History," *Bulletin of the History of Medicine* 8 (1940): 497–508.

119. Westermarck, *History of Marriage,* 2:56.

120. Felix Theilhaber, "Die Genealogie einer jüdischen Familie in Deutschland: Das Geschlecht Samson aus Wolfenbüttel," *Archiv für Rassen- und Gesellschafts-Biologie* 4 (1912): 207–13. See also the discussion of such marriages in Helene Deutsch, *Confrontations with Myself: An Epilogue* (New York: W. W. Norton, 1973), 52.

121. Karl Abraham, "Über neurotische Exogamie: Ein Beitrag zum den Übereinstimmung im Seelenleben der Neurotiker und der Wilden," *Klinische Beiträge*

zur Psychoanalyse aus den Jahren 1907–1920, Internationale Psychoanalytische Bibliothek 10 (Leipzig: Internationaler Psychoanalytischer Verlag, 1921), 227–30 (in the Freud Library, London).

122. Otto Fenichel, "Elements of a Psychoanalytic Theory of Anti-Semitism," in *Anti-Semitism: A Social Disease,* ed. Ernst Simmel (New York: International Universities Press, 1946), 11–33, here 27.

123. William I. Thomas and Florian Znaniecki, *The Polish Peasant in Europe and America,* 5 vols. (Chicago: University of Chicago Press, 1918–20), 2:1241, 1243.

124. Artur Dinter, *Die Sünde wider das Blut: Ein Zeitroman* (Leipzig: Matthes und Thost, 1918). See Kater, *Doctors under Hitler,* 177–83, and von Braun, *Die schamlose Schönheit,* 101–4.

125. Hugo Bettauer, *Die Stadt ohne Juden: Ein Roman von Übermorgen* (1922; Salzburg: Hannibal, 1980), 118.

126. Albert Moll, "Die sexuelle Abstinenz," in his *Handbuch der Sexualwissenschaften,* 2 vols. (Leipzig: F. C. W. Vogel, 1926), 2:1080.

127. Westermarck, *History of Marriage,* 2:57.

128. *Der Untergang Israels von einem Physiologen* (Zurich: Verlags-Magazin/J. Schabelitz, 1894).

129. Felix A. Theilhaber, *Der Untergang der deutschen Juden: Eine volkswirtschaftliche Studie,* 2d ed. (Berlin: Jüdischer Verlag, 1921). On the general background of such arguments see D. E. C. Eversely, *Social Theories of Fertility and the Malthusian Debate* (Oxford: Clarendon Press, 1959), and E. P. Hutchinson, *The Population Debate: The Development of Conflicting Theories up to 1900* (Boston: Houghton Mifflin, 1967). On Theilhaber see H. Lehfeldt, "Felix A. Theilhaber—Pioneer Sexologist," *Archives of Sexual Behavior* 15 (1986): 1–12.

130. Arthur Ruppin, *Die Juden der Gegenwart* (Berlin: Jüdischer Verlag, 1904).

131. Arthur Ruppin, *The Jews of the Modern World* (London: Macmillan, 1934), 76.

132. *Protokolle der Wiener Psychoanalytischen Vereinigung,* 3:259–60; translation from *Minutes of the Vienna Psychoanalytic Society,* 3:273–74.

133. Max Marcuse, "Zum Untergang der deutschen Juden," *Zeitschrift für Sexualwissenschaft* 14 (1927): 279–80.

134. H. Rost, "Konfession und Geburtenfrequenz," *Soziale Kultur* 8 (1912): 460.

135. Raphael Becker, "Zur Frage der Mischehe und Verwandtenehe," *Zeitschrift für Demographie und Statistik der Juden* 1 (1924): 21–23, 51–54.

136. Max Marcuse, "Die christlich-jüdische Mischehe," *Sexual-Probleme* 7 (1912): 691–749, here 713.

137. Gustav Jaeger, *Die Entdeckung der Seele* (Leipzig: Ernst Günther, 1880), 141 (in the Freud Collection, New York).

138. Leo Sofer, "Über die Entmischung der Rassen," *Zeitschrift für Demographie und Statistik der Juden* 2 (1905): 9–10, as well as his "Über Vermischung

und Entmischung der Rassen," *Politisch-Anthropologische Revue* 1 (1902): 435–38.

139. Werner Sombart, *Die Zukunft der Juden* (Leipzig: Duncker und Humblot, 1912), 45.

140. Francis Galton, *Inquiries into Human Faculty and Its Development* (New York: Macmillan, 1883), 305. See *SE* 4:139, 293, 5:494, 649.

141. Sombart, *Die Zukunft der Juden,* 44.

142. S. R. Steinmetz, "Das persönliche Element in der Rassenkreuzung," *Zeitschrift für Sexualforschung* 1 (1915): 28–32.

143. See David H. Spain et al., "The Westermarck-Freud Incest Theory Debate: An Evaluation and Reformulation," *Current Anthropology* 28 (1987): 623–35, and M. L. Rodrigues de Areia and David H. Spain, "On the Westermarck-Freud Incest Theory Debate," *Current Anthropology* 29 (1988): 313–14.

144. W. W. Kopp, "Beobachtung an Halbjuden in Berliner Schulen," *Volk und Rasse* 10 (1935): 392.

145. M. Lerche, "Beobachtung deutsch-jüdischer Rassenkreuzung an Berliner Schulen," *Die Medizinische Welt* 1 (September 17, 1927): 1222. In long letters to the editor, the Jewish sexologist Max Marcuse strongly dismissed the "anti-Jewish" presuppositions of Lerche's views, while at the same time Professor O. Reche of the University of Leipzig saw in Lerche's piece a positive contribution to racial science (*Die Medizinische Welt* 1 [October 15, 1927]: 1417–19). Lerche responded to Marcuse's call for a better science of race to approach the question of the *Mischling* with her own claim that her work was at best the tentative approach of a pedagogue. She also disavowed any "anti-Jewish bias" in her study (*Die Medizinische Welt* 1 [November 12, 1927]: 1542).

146. Wilhelm Stekel, "A Case of Orthopedic Fetishism," in his *Sexual Aberrations: The Phenomena of Fetishism in Relation to Sex,* trans. S. Parker, 2 vols. (London: John Lane/Bodley Head, 1930), 1:147–280.

147. Jones, *Life and Work,* 1:174.

148. Sally Shuttleworth, *George Eliot and Nineteenth-Century Science: The Make-Believe of a Beginning* (New York: Cambridge University Press, 1984), as well as more specifically her essay, "The Language of Science and Psychology in George Eliot's *Daniel Deronda,*" in *Victorian Science and Victorian Values: Literary Perspectives,* ed. James Paradis and Thomas Postlewait (New York: New York Academy of Sciences, 1981), 269–98. See Mary Wilson Carpenter, "'A Bit of Her Flesh': Circumcision and 'The Signification of the Phallus' in Daniel Deronda," *Genders* 1 (1988): 1–23. On Freud and Eliot see Peter Brückner, *Sigmund Freuds Privatlektüre* (Cologne: Verlag Rolf Horst, 1975), 106–10.

149. Joseph Wortis, *Fragments of an Analysis with Freud* (New York: Jason Aronson, 1984), 144.

150. Ellis, *Studies in the Psychology of Sex,* 6:6.

151. Krafft-Ebing, *Psychopathia Sexualis,* 25. Politically Krafft-Ebing was a liberal. He contributed a notable attack on anti-Semitism to a collection of such statements made by leading public figures of the turn of the century. See *Freiheit,*

Liebe, Menschlichkeit! Ein Manifest des Geistes von hervorragenden Zeitgenossen (Berlin: J. van Groningen, 1893), 47.

152. A. J. Storfer, *Zur Sonderstellung des Vatermordes: Eine rechtsgeschichtliche und völkerpsychologische Studie,* Schriften zur angewandten Seelenkunde 12 (1911; Nendeln: Kraus Reprint, 1970). Storfer was a member of the inner circle of Freud's intellectual world and was in charge of many of the publications for the Viennese Psychoanalytic Society. See *SE* 11:204, 13:9. On the general exclusion of any discussion of the Jews in the ethnological literature of the time see Howard Eilberg-Schwartz, *The Savage in Judaism: An Anthropology of Israelite Religion and Ancient Judaism* (Bloomington: Indiana University Press, 1990), 141–76.

153. Jeffrey Moussaieff Masson, ed., *The Complete Letters of Sigmund Freud to Wilhelm Fliess, 1887–1904* (Cambridge: Harvard University Press, 1985), 252. Hereafter cited as *Freud-Fleiss.*

154. On the question of incest see Madelon Sprengnether, *The Spectral Mother: Freud, Feminism, and Psychoanalysis* (Ithaca, N.Y.: Cornell University Press, 1990), 86–119. Compare Pierre Watte, "Quelques interprétations anthropologiques récentes des interdits oedipiens," *Cahiers de l'Institut de Linguistique de Louvain* 4 (1977): 103–20.

155. This was powerfully argued specifically concerning the Jews in most of the medical literature of the time concerning "inbreeding" and "crossbreeding." See the summary of this literature in Felix Peipers, "Consanguität in der Ehe und deren Folgen für die Descendenz," *Allgemeine Zeitschrift für Psychiatrie und Psychisch-Gerichtliche Medicin* 58 (1901): 793–862.

156. Rüdiger Herren, *Freud und die Kriminologie: Einführung in die psychoanalytische Kriminologie* (Stuttgart: Ferdinand Enke, 1973), 119–35.

157. Max Marcuse, *Von Inzest* (Halle: Carl Marhold, 1915).

158. Ellis, *Studies in the Psychology of Sex,* 7:523.

159. John Lubbock, *The Origin of Civilization and the Primitive Conditions of Man* (1870; Chicago: University of Chicago Press, 1978), 108. See *SE* 13:13, 111.

160. Émile Durkheim, "La prohibition de l'inceste et ses origines," *Année Sociologique* 1 (1898): 1–70. This has been reprinted in Jean Duvignaud, ed., *Émile Durkheim, Journal Sociologique* (Paris: Presses Universitaires de France, 1969); the discussion of the greater mortality of the Jews owing to their higher suicide rate as well as the greater incidence of insanity among the Jews is found on pp. 68–69. On the parallels of Freud and Durkheim see Talcott Parsons, "The Superego and the Theory of Social Systems," in his *Social Structure and Personality* (New York: Free Press, 1964), 17–33.

161. Émile Durkheim, *Le suicide: Étude de sociologie* (Paris: Alcan, 1897), 39 (on the insanity rates of the Jews); 149–73 (on the rate of suicide).

162. See, for example, T. G. Masaryk, *Der Selbstmord als sociale Massenerscheinung der modernen Civilization* (Vienna: C. Konegen, 1881), 223, and Enrico Morselli, *Der Selbstmord* (Leipzig: F. A. Brockhaus, 1881), 139.

163. Charles Darwin, *The Variation of Animals and Plants under Domestication,* 2 vols. (London: John Murray, 1868), 2:92–126.

164. Ritvo, *Darwin's Influence on Freud,* 105.

165. Charles Darwin, *The Descent of Man,* 2d ed. (London: John Murray, 1874), 524.

166. Darwin, *Variation,* 2:104.

167. George H. Darwin, *Die Ehen zwischen Geschwisterkindern und ihre Folgen,* trans. Dr. v. d. Velde (Leipzig: W. Engelmann, 1876).

168. Joseph Jacobs, "Consanguinity," in *The Jewish Encyclopedia,* 4:230.

169. See the debate following the presentation of Joseph Jacobs, "On the Racial Characteristics of Modern Jews," *Journal of the Anthropological Institute* 16 (1886): 23–63, here 61.

170. Wilhelm Stekel, *Die Träume der Dichter: Eine vergleichende Untersuchung bei Dichtern, Neurotikern und Verbrechern* (Wiesbaden: Bergmann, 1912), 27–28.

171. Sarah Kofman, *The Enigma of Woman: Woman in Freud's Writings,* trans. Catherine Porter (Ithaca, N.Y.: Cornell University Press, 1985), 85.

172. Karl Abraham, "Die Stellung der Verwandtenehe in der Psychologie der Neurosen," in *Klinische Beiträge zur Psychoanalyse aus den Jahren 1907–1920,* 45–52.

173. *Sigmund Freud–Karl Abraham, Briefe, 1907–1926,* ed. Hilda C. Abraham and Ernst L. Freud (Frankfurt am Main: Fischer, 1980), 65; translation from *A Psycho-Analytic Dialogue: The Letters of Sigmund Freud and Karl Abraham, 1907–1926,* ed. Hilda C. Abraham and Ernst L. Freud, trans. Bernard Marsh and Hilda C. Abraham (London: Hogarth Press, 1965), 56.

174. Sachs, *Freud: Master and Friend,* 113.

175. *Protokolle der Wiener Psychoanalytischen Vereinigung,* 1:78; translation from *Minutes of the Vienna Psychoanalytic Society,* 1:83.

176. Alfred Meisl, "Hunger und Liebe: Analytische Studien über die Elemente der psychischen Funktion," *Wiener Klinische Rundschau* 21 (1907): 269–71.

177. See the chapter "Jüdische Geschwister," in Else Croner, *Die moderne Jüdin* [*sic*] (Berlin: Axel Juncker, 1913), 66–72.

178. Gustave Aimable Asselin, *L'état mental des parricides: Étude médico-légale* (Paris: Baillière, 1902).

179. Paul Kovalevsky, *La psychologie criminelle* (Paris: Vigot Frères, 1903), 345.

180. Paul Kovalevsky, "Zur Psychologie des Vatermords," *Monatsschrift für Kriminalpsychologie und Strafrechtsreform* 1 (1904): 309–19, here 319.

181. Arnold Kutzinki, "Über nervöse Entartung bei den Juden," *Ost und West* 12 (1912): 907–10.

182. Concerning the psychoanalytic reading of the meaning of the circumcised Jewish body see Frank Zimmerman, "Origin and Significance of the Jewish Rite of Circumcision," *Psychoanalytic Review* 38 (1951): 103–12, Ernest Fraenkel, "La circoncision chez les juifs peut-elle s'expliquer comme une castration atténuée, infligée à ses fils par le chef de la horde?" *Psyché-Paris* 7 (1952): 367–85,

and Bruno Bettleheim, *Symbolic Wounds: Puberty Rites and the Envious Male* (Glencoe, Ill.: Free Press, 1954).

183. Georg Fuchs, *Wir Zuchthäusler: Erinnerungen des Zellengefangenen Nr. 2911. Im Zuchthaus geschrieben* (Munich: Albert Langen, 1931).

184. *SE* 22:252. See K. R. Eissler, "A Hitherto Unnoticed Letter by Sigmund Freud," *International Journal of Psycho-Analysis* 42 (1961): 199–200.

185. Paul Lawrence Rose, *Revolutionary Antisemitism in Germany from Kant to Wagner* (Princeton: Princeton University Press, 1990), 44–50, 252–62.

186. Voltaire, *Philosophical Dictionary,* ed. Theodor Besterman (Harmondsworth, England: Penguin, 1971), 256–57.

187. Erika Weinzierl, "Katholizismus in Österreich," in *Kirche und Synagoge: Handbuch zur Geschichte von Christen und Juden,* ed. Karl Heinrich Rengstorf and Siegfried von Kortzfleisch, 2 vols. (Stuttgart: Ernst Klett, 1970), 2:483–531, here 507–13.

188. The debate and texts of the fin de siècle as well as the background material are documented by Hugo Hayn, *Übersicht der (meist in Deutschland erschienenen) Litteratur über die angeblich von Juden verübeten Ritualmorde und Hostienfrevel* (Jena: H. W. Schmidt, 1906). See Alan Dundes, "The Ritual Murder or Blood Libel Legend: A Study of Anti-Semitic Victimization through Projective Inversion," *Temenos* 25 (1989): 7–32, for a critical survey of the literature on the topic.

189. Americus Featherman, *Social History of the Races of Mankind,* 7 vols. (London: Kegan Paul, Trench, Trübner, 1891), 4:597. See *SE* 11:195.

190. Bracha Rivlin, "1891: Blood-Libel in Corfu," *Jewish Museum of Greece Newsletter* 27 (1989): 1–7. Lectures on the Corfu riots were held in Germany and Austria in 1891. See Ludwig Gorel, *Das Blutmärchen: Seine Entstehung und Folgen bis zu den jüngsten Vorgängen auf Korfu* (Berlin: J. Gnadenfeld, 1891).

191. Hermann L. Strack, *Der Blutaberglaube in der Menschheit, Blutmorde und Blutritus: Zugleich eine Antwort auf die Herausforderung des "Osservatore Cattolico"* (Munich: C. H. Beck, 1882); cited from the revised translation, *The Jew and Human Sacrifice,* trans. Henry Blanchamp (London: Cope and Fenwick, 1909), 212–35.

192. *Die Fackel,* October 1899, 23–26.

193. T. G. Masaryk, *Die Notwendigkeit der Revision des Polnaer Mordes* (Prague: Die Zeit, 1899).

194. Larry Wolff, *Postcards from the End of the World: An Investigation into the Mind of Fin-de-Siècle Vienna* (London: Collins, 1989), 102–10.

195. Rudolf Kleinpaul, *Menschenopfer und Ritualmorde* (Leipzig: Schmidt und Günther, 1892), 1–2.

196. See the review by Hans Gross of Maximilian Paul-Schiff, *Der Prozess Hilsner: Aktenauszug* (Vienna: Buchhandlung, 1908); *Archiv für Kriminal-Anthropologie und Kriminalistik* 29 (1908): 314. See *SE* 5:396.

197. August Rohling, *Die Polemik und die Menschenopfer des Rabbinismus* (Paderborn: Verlag der Bonifacius-Druckerei, 1883).

198. Jones, *Life and Work,* 1:190.

199. Hippolyte Bernheim, *Die Suggestion und Ihre Heilwirkung,* trans. Sigmund Freud (Leipzig: Franz Deuticke, 1888), 152–54. For the historical context of this analysis, see Andrew Handler, *Blood Libel at Tiszaeszlar* (New York: Columbia University Press, 1980).

200. Kleinpaul, *Menschenopfer und Ritualmorde.*

201. On this question see Stefan Lehr, *Antisemitismus: Religiöse Motive im sozialen Vorurteil* (Munich: Kaiser, 1974), as well as Gavin I. Langmuir, *Toward a Definition of Anti-Semitism* (Berkeley and Los Angeles: University of California Press, 1990).

202. Kleinpaul, *Menschenopfer und Ritualmorde,* 9–13.

203. *Freud-Fliess,* 227.

204. Theodor Reik, "Die Pubertätsriten der Wilden: Über einige Übereinstimmungen im Seelenleben der Wilden und der Neurotiker," *Imago* 6 (1915–16): 125–44, 189–222.

205. Fritz Wittels, *Sigmund Freud: His Personality, His Teaching, and His School,* trans. Eden Paul and Cedar Paul (London: George Allen and Unwin, 1924), 163. This edition, rather than the original German one, reflects Freud's notes and corrections of Wittels's text.

206. W. Robertson Smith, *Lectures on the Religion of the Semites* (London: Adam and Charles Black, 1894), 344. See *SE* 13:132–40, 143, 147, 151–52, 17:262, 20:67–68; 23:82–83, 130–32.

207. Herbert Spencer, *The Principles of Sociology,* 3 vols. (New York: D. Appleton, 1900–1901), 3:26. See *SE* 13:77, 93, 110.

208. Dr. Hacker, "Die Beschneidung der Juden, ein Überrest der Barbarei dieses Volkes, und ein Ersatz für seine früheren Menschenopfer," *Medicinischer Argos* 5 (1843): 375–79. Freud evokes the ethnopsychological image of cannibalism in his discussion of masochism as self-hatred, *SE* 7: 159.

209. On the social context of this word see Ken Frieden, *Freud's Dream of Interpretation* (Albany: State University of New York Press, 1990), 122–25.

210. As much as I would like to believe that Mark Twain was the forgotten source of this comment, I am not convinced by the reading provided by Marion A. Richmond, "The Lost Source in Freud's 'Comment on Anti-Semitism': Mark Twain," *Journal of the American Psychoanalytic Association* 28 (1980): 563–74. Although Freud was a great fan of Twain and heard him read in Vienna, there are simply too many disparities between Freud's account of his source and the Twain essay.

211. See "The Jewish Essence: Anti-Semitism and the Body in Psychoanalysis," in Gilman, *Jew's Body,* 194–209.

Conclusion: The Life of a Myth

1. See the overall discussion of the problems of psychoanalytic epistemology as well as the role of countertransference in Carlo Strenger, *Between Hermeneutics and Science: An Essay on the Epistemology of Psychoanalysis* (Madison,

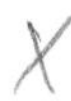

Conn.: International Universities Press, 1991). On the history of transference and countertransference see U. H. Peters, "Transference," in *Introducing Psychoanalytic Theory,* ed. Sander L. Gilman (New York: Brunner/Mazel, 1982), 77–115.

2. Judith Dupont, ed., *The Clinical Diary of Sándor Ferenczi,* trans. Michael Balint and Nicola Zarday Jackson (Cambridge: Harvard University Press, 1988).

3. Theodor Billroth, *Über das Lehren und Lernen der medicinischen Wissenschaften an den Universitäten der deutschen Nation nebst allgemeinen Bemerkungen über Universitäten: Eine culturhistorische Studie* (Vienna: Carl Gerold's Sohn, 1876), 146–54. On the response to Billroth on the part of the German-Jewish writer Bertold Auerbach, see Paul Lawrence Rose, *Revolutionary Antisemitism in Germany from Kant to Wagner* (Princeton: Princeton University Press, 1990), 238–39. Billroth's image of the Eastern Jewish medical student remained a "classic" characterization, according to the *Ostdeutsche Rundschau* in 1911, well after its author had radically altered his own view. See Christoph Stölzl, *Kafkas böses Böhmen: Zur Sozialgeschichte eines Prager Juden* (Munich: Text und Kritik, 1975), 44. The quotation on the state of the medical school in the 1930s is from Esther Menaker, *Appointment in Vienna: An American Psychoanalyst Recalls Her Student Days in Pre-War Austria* (New York: St. Martin's Press, 1989), 45.

4. See the general discussion of this topic in Joseph Sandler, ed., *Projection, Identification, Projective Identification* (London: Karnac, 1989), 1–26.

5. Heinrich Racker, *Transference and Countertransference* (New York: International Universities Press, 1968).

6. Heinz Hartmann, *Ego Psychology and the Problem of Adaptation* (New York: International Universities Press, 1939).

7. Rafael Moses, "Projection, Identification, Projective Identification: Their Relation to the Political Process," in Sandler, *Projection,* 133–51, here 136.

8. Melanie Klein, "Notes on Some Schizoid Mechanisms," *International Journal of Psycho-Analysis* 27 (1946): 99–110, here 102.

9. Sigmund Freud and C. G. Jung, *Briefwechsel,* ed. William McGuire and Wolfgang Sauerländer (Frankfurt am Main: Fischer, 1974), 426–27; translation in *The Freud/Jung Letters,* ed. William McGuire, trans. Ralph Manheim and R. F. C. Hull (Princeton: Princeton University Press, 1974), 386–87.

10. Regina Markell Morantz-Sanchez, *Sympathy and Science: Women Physicians in American Medicine* (New York: Oxford University Press, 1985).

11. William E. Cross, Jr., *Shades of Black: Diversity in African-American Identity* (Philadelphia: Temple University Press, 1991).

12. Nancy Stepan and Sander L. Gilman, "Appropriating the Idioms of Science: Some Strategies of Resistance to Biological Determinism," in *The Bounds of Race,* ed. Dominick La Capra (Ithaca, N.Y.: Cornell University Press, 1991), 72–103.

13. Menaker, *Appointment in Vienna,* 48.

14. See Eugene Levy, " 'Is the Jew a White Man?' Press Reaction to the Leo Frank Case, 1913–1915," *Phylon* 35 (1974): 212–22.

15. Carl G. Jung, *Collected Works,* ed. Herbert Read et al., trans. R. C. F. Hull, 20 vols. (London: Routledge and Kegan Paul, 1957–79), 10:13, See Aryeh Maidenbaum and Stephen Martin, eds., *Lingering Shadows: Jungians, Freudians, and Anti-Semitism* (Boston: Shambhala, 1991), and Victor Brome, *Freud and His Disciples: The Struggle for Supremacy* (London: Caliban Books, 1984), 142–53, for a discussion of this material. See also Aniela Jaffé, *From the Life and Work of C. G. Jung,* trans. R. F. C. Hull (London: Hodder and Stoughten, 1972), 78–98, for a Jewish defense of Jung's relation to anti-Semitism, as well as the issue entitled "Jung face au nazisme" of the *Cahiers de Psychologie Jungienne* 12 (1977) for the facts of Jung's anti-Semitism and a possible reading of them. For the earlier relationship see also Duane Schultz, *Intimate Friends, Dangerous Rivals: The Turbulent Relationship between Freud and Jung* (Los Angeles: J. P. Tarcher; New York: Distributed by St. Martin's Press, 1990).

16. Quoted by Mortimer Ostow in a "Letter to the Editor," *International Review of Psycho-Analysis* 4 (1977): 377.

17. Andrew Samuels, "National Psychology, National Socialism, and Analytic Psychology: Reflections on Jung and Anti-Semitism," *Journal of Analytic Psychology* 37 (1992): 3–28 and 127–48.

18. Sander L. Gilman, *The Jew's Body* (New York: Routledge, 1991).

19. Fritz Stern, *Gold and Iron: Bismarck, Bleichröder, and the Building of the German Empire* (New York: Alfred A. Knopf, 1977).

INDEX

Page numbers in **boldface** type refer to illustrations.

common mental construction 83, 199, 212

INDEX

Dolchstoß legend — 119